~

Cardiovascular Physiology

Third Edition

R. David Baker

The University of Texas Medical Branch

Galveston

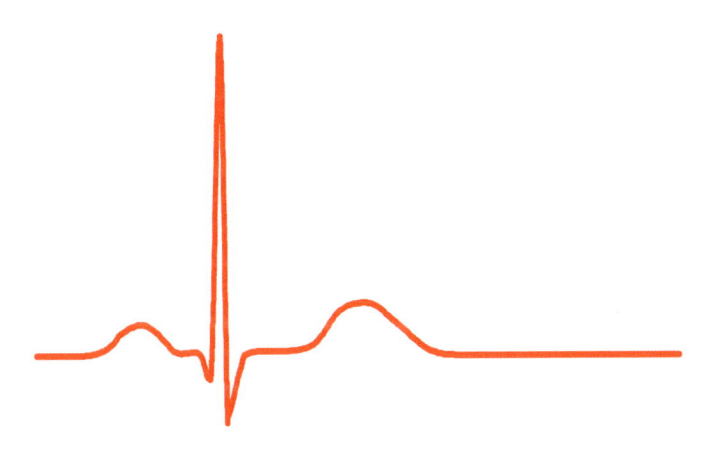

Strand Street Press

First Edition: Copyright © 2003 by R. David Baker, Strand Street Press, Galveston, TX. All rights reserved.

First Edition, 2nd printing with corrections: June 2004, Strand Street Press, Galveston, TX.

Second Edition: Copyright © 2006 by R. David Baker, Strand Street Press, Galveston, TX. All rights reserved.

Third Edition: Copyright © 2012 by R. David Baker, Strand Street Press, Galveston, TX. All rights reserved.

The author and publisher welcome use of the original graphics in this book by educators. When used for local, noncommercial teaching purposes, appropriate acknowledgment of the source automatically gains permission. When used in any commercial medium, formal permissions must be obtained. Requests for permissions should be addressed to R. D. Baker, UTMB, Rt. 1069, Galveston, TX, 77555.

Library of Congress Control Number: 2003093686

ISBN: 0-9741653-6-0

The drawing on the front cover is from the *Medical Illustration Library*, Sobotta Cardiology/Pulmonology Anatomy Collection, 1996, Williams & Wilkins.

Preface

This textbook is intended primarily for medical students. It has arisen from many years of teaching first and second year medical students at The University of Texas Medical Branch at Galveston..

There is also an electronic edition on CD that runs under Windows. It has interactive and multimedia features, and also includes a condensed version of the main text that can be useful for review. Most of the links to hypertext, animations, *etc.* have been retained in the print version so that the reader knows what's in the electronic version. Unfortunately, clicking in the print book probably won't work.

Each reference to a figure (*i.e.* Figure 1) generally comes at the head of the paragraph dealing with that particular figure rather than embedded within the paragraph, as is traditionally the case. I think this makes it easier to identify the text that is relevant to each figure.

I am extremely grateful to the late Dr. Malcolm Brodwick for essential encouragement and many helpful suggestions. This book is dedicated to him.

I would appreciate feedback concerning errors and ideas for improvement.
rdbaker@utmb.edu

David Baker
May 2012

Contents

Page

Chapter 1: Introduction to Cardiovascular Physiology 1
Part 1: Some General Features of the Cardiovascular System
Part 2: Some Important Terminology
Part 3: Global Control of the Cardiovascular System
Part 4: Table of Normal Values for the Cardiovascular System

Chapter 2: Cardiac Muscle: Structure and Mechanism of Contraction 9
Part 1: Structure of Working Myocardium
Part 2: Mechanism of Contraction

Chapter 3: Cardiac Muscle: Excitation 19
Part 1: Excitatory System of the Heart
Part 2: Excitation-Contraction Coupling
Part 3: Action Potentials of Working Myocytes
Part 4: Action Potentials of Pacemaking Cells and Automaticity

Chapter 4: Cardiac Muscle: Regulation of Contraction 33
Part 1: Intrinsic Regulation of Contraction
Part 2: Effects of Extrinsic Agents on Contraction

Chapter 5: The Cardiac Cycle 43
Part 1: The Motions of the Heart
Part 2: The Phases of the Cardiac Cycle
Part 3: The Events of the Cardiac Cycle
Part 4: Left Ventricular Pressure-Volume Loops

Chapter 6: Electrocardiography 53
Part 1: Basic Principles
Part 2: Frontal-Plane Electrocardiography
Part 3: The Chest Leads and the Standard Twelve Lead Electrocardiogram
Part 4: Arrhythmias

Chapter 7: Regulation of Stroke Volume 63
Part 1: Effect of Afterload on Stroke Volume
Part 2: Effect of Preload on Stroke Volume
Part 3: Effect of Contractility on Stroke Volume
Part 4: Automatic Compensations for Changes in Afterload
Part 5: Effects of Exercise on Stroke Volume
Part 6: The Curious Effect of High Heart Rates on Stroke Volume and Cardiac Output

Chapter 8: Regulation of Cardiac Output 73
Part 1: Introduction to Guyton Diagrams
Part 2: Increased Cardiac Output during Exercise
Part 3: Effect of Postural Changes on Cardiac Output
Part 4: A Simulation of Cardiovascular Control

Chapter 9: Myocardial Energetics 81
Part 1: ATP Supply
Part 2: ATP Use
Part 3: Myocardial Hypoxia

Chapter 10: Responses of the Heart to Chronic Overload 91

Chapter 11: Principles of Blood Flow 95
Part 1: General Principles of Fluid Flow through Tubes
Part 2: Special Features of Blood Flow through Tubes
Part 3: Special Features of Blood Flow through Microvessels
Part 4: Blood Flow through Vascular Beds

Chapter 12: Vascular Smooth Muscle 107
Part 1: Structure and Mechanism of Contraction
Part 2: The Membrane Potential and Ion Channels
Part 3: Mechanisms for Modulating Tone in Vascular Smooth Muscle
Part 4: Specific Endogenous Agonists
Part 5: Vasodilator Drugs

Chapter 13: The Systemic Arterial System 123
Part 1: Mean Arterial Pressure
Part 2: The Arterial Pulse
Part 3: Some Variations in Arterial Pressures
Part 4: Blood Flow in the Large Arteries
Part 5: Transmission of the Arterial Pulse Wave

Chapter 14: The Systemic Venous System 131
Part 1: Venous Pressure
Part 2: The Venous Pulse
Part 3: The Venous System is a Variable Blood Reservoir
Part 4: Venous Pumps

Chapter 15: Neuro-Humoral-Renal Control of the Circulation 137
Part 1: The Baroreceptor Reflexes
Part 2: Control of Renal NaCl and Water Output
Part 3: Long-Term Control of Blood Volume, MAP, and CVP
Part 4: Responses to Acute Hypovolemia (Hemorrhage)
Part 5: Other Cardiovascular Situations and Responses

Chapter 16: Control of Regional Blood Flow 155
Part 1: Principles and Mechanisms for Control of Regional Blood Flow
Part 2: Control of Cerebral Blood Flow
Part 3: Control of Skeletal Muscle Blood Flow
Part 4: Coronary Blood Flow

Chapter 17: Transvascular Movements of Solutes and Water 167
Part 1: The Exchange Vessels
Part 2: Transendothelial Diffusion of Solutes
Part 3: Transendothelial Fluid Flow
Part 4: The Lymphatic System
Part 5: The Blood-Brain Barrier (BBB)

Chapter 18: Cardiovascular Effects of Aging 179
Part 1: Introduction
Part 2: Effects of Aging on Some Basic Properties of the Cardiovascular System
    in Healthy People at Rest
Part 3: Hemodynamic Changes in Healthy People at Rest
Part 4: Exercise in Aging and the Effects of Exercise Training
Part 5: Responses to Postural Changes and Hypovolemia

Index 195

Chapter 1

Introduction to Cardiovascular Physiology

The cardiovascular system is for conveying materials and heat from one place in the body to another. Materials include the respiratory gases, nutrients, metabolic wastes, hormones, cytokines, components of the clotting and fibrinolytic systems, blood cells, etc.

This chapter presents some general information about the cardiovascular system. Preliminary remarks about the control of cardiac output are included. A table of normal values is provided for reference.

Part 1: Some General Features of the Cardiovascular System

Topic 1: The Heart Consists of Two Pumps

Figure 1
The right heart pumps blood through the pulmonary vessels to the left heart, while the left heart pumps blood through the systemic circuit back to the right heart. Both pumps share the same timing device, the SA node; therefore, they beat almost simultaneously. First, both atria contract. Then, after a brief delay, both ventricles contract. Contraction of the heart is called systole; filling of the heart with blood while it is relaxed is called diastole. These terms can be applied to the atria (*e.g.* atrial systole), but when not so qualified always refer to the ventricles.

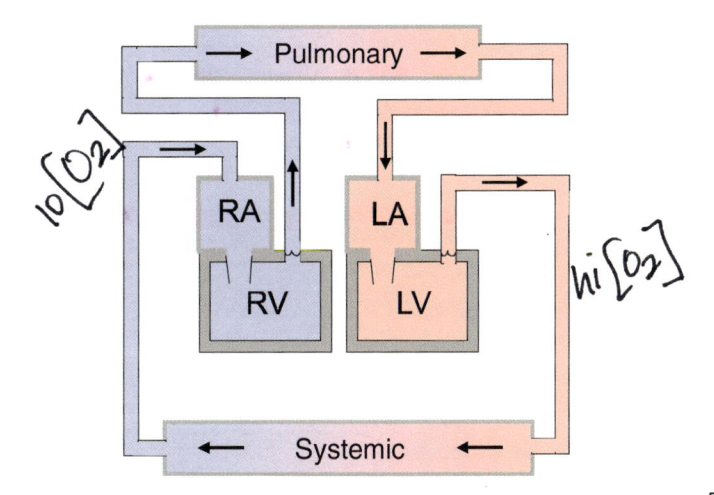

Figure 1. Simple diagram of the cardiovascular system. RA = right atrium, RV = right ventricle, LA = left atrium, LV = left ventricle.

Topic 2: The Cardiovascular System is Laid out as a Series of Components

Figure 2
The blood vessels are laid out in two series circuits: the systemic circuit and the pulmonary circuit. The systemic circuit provides blood to most of the organs of the body. The pulmonary circuit provides blood to the lungs.

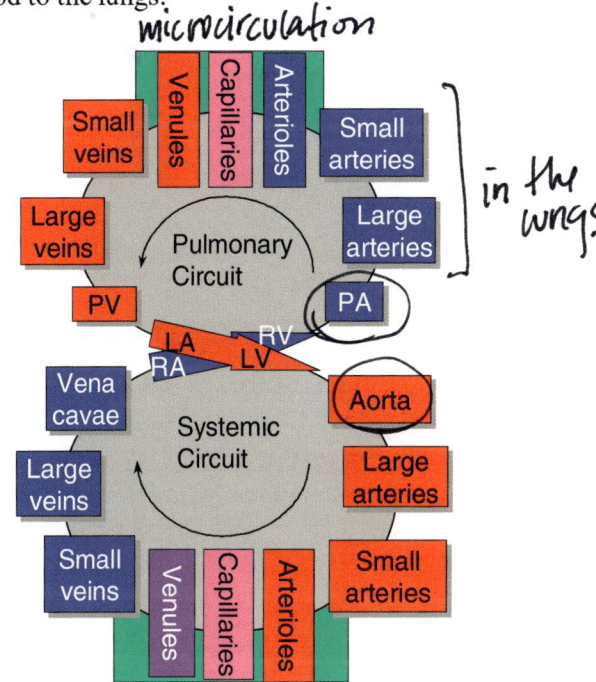

Figure 2. The series components of the cardiovascular system. The components backed by green constitute the microcirculation. The microcirculation includes the smallest arteries, arterioles, capillaries, venules, and smallest veins. PA = pulmonary arteries, PV = pulmonary veins.

General Functions of the Components

Arteries: The progressively branching tree of arteries is the conduit for blood as it flows under high pressure from the ventricles to the capillaries. During ventricular systole, blood expands the arteries and the pressure in them rises. During ventricular diastole, this pressure continues to force blood through the microcirculation to the veins although the ventricles are no longer ejecting blood.

Precapillary resistance vessels: The smallest arteries, together with the arterioles, are called the precapillary resistance vessels. Most of the resistance to flow around the systemic or pulmonary circuits is located in the precapillary resistance vessels and in the capillaries themselves. The caliber of the precapillary resistance vessels and, therefore, the resistance to flow through them, is adjustable by contraction or relaxation of smooth muscle in their walls. Thus, the precapillary resistance vessels act as valves that control regional blood flow and total peripheral resistance.

Capillaries and venules: Net movement of materials into and out of the vascular system takes place almost exclusively across the endothelium of the capillaries and venules. True capillaries have no smooth muscle and cannot actively change caliber.

Veins: The progressively debranching tree of veins is the conduit for blood as it flows under low pressure back to the atria. Far more interesting, however, is the reservoir function of the venous system. The veins contain most of the blood in the entire vascular system. The volume of blood the veins can hold at a given pressure is called the venous capacity. Venous capacity can be adjusted by contraction or relaxation of venous smooth muscle. Changes in venous capacity are extremely important in controlling arterial pressure and cardiac output, as we shall see in later chapters.

Topic 3: Branching and Debranching

In both the pulmonary and systemic circuits, along the arterial trees, the vessels progressively branch. At each branch the resulting vessels become narrower but more numerous than the stem vessel. Additional branching occurs in the systemic and pulmonary microcirculations resulting in several billion capillaries. Debranching occurs along systemic and pulmonary venous systems to the atria.

Topic 4: The Systemic Circulatory System is Laid Out as a Parallel Arrangement of Vascular Beds through the Organs

Figure 3

In the systemic circuit, the vascular beds through most of the organs are arranged in parallel with each other as illustrated in the figure. The resistance to blood flow through each systemic vascular bed is adjustable, mainly by constriction or relaxation of arterioles and other precapillary resistance vessels.

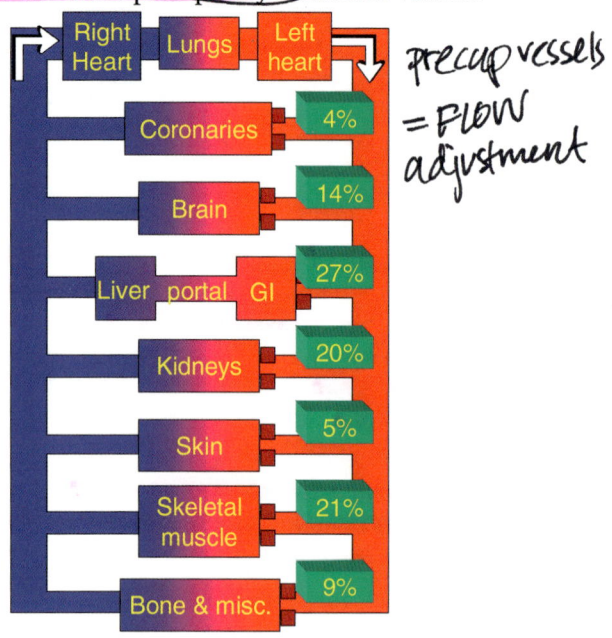

Figure 3. The parallel arrangement of systemic vascular beds. The constrictions leading into each vascular bed represent precapillary resistance vessels (terminal arteries and arterioles). Most of the resistance to blood flow resides in these structures. Changes in caliber of the precapillary resistance vessels control total resistance to flow in the systemic system as well as specific resistance to flow in each individual vascular bed. The percentage of total cardiac output flowing through each bed is shown for a normal person at rest.

Topic 5: The Cross-Sectional Area of the Series Components of the Systemic System

Figure 4

The cross-sectional area of any one branch is smaller (except for capillary branching) than that of the stem from which it branched. However, since branching results in more vessels, the resulting total cross-sectional area is greater than that of the stem vessel. Consequently, the total cross-sectional area of the successive parts of the systemic vascular system progressively increases to the level of the venules and then decreases again to the *vena cavae*.

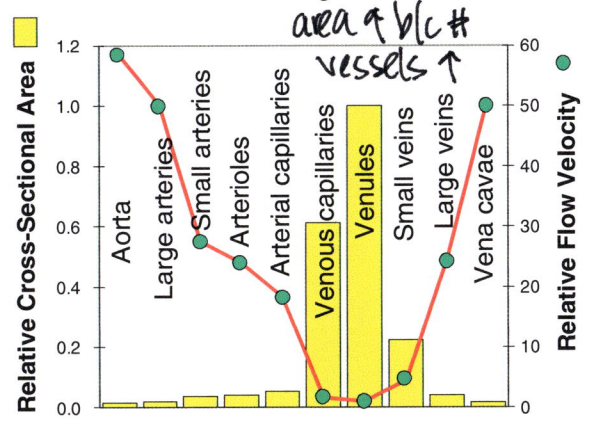

Figure 4. Relative total cross-sectional area and velocity of blood flow for the series components of the systemic system. All values are in comparison to those of the venules.

Topic 6: The Velocity of Blood Flow through the Series Components of the System

See Figure 4 again

For a given rate of blood flow (*e.g.* in liters/min), the velocity of flow (cm/sec) is inversely proportional to the total cross-sectional area. Therefore, the velocity of blood flow is least in the venules and greatest in the large arteries – just the inverse of the cross-sectional area distribution. A distinction is made between arterial capillaries and venous capillaries, since in many microcirculatory beds the capillaries branch. Each branch (a venous capillary) is generally of larger diameter than its stem (an arterial capillary). Consequently, the total cross-sectional area of venous capillaries is far greater than that of arterial capillaries, and the velocity of blood flow is correspondingly less. Note that the greatest total cross-sectional area and, therefore, the least velocity are at the level of the venules, not the capillaries (as is commonly supposed).

Topic 7: Distribution of Blood Volume in the Cardiovascular System

Figures 5, 6, and 7

These figures contain the relevant information regarding distribution of blood volume.

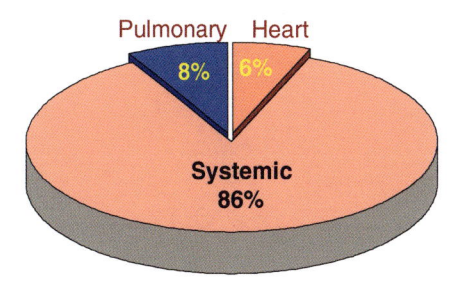

Figure 5. Distribution of total blood volume in the entire vascular system.

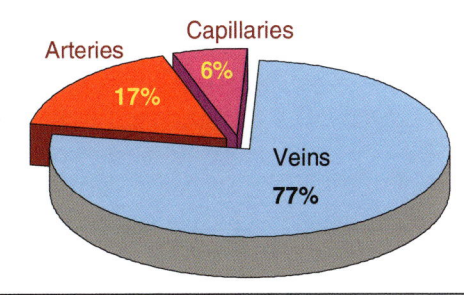

Figure 6. Distribution of blood volume in the systemic vascular system. In this case the arteries include the arterioles and the veins include the venules.

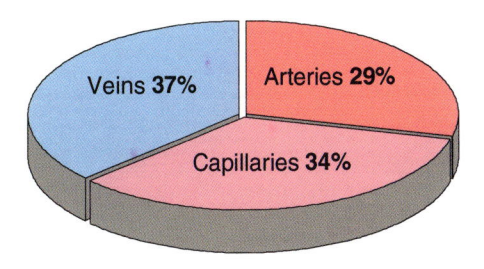

Figure 7. Distribution of blood volume in the pulmonary vascular system. The arteries include the arterioles and the veins include the venules.

Topic 8: Distribution of Resistance to Flow in the Systemic Vascular System

Figure 8

The arterioles have, by far, the highest total resistance to flow. Furthermore, the resistance through the arterioles is adjustable (by smooth muscle contraction), and can be adjusted independently in the various organs of the body. Consequently, the arterioles bear the main responsibility for regulating the resistance to flow through each vascular bed.

4   Chapter 1

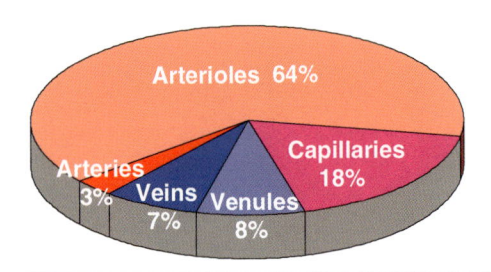

Figure 8. Distribution of resistance to blood flow in the systemic vascular system.

It may seem odd that the arterioles, arranged in parallel with each other, have a greater total resistance to flow than the large arteries while also having a greater total cross-sectional area. It might seem that greater cross-sectional area would lead to lower resistance. The explanation for this apparent inconsistency lies in the fact that each individual arteriole is so skinny. As explained in Chapter 11, resistance is reciprocally related to the fourth power of the radius, while cross-sectional area depends on radius squared.

Topic 9: Distribution of Pressures in the Cardiovascular System

Figure 9
Most of the drop in pressure from arterial to venous sides of the systemic and pulmonary systems occurs in the microcirculation since this is where most of the resistance to flow is located. Within the microcirculation, most of the pressure drop occurs in the arterioles.

The pulsations with each heartbeat are of greatest amplitude in the ventricles. In the systemic arterial tree, the pulsation amplitude gradually increases along the large arteries, but then gradually diminishes to nearly zero in the capillaries.

The table in Part 4 of this chapter provides, for reference, a detailed list of normal cardiovascular pressures.

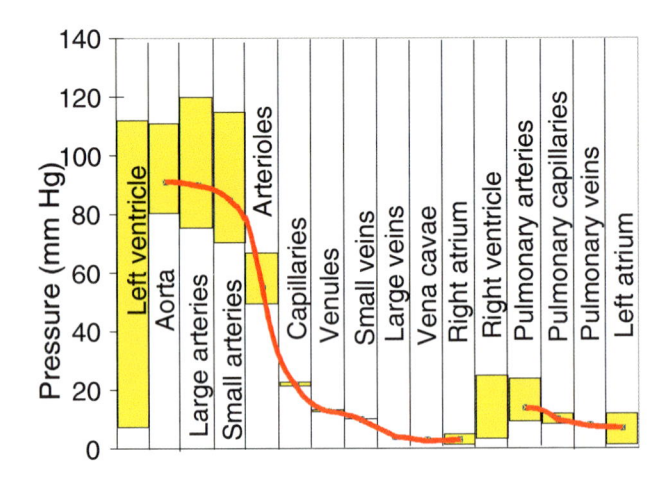

Figure 9. Distribution of pressures in the cardiovascular system. In addition to the distribution of mean pressures (red line), this figure shows the amplitude of the pressure fluctuations that occur with each beat of the heart. The top of each bar indicates peak-systolic pressure, and the bottom of each bar indicates end-diastolic pressure.

Part 2: Some Important Terminology

Topic 1: Terminology related to the Heart and Cardiac Output

Cardiac output, CO: The volume of blood ejected by the left ventricle into the aorta, or by the right ventricle into the pulmonary artery, per minute. CO is usually given in liters/min, but sometimes in ml/min. [Note: the average rate of blood flow is the same in all series components of the cardiovascular system. In other words, the cardiac output, arterial flow rate, microcirculatory flow rate, and venous return are all the same (except during brief transients). Since the heart provides the dramatic pumping action, circulatory flow rate is usually called cardiac output.

Cardiac index, CI: Cardiac output divided by body

surface area. Calculation of CI is the most common way to normalize data among individuals of various sizes.

Stroke volume, SV: The volume of blood ejected from either the left or the right ventricle during a single beat. Although there can be momentary differences in stroke volume between left and right ventricles, on the average they must, of course, be identical. Stroke volume is the difference between ventricular end-diastolic volume and ventricular end-systolic volume.

Stroke index, SI: Stroke volume divided by body surface area.

Ventricular end-systolic volume: The volume of

blood remaining in a ventricle at the end of systole.

Ventricular end-diastolic volume: The volume of blood in a ventricle at the end of diastole, just before systole.

Ejection fraction: Stroke volume divided by ventricular end-diastolic volume.

Cardiac contractility: Intrinsic muscular strength at any given sarcomere length. Increased contractility results in increased active tension and increased shortening velocity at any sarcomere length. The changes in active tension and shortening velocity that result directly from changes in sarcomere length do not strictly qualify as changes in contractility (see Chapter 4, Part 2 for an elaboration of this definition).

Preload: The passive tension in a muscle before it begins to contract. Preload for any cardiac chamber is determined by the volume of blood it contains just before it contracts.

Afterload: The active tension a muscle must generate in order to shorten. Afterload for any cardiac chamber is determined mainly by the pressure it must pump against. For example, the afterload for the left ventricle is mainly determined by the pressure in the aorta. When an outflow valve fails to open properly, resistance to flow of blood out of the chamber can increase the afterload; examples are aortic stenosis and mitral stenosis.

Topic 2: Terminology Related to the Systemic Vascular System

Mean arterial pressure, MAP: The pressure in a large artery averaged over the entire cardiac cycle. Clinically, MAP is usually measured in the brachial artery.

Central venous pressure, CVP: The mean pressure in the large intrathoracic veins and right atrium. The mean pressure is essentially the same in all these locations in a reclining subject.

Total peripheral resistance, TPR: Resistance to flow is defined as the pressure difference that drives flow, divided by the flow rate. Therefore, total peripheral resistance is defined by:

$$TPR = (MAP - CVP) / CO$$

The term systemic vascular resistance (SVR) is often used and is synonymous with TPR.

Arterial and venous compliances: Compliance of a closed chamber is defined as the slope of the pressure-volume relationship, dV/dP. It measures the ease of inflating the chamber at any given pressure.

Venous capacity (capacitance): The volume of blood in the venous system at any given pressure.

Part 3: Global Control of the Cardiovascular System

Topic 1: Introduction

The general performance of the cardiovascular system is reflected in how well it regulates cardiac output, mean arterial pressure, and central venous pressure. Regulation of these quantities is accomplished by adjustments in:
- Heart rate
- Cardiac contractility
- Total peripheral resistance
- Total blood volume
- Venous capacity

These independently adjustable variables operate together to determine cardiac output, mean arterial pressure, and central venous pressure.

The settings of these parameters are influenced by autonomic nervous activity, hormones, disease, aging, *etc*. Most of the drugs used to treat major cardiovascular disorders such as hypertension, heart failure, and angina act, directly or indirectly, on one or more of these independently adjustable parameters.

The mechanisms by which alterations in the primary adjustable parameters control cardiac output, mean arterial pressure, and central venous pressure will be discussed in later chapters. What follows here is a brief overview.

Topic 2: Arterial and Venous Blood Volumes are Determined by the Primary Adjustable Parameters

Whenever the value of one of the primary adjustable parameters is altered, arterial and venous blood volumes change. Increases in volume cause increases in pressure, just like inflating an inner tube.

Figure 10

In this figure, the circulatory system is modeled in the simplest possible way. The model has only four components, the pump-oxygenator (heart and lungs), the systemic arteries, the systemic veins, and the total peripheral resistance. All of the resistance to flow around the circuit is lumped into the latter component.

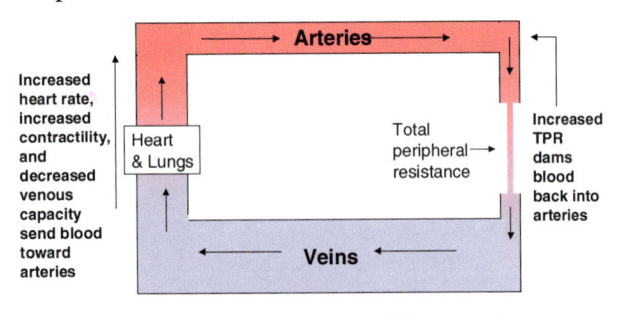

Figure 10. The above diagram summarizes the alterations that result in more blood in the arteries, thereby elevating MAP.

When heart rate and/or contractility are increased, the heart becomes a more effective pump and blood is shifted from veins to arteries. Arterial pressure rises while venous pressure falls.

When total peripheral resistance increases, blood is dammed back into the arteries – the upstream volume and pressure increase and the downstream volume and pressure decrease.

When venous capacity decreases (due to venous smooth muscle contraction or to compression of the veins), blood is shifted (*via* the heart) from veins to arteries. Mean arterial and venous pressures both increase.

When total blood volume increases, both arterial and venous volumes increase (about equally) and pressure rises everywhere.

Of course, alterations of the adjustable parameters in the opposite directions have the opposite effects.

Topic 3: The Determinants of Cardiac Output

Figure 11

Cardiac output is the product of stroke volume and heart rate. This statement is true but simplistic since stroke volume is not itself a primary adjustable parameter.

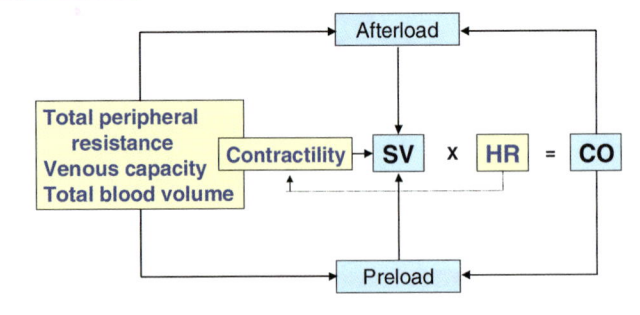

Figure 11. The determinants of cardiac output. The primary adjustable parameters are in blue letters with yellow background.

Contractility, preload, and afterload determine stroke volume. Of these, only contractility is a primary adjustable parameter of the cardiovascular system. Preload and afterload are determined directly by total peripheral resistance, venous capacity, and total blood volume. Heart rate and contractility also influence preload and afterload *via* their effects on cardiac output. There is also an effect of heart rate on contractility. All of this will be discussed in later chapters.

Topic 4: Cardiac Output is Closely Adjusted to Meet Metabolic Demands for Oxygen

Variations in cardiac output among normal individuals at rest are determined largely by variations in basal metabolic rate. Basal metabolic rate in normal people is closely related to body surface area (since heat loss is dependent upon surface area). Consequently, for normalizing data among individuals, cardiac output is divided by body surface area to get the cardiac index. Changes in cardiac output during exercise are closely related to changes in the intensity of aerobic metabolism.

Introduction to Cardiovascular Physiology

Part 4: Table of Normal Values for the Cardiovascular System: Recumbent Adult Humans

	Mean	Range
Heart rate, HR (beats/min)	70	53-89 *
Flows and Volumes		
Cardiac output, CO (L/min)	5.8	4.8-7.1
Cardiac index, CI (L/min/m^2)	3.4	2.8-4.2
Stroke volume, SV (ml)	80	51-110
Stroke index, SI (ml/m^2)	47	30-65
Ejection fraction	0.67	
Total Blood volume, TBV (L)	5.0	
Pressures in Heart (mmHg)		
Right atrial (mean), MRAP	2	-1 to 8
Right vent. (peak systolic)	25	15-28
Right vent. (end-diastolic)	2	0-8
Left atrial (mean), MLAP	7	4-12
Left vent. (peak-systolic)	112	
Left vent. (end-diastolic)	7	4-12
Pressures in Systemic System (mmHg)		
Aorta (mean)	91	
Aorta (peak-systolic)	111	
Aorta (end-diastolic)	80	
Brachial artery (mean)	90	70-105
Brachial artery (peak-systolic)	120	90-140
Brachial artery (end-diastolic)	75	60-90
Capillaries (mean)	22	
Venules (mean)	13	
Pressures in Pulmonary System (mmHg)		
Pulmonary artery (mean)	14	10-22
Pulmonary artery (peak-systolic)	24	15-28
Pulmonary artery (end-diastolic)	9	5-16
Capillaries (mean)	12	
Pulmonary veins (mean)	8	
Resistances to Blood Flow (dyne-sec/cm^5)		
Total peripheral, TPR	1231	900-1400
Systemic arteriolar	938	600-900
Total pulmonary	97	150-250
Pulmonary arteriolar	28	45-120

* Normal range for HR, but the clinical standard for <u>abnormality</u> is < 60 (bradycardia) and > 100 (tachycardia)

Source:
Most (but not all) of these values are from R.C. Schlant and E.H. Sonnenblick, *Normal Physiology of the Cardiovascular System*, in Hurst's, The Heart: Arteries and Veins, 8th Edition, Edited by R.C. Schlant and R.W. Alexander, McGraw-Hill, 1994, Table 5.3, p. 141.

Pressure conversions:
Usually millimeters of mercury (mmHg) are used for cardiovascular pressures.
  1 mmHg = 133.3 Pascals
  1 mmHg = 1333 dynes/cm^2
  1 mmHg = 0.736 cmH$_2$O
  760 mmHg = 1 atmosphere

Resistance conversions:
Various units of flow resistance are used, but cgs units are probably the most common.
In the cgs system, flow resistance is in dyn·sec/cm^5
  1332 dyn·sec/cm^5 = 1 mmHg/(ml/sec)
                    = 1 peripheral resistance unit (PRU)
  80 dyn·sec/cm^5 = 1 mmHg/(L/min) = 1 R unit

Chapter 2

Cardiac Muscle: Structure and Mechanism of Contraction

Here we study the mechanism of cardiac muscle contraction. Previous knowledge of skeletal muscle should be very helpful.
Part 1 reviews the structure of myocardial cells. Detailed knowledge of myofibril structure (course, fine, and molecular) is essential for understanding the mechanism of contraction.
Part 2 discusses the mechanism of contraction.

Part 1: Structure of Working Myocardium

Topic 1: Cardiac Myocytes

Figure 1
Cardiac myocytes (muscle cells) are much smaller than skeletal muscle myocytes. They have very few nuclei (however, usually more than one). The nuclei are centrally placed among the myofibrils. Bundles of myofibrils tend to have different lengths often giving the ends of the cell a staggered or stair-step appearance. Cardiomyocyte dimensions vary considerably. Ventricular myocytes average about 100 µm long and 15 µm across. Atrial myocytes are somewhat longer and skinnier.

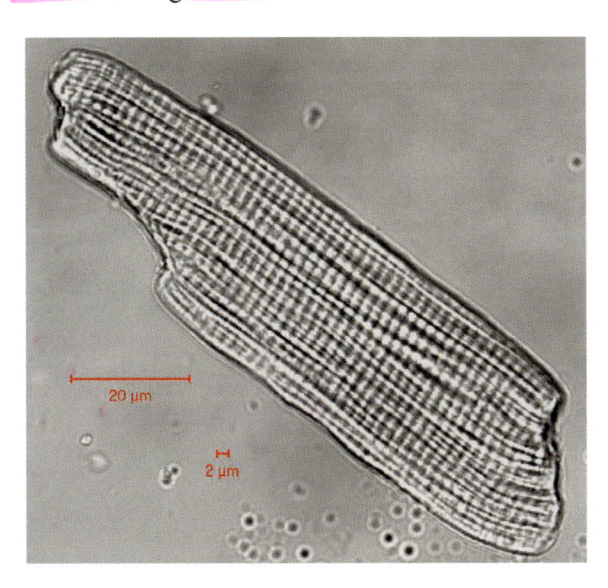

Figure 1. Isolated ventricular myocyte from rat heart. Heart was enzymatically treated to free individual cells. Cross striations are evident. Sarcomere length in this relaxed cell is 1.90 µm. The myofibrils appear in groups having different lengths. Courtesy of Dr. Phillip Palade (myocyte preparation) and Dr. Leoncio Vergara (imaging); Dept. of Physiology and Biophysics, UTMB, Galveston, TX.

Figure 2
The myofibrils are the contractile component. They run longitudinally in the myocyte, separated from each other by rows of mitochondria and membranes of the sarcoplasmic reticulum. You are urged to look at microanatomy texts for electron micrographs of cardiac muscle cells.

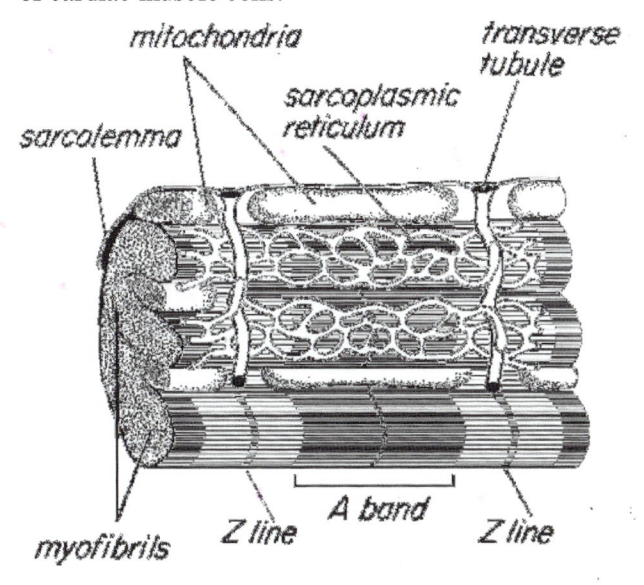

Figure 2. General relationships among myofibrils, sarcolemma, T tubules, sarcoplasmic reticulum, and mitochondria in cardiac muscle.
Drawing by Dr. Donald Stubbs, Dept. of Physiology & Biophysics, UTMB, Galveston, TX

Topic 2: Connections between Myocytes at Intercalated Disks

Figure 3
At their tips, myocytes neatly fit to each other along a dark line called the intercalated disk. Intercalated disks often have a stair step appearance since the ends of the cells are often staggered. Thus, there are both transverse and longitudinal regions of the intercalated disks.

Frequently, bundles of myofibrils at the periphery of the myocyte are much shorter than the maximum cell length. These bundles end in intercalated disks that join to laterally adjacent cells. Usually each cell connects to several other cells, and a network is formed.

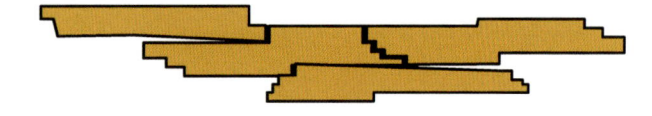

Figure 3. Each cardiac muscle cell is attached at intercalated disks to several other cells. This arrangement gives the appearance of branching. True branching is said to be rare although it is commonly depicted in textbooks.

At each end of each myofibril, the thin filaments are anchored to the sarcolemma *via* a layer of poorly defined amorphous material. This layer appears as the dense transverse part of the intercalated disk. Along the longitudinal parts of the intercalated disk, adjacent cells are mechanically connected to each other by desmosomes, and electrically connected to each other by gap junctions.

Gap junctions provide pathways from cell to cell having very low electrical resistance. These pathways allow rapid electrical transmission of action potentials from one cell to the next. Since each ventricular cell is electrically connected to several of its neighbors, the entire ventricular myocardium is an electrically interconnected network of cells. Such a network is sometimes called an electrical syncytium. Atrial cells are likewise connected to each other electrically.

The atrial and ventricular cell networks are largely insulated from each other by the fibrous skeleton of the heart (base of the heart). Normally, the only electrical pathway between the atria and ventricles is the bundle of His, which penetrates through the central fibrous body (see Chapter 5, Figure 1).

Topic 3: Arrangement of Myocyte Networks

The atrial and ventricular myocyte networks are attached to the fibrous skeleton of the heart. It was formerly thought that myocytes in the free walls of the ventricles are arranged as distinct sheets that spiral to and from the apex at various pitches. While this arrangement is drawn in many textbooks, it is apparently not real. Instead, the entire ventricular myocardium is an interconnected network whose cells lie at different angles depending on location. Myocytes at either the endocardial or the epicardial surfaces lie approximately parallel to the base-to-apex axis of the heart. Away from either surface, myocytes lie at progressively increasing angles to this axis until, midway between endocardial and epicardial surfaces, myocytes lie approximately perpendicular to the base-to-apex axis. There are thickenings of ventricular muscle around the orifices of valves and at the apex. On the endocardial surface, the network of myocytes forms the trabeculae carnae and projects at specific locations to form the papillary muscles.

Topic 4: Myofibrils – Course Structure

Figure 4
Myofibrils are striated, and all the striations have names as indicated in this figure. The sarcomere is the structural and contractile unit of a myofibril. A sarcomere runs from one Z line to the next. In the

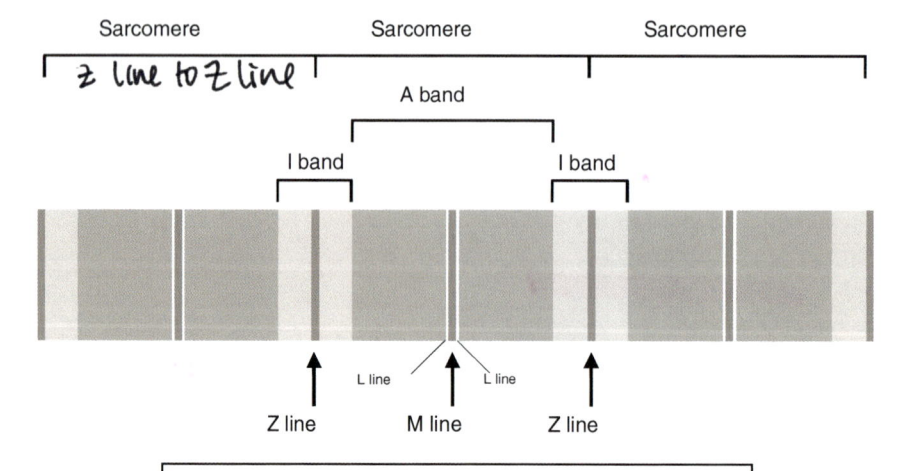

Figure 4. Diagram of sarcomere structure.

Cardiac Muscle: Structure and Mechanism of Contraction

order of 50 sarcomeres, connected end-to-end at their Z lines, make a ventricular myofibril. A relaxed sarcomere that is neither contracting nor being stretched is approximately 1.9 µm long. This length is called its slack length.

A few hundred myofibrils line up in each cardiomyocyte, connected to each other at the level of Z lines by desmin intermediate filaments. Thus, the striations in all the myofibrils are in register with each other giving the entire myocyte a striated appearance.

desmin connects myofibrils

Topic 5: Myofibrils – Fine Structure

Figure 5
The principal structural elements of each sarcomere are thick filaments, thin filaments, and Z lines. The thick filaments are centered in each sarcomere and are connected to each other at the M line. They are about 1.6 µm long.

Thin filaments are attached to Z lines and project into each sarcomere toward its center. Their length averages about 1.05 µm. Therefore, at slack length, the average thin filament extends just past the M line into the other half of the sarcomere, slightly overlapping thin filaments from the next Z line. Each thick filament is surrounded by six thin filaments.

I bands are regions that have thin filaments but no thick filaments. A bands contain both thick and thin filaments.

Effect of Stretch
If tension is applied to the ends of a relaxed myofibril, its sarcomeres all become longer. The Z lines move farther apart. Since the thin filaments are attached to Z lines, they slide out alongside the thick filaments resulting in less overlap between the two. This process increases the length of the I bands. As a myofibril is stretched, it not only gets longer, but it also gets thinner. The myofibril and all of its sarcomeres remain at constant volume.

As a cardiac chamber fills with blood during diastole, longitudinal tension is applied to all of its myocytes and, therefore, to all of its myofibrils. The sarcomeres elongate and get skinnier. In a normal person at rest, diastolic filling stretches sarcomeres to approximately 2.2 µm. Under conditions of increased diastolic filling, cardiac sarcomeres can be stretched to a maximum of about 2.4 µm.

Effect of Shortening
During a shortening contraction, the thin filaments are pulled toward the other half of the sarcomere by the thick filaments. Consequently, the Z lines are

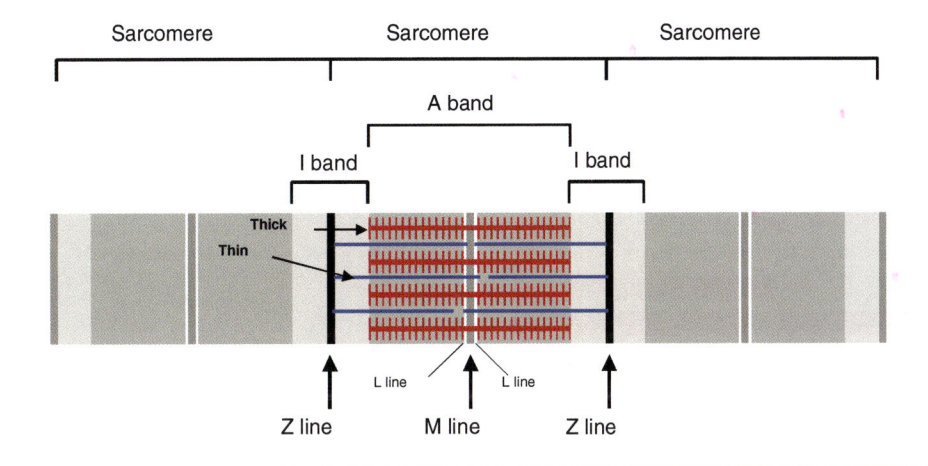

Figure 5. Each sarcomere is constructed of Z lines, thick filaments (red), and thin filaments (blue). The thick filaments have projections at regular intervals that extend nearly to the thin filaments. There are about 300 such projections on each thick filament. Note that the thin filaments in cardiac muscle are not all exactly the same length as they are in skeletal muscle. [This illustration is drawn to scale except that in the vertical direction the thick and thin filaments are shown about 10-fold thicker than they really are.]

pulled closer to each other and the I bands decrease in length. The sarcomeres get shorter and fatter, again retaining constant volume. They ordinarily do not get shorter than about 1.8 μm.

Interactive Sliding Filaments
[Special: Length-Tension Relationship]
[Available in electronic edition of this textbook]
This special shows the effect of changing sarcomere length on passive tension and on active isometric tension. Cardiac muscle is compared to skeletal muscle. For now, there is no need to plot tensions. Simply change sarcomere length between 1.8 and 2.4 μm by moving the slider. Examine the sarcomere model to see the complete range of filament interdigitation.

Here is another little model to play with. Move the sarcomere halves through their normal range of motion.
[Special: Sliding filaments]

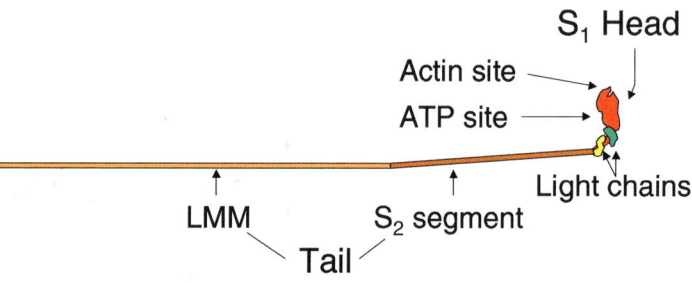

Figure 6. The components of muscle myosin.

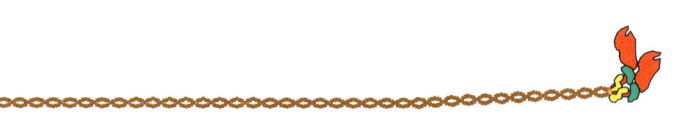

Figure 7. Double myosin (myosin-II).

Topic 6: Myofibrils – Molecular Structure

Thick Filaments
Figure 6
Thick filaments are constructed mainly from myosin. The major component of myosin is a long polypeptide, the myosin heavy chain. The myosin heavy chain has a long α helical tail and a pear-shaped head. The head, called S_1, is an ATPase. The tail has two parts called S_2 and light meromyosin (LMM). Two shorter polypeptide chains are wrapped around the stem of S_1; these are called the essential light chain and the regulatory light chain respectively.

Figure 7
The tails of two heavy chains are wrapped around each other to form the complete myosin molecule (called myosin-II). Thus, each complete myosin molecule has two heavy chains (with two S_1 heads), each of which has two light chains.

Figure 8
Thick filaments are hollow tubes. The LMM segments of about 300 myosin tails associate with each other longitudinally to form the rim of each thick filament. Double S_1 heads project radially from the thick filament surface at regular intervals. The length of an S_1 head is 16.5 nm, which is almost long enough to reach a nearby thin filament. The S_2 segments of myosin tails can lift slightly off the thick filament surface. Thus, the distance the S_1 heads project out from the surface is variable.

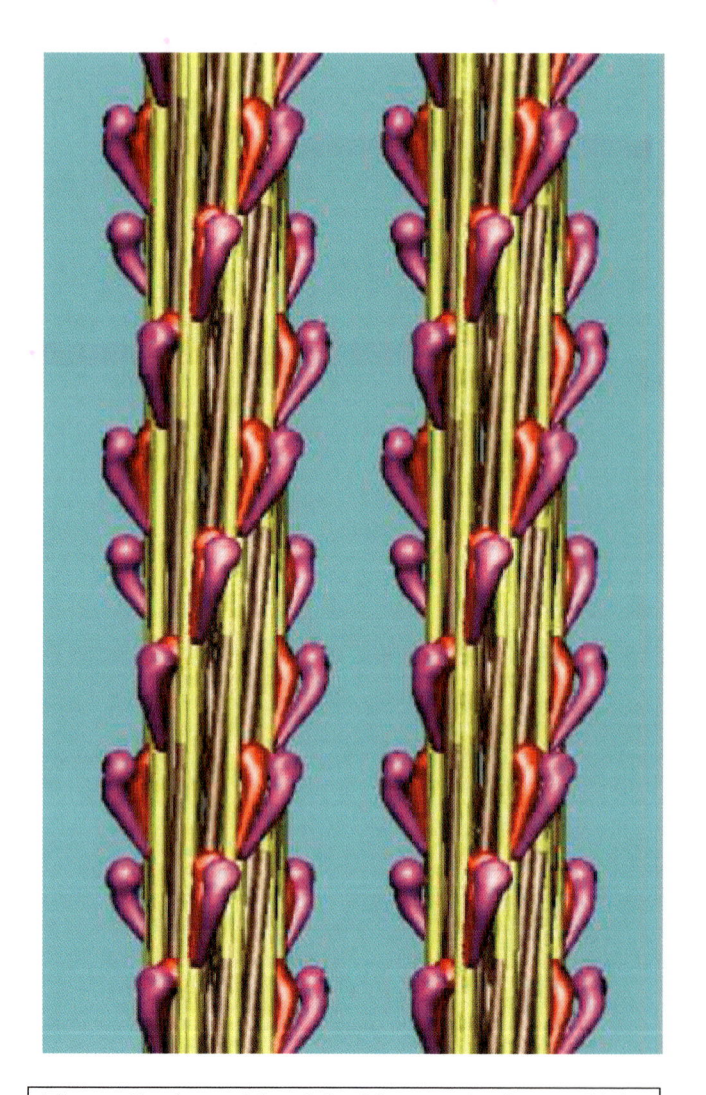

Figure 8. Assembly of double myosins into a thick filament tube. Stereo pair from L. Skubiszak and L. Kowalczyk, website no longer available.

Cardiac Muscle: Structure and Mechanism of Contraction 13

no S₁ heads or M bands

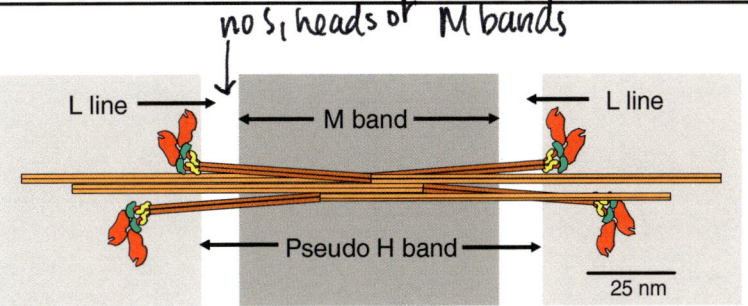

Figure 9. Self-assembly of double myosin tails to form a thick filament. Only four double myosins at the center of a thick filament are depicted here. Their tails stick to each other side-to-side with the heads toward the eventual ends of the thick filament. A complete thick filament is made by insertion of more double myosins at each end of the growing filament, eventually forming a tube about 1.6 µm long. Notice that this arrangement of myosin molecules leaves a central bare region where there are no S₁ heads. This region is called the pseudo H band. It consists of the M line sandwiched between two light lines called L lines. The L lines are light because of the absence of S₁ heads and of M band proteins.

Figure 9
Myosin molecules point in opposite directions in the two halves of the thick filament. Therefore, there is a short region at the center of each thick filament where there are no S₁ projections. This bare region accounts for the L lines at each edge of the M line.

Thin Filaments
Figure 10
The main proteins of thin filaments are α-actin, tropomyosin, and troponin. Globular subunits of α-actin (5.5 nm in diameter) stick together in long chains. Two such chains wind around each other in a double helix to form the core of each thin filament. Actin subunits have sites that can bind myosin S₁ heads.

Tropomyosin molecules (42 nm long) are bound to actin along each chain of the actin double helix. Each tropomyosin molecule spans about 7.5 actin subunits and slightly overlaps with the next tropomyosin molecule. At rest, the tropomyosin molecules physically cover the sites on actin that could otherwise bind myosin S₁ heads.

Troponin consists of three subunits called TnC, TnI, and TnT. A troponin complex is attached at one end of each tropomyosin molecule. In Chapter 3 we will see how a Ca^{++}-induced change in conformation of the troponin-tropomyosin complex triggers contraction.

Figure 10. Structure of thin filaments. Only the troponin-tropomyosin complexes that are related to one of the two actin chains are depicted here. Actual thin filaments are about 6 times this long, *i.e.* about 6 times as many subunits.

Z lines
Figure 11
Thin filaments from adjacent sarcomeres overlap each other in the Z lines as shown in Figure 11. Their plus ends are capped by a protein called CapZ. They are attached to each other at regular intervals by α–actinin. *attach thin fils to e/o*

Other Proteins
Figure 12
Titin: Molecules of the giant protein, titin, are also attached to the Z lines. They extend from each Z line all the way to the center of the sarcomere where they are attached to the M line. In the region of the A band, they attach to the surface of thick filaments. In the region of the I band, titin molecules are very springy. This arrangement holds the thick filaments exactly in the center of the A band.

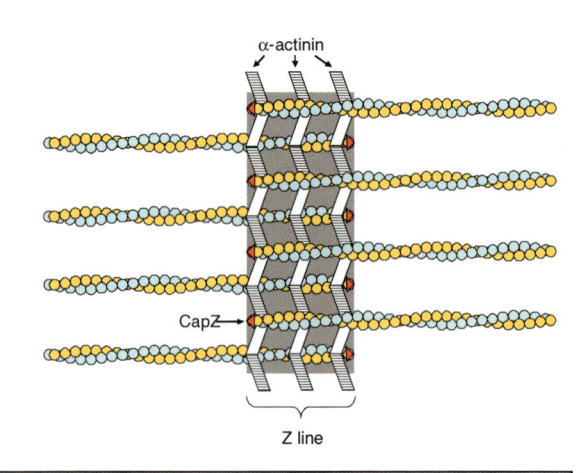

Figure 11. Structure of Z lines.

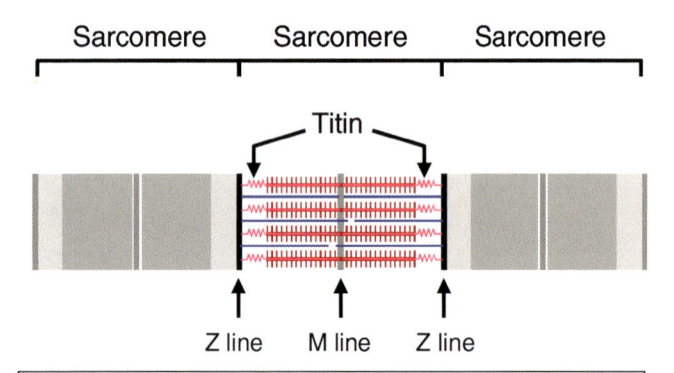

Figure 12. Arrangement of titin in the sarcomere.

Myosin-binding protein C: Molecules of myosin-binding protein C are attached to thick filaments, binding to both myosin and titin. They extend transversely out from each thick filament at 43 nm intervals. When myosin-binding protein C is phosphorylated, it makes the S_1 heads of myosin move slightly farther from the thick filament backbone, closer to nearby thin filaments.

M-protein and myomesin: These proteins are in the M line; they connect the centers of adjacent thick filaments to each other.

Topic 7: Membranes of the Myocyte

See Figure 2 again
The Sarcolemma and T Tubules
The surface membrane of muscle cells is called the sarcolemma. It invaginates at regular intervals, approximately at the location of Z lines, to form transverse tubules (T tubules). The T tubules extend into the interior of the myocyte, coursing around the myofibrils. In ventricular myocytes, branches from the T tubules extend longitudinally between some of the myofibrils. These branches connect with each other forming an intracellular network of membranes called the transverse-axial tubular system. In atrial myocytes, the system of T tubules is not as well developed as it is in ventricular myocytes, and has no axial component. Hereafter we will refer to the transverse-axial tubular system simply as T tubules.

Action potentials that travel along the sarcolemma continue along T tubules into the interior of the cell. These membranes are equipped with all the ion channels necessary for conducting action potentials including Na^+ channels, K^+ channels, and Ca^{++} channels.

The sarcolemma and T tubule membranes are also equipped with various primary pumps and carriers, which will be important in our story of excitation in the next chapter). Of course, they possess the ubiquitous Na^+-K^+ pump, which is responsible for maintaining the intracellular concentrations of Na^+ and K^+ out of equilibrium with their extracellular concentrations. They also possess the Na^+-Ca^{++} exchanger and the primary Ca^{++} pump that are responsible for extruding Ca^{++} from the cell. The L-type Ca^{++} channel is also present. DHP

A very small transmembrane protein called phospholemman is also present in the sarcolemma. This protein helps regulate the Na^+-K^+ pump and the Na^+-Ca^{++} exchanger, and maybe even the L-type Ca^{++} channel. Its role in responses to β_1-adrenergic stimulation will be mentioned in Chapter 4.

The Sarcoplasmic Reticulum
The sarcoplasmic reticulum (SR) of cardiac muscle forms a complex system of tubes, the network SR, which surrounds each myofibril. Near the Z lines, some of these tubes enlarge into saccules called the junctional SR, which make many close contacts with the T tubules. Junctional SR also makes close contacts with the sarcolemma.

The membranes of network SR are densely studded with primary Ca^{++} pumps called SERCA (short for SR/ER Ca-ATPase), which continuously pump Ca^{++} out of the cytoplasm into the lumen of the network SR. This Ca^{++} diffuses through the lumen of the network SR to the junctional SR where a large fraction of it is loosely bound to a protein called calsequestrin. At rest, the concentration of Ca^{++} in the cytoplasm is kept very low (roughly 0.1 µM).

A protein called phospholamban is closely associated with SERCA. Phospholamban exerts an inhibitory effect on these pumps. When phospholamban is phosphorylated, the inhibitory effect is relieved and the Ca^{++} pumps operate faster. The role of this process in control of contraction will be discussed in Chapter 4.

The membranes of junctional SR are equipped with Ca^{++}-release channels (CRCs), also called ryanodine receptors. The role of CRCs in the initiation of contraction will be described in Chapter 3.

Topic 8: Connections with the Extracellular Matrix

Figure 13
There are two types of protein complexes that attach the Z lines and the cortical actin cytoskeleton to the extracellular connective tissue matrix. These are 1) the dystroglycan/dystrophin complex, and 2) the β1-integrin complex.

The Dystroglycan/Dystrophin Complex
β-dystroglycan spans the sarcolemma. Just outside the membrane it attaches to α-dystroglycan, which in turn connects to laminin within the basal lamina. Laminin helps hold the extracellular matrix together. On the cytoplasmic side of the sarcolemma, β-dystroglycan attaches to dystrophin, which in turn makes many connections in the cortical cytoskeleton. Along its N-terminal domain, a dystrophin strand can make as many as 24 connections with a single γ-actin filament; this stiffens the actin filaments and strengthens the cortical cytoskeleton. Near its C-terminal end, dystrophin connects to α-actinin, which in turn connects to cortical actin filaments. The latter can attach to the α-actinin of Z lines, thus gluing the Z lines of peripheral myofibrils to the dystroglycan/dystrophin complex and hence to the extracellular matrix.

Dystrophin also binds a group of cortical cytoplasmic proteins called syntrophins and another called dystrobrevin. The latter is notable for its ability to bind desmin, thereby providing an additional connection between peripheral myofibrils and the dystroglycan/dystrophin complex.

There are some additional transmembrane proteins in the dystroglycan/dystrophin complex (the sarcoglycans and sarcospan), which may help hold the whole thing together (?).

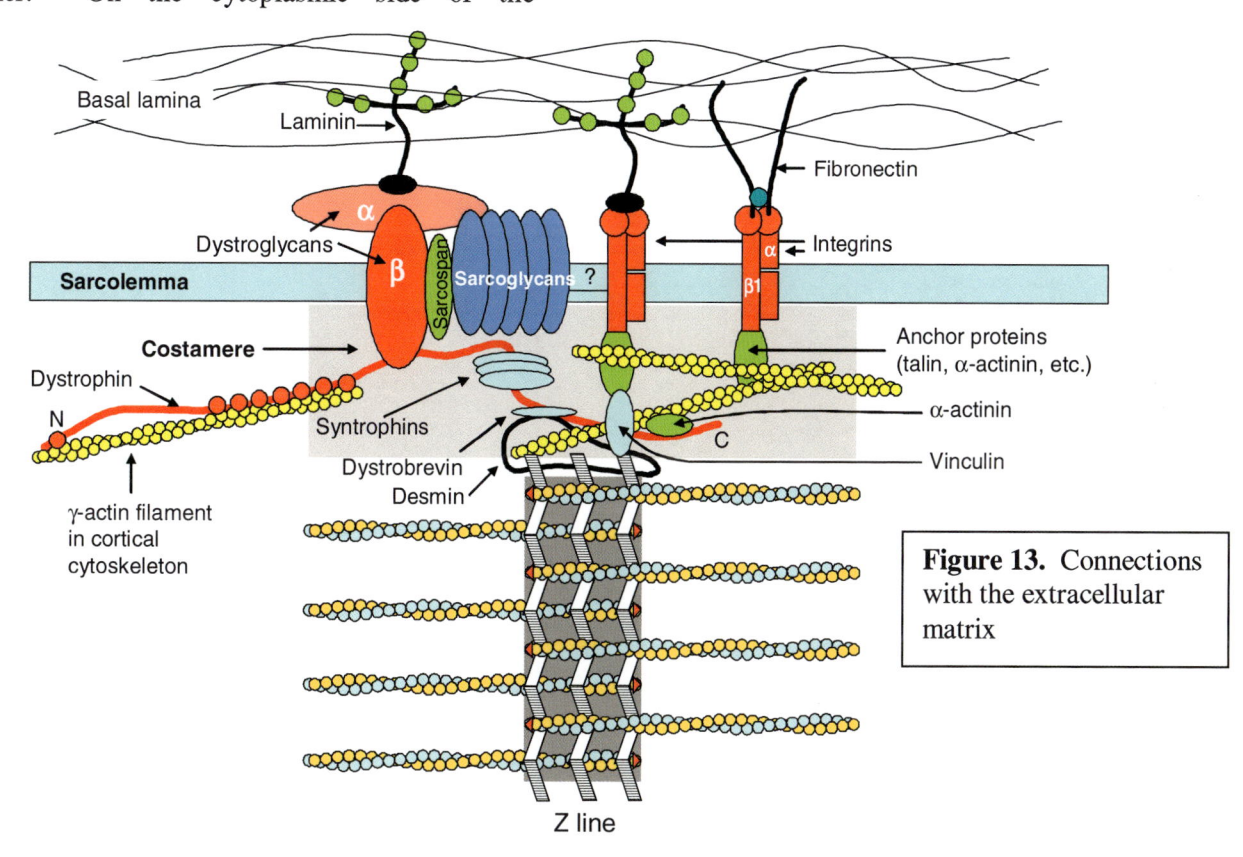

Figure 13. Connections with the extracellular matrix

The β1-Integrin Complex

β1-integrins (complexed with various α–integrins) span the membrane. Just outside the membrane, these integrins connect to components of the basal lamina, including laminin, fibronectin, and collagen. Near the inner surface of the membrane, β1-integrins connect to γ-actin filaments *via* various anchor proteins. The cortical actin filaments connect to α-actinin in the Z lines. Thus, the Z lines of peripheral myofibrils are glued to β1-integrins and beyond.

Topic 9: Costameres

Figure 14

The components of the dystroglycan/dystrophin complexes and the β1-integrin complexes are located, for the most part, at the level of Z lines. They form circumferential, rib-like structures on the inner surface of the sarcolemma called costameres, which can be seen using fluorescent-labeled antibodies to costameric components such as vinculin or γ-actin. Figure 14 diagrams this arrangement. Note that it is only the outermost myofibrils that directly connect to costameres.

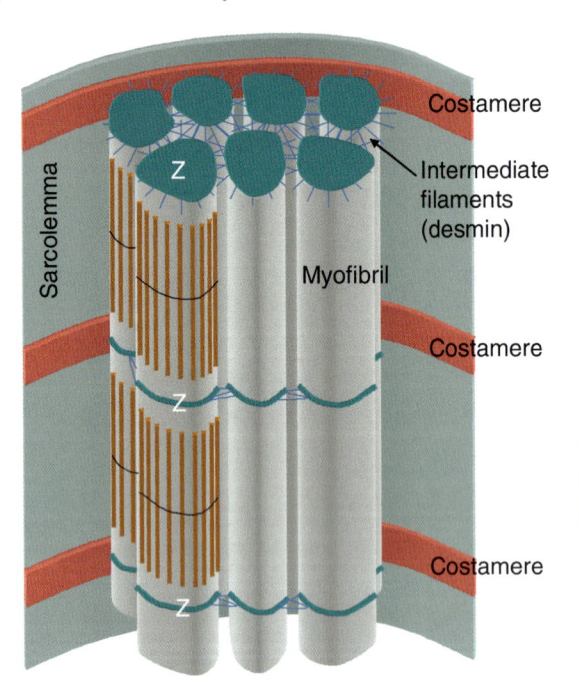

During contraction, shearing between sarcomeres and the sarcolemma and between the sarcolemma and the extracellular matrix must be avoided as much as possible. The costameric connections between Z lines and the extracellular matrix are essential for protecting the sarcolemma against damage due to shearing. As sarcomeres shorten, Z lines come closer together and, due to costameric connections, the sarcolemma tends to pucker between Z lines rather than tear.

In addition, shearing between adjacent cells must be minimized. The extracellular matrix is connected to all surrounding cells *via* dystroglycan/dystrophin and β1-integrin complexes. Thus, the Z lines of adjacent cells are all connected to each other; this tends to minimize cell-to-cell shearing.

Topic 10: Muscular Dystrophy

Defects in costameric components cause muscular dystrophy, presumably due to sarcolemmal damage. The most severe and most common muscular dystrophy in humans, Duchenne muscular dystrophy, is caused by absence of dystrophin. Cardiac involvement is common. A milder form, called Becker muscular dystrophy, is caused by a deficiency in dystrophin. Defects in most of the other costameric components can lead to other forms of muscular dystrophy or to fetal death due to muscle disease.

Figure 14. The relationship of Z lines to each other and to costameres (highly diagrammatic).

Cardiac Muscle: Structure and Mechanism of Contraction

Part 2: Mechanism of Contraction

Topic 1: Introduction

Now the stage is set. The cast of characters has been introduced, and we are ready for the action.

Contraction results from a cyclic reaction involving myosin, actin, and ATP, during which the S_1 heads of myosin force thin filaments toward the other half of the sarcomere. Since thin filaments are attached to Z lines, the Z lines are drawn closer together. As the sarcomeres shorten, they also get thicker (retaining constant volume). Neither thick nor thin filaments change appreciably in length.

Topic 2: The Resting State

At rest, S_1 has ADP and P attached and has a pronounced curvature. S_1 cannot bind to actin since the binding sites on actin are physically covered by tropomyosin. On occasion, even at rest, ADP and P dissociate from S_1. Whenever this event occurs, S_1 suddenly and forcefully straightens out. This would be a power stroke if S_1 were attached to actin, but at rest these unbending motions (which occur only about once a minute) are unproductive.

Topic 3: The Trigger for Contraction

Tropomyosin can take alternative positions along the actin chain. At rest, tropomyosin is positioned so that it covers the S_1 binding sites on actin. An excitatory event causes tropomyosin to move slightly (a little further into the groove formed by the actin double helix), thereby uncovering the S_1 binding sites on actin. This movement of tropomyosin triggers contraction. The process by which tropomyosin movement is regulated by Ca^{++} and the troponin complex will be discussed in Chapter 3.

Topic 4: The Power Stroke

Figure 15
As soon as tropomyosin moves out of the way, S_1 can bind to actin (top panel). Actually, each S_1 binds to two adjacent actin subunits. When S_1 is attached to actin, it is called a crossbridge. The attachment forms an angle of about 45° between actin and S_1. This attachment is stiff; *i.e.*, little or no rotation can take place.

Once the crossbridge forms, ADP and P immediately dissociate from S_1, and S_1 forcefully unbends. Now the power stroke is productive; it generates longitudinal force between thick and thin filaments.

The stem of S_1 is flexible. In addition, rotation can occur between S_1 and S_2. But the angle of attachment between S_1 and actin is fixed. Thus, the power stroke drives the thin filament toward the other half of the sarcomere (toward the left in the figure).

Each individual power stroke can generate roughly 2 pN of force, and can move the thin filament approximately the diameter of one actin monomer (5.5 nm). In the active state, the biochemical-mechanical crossbridge cycle repeats several orders of magnitude more frequently than at rest. Thus, ATP is used at a greatly increased rate.

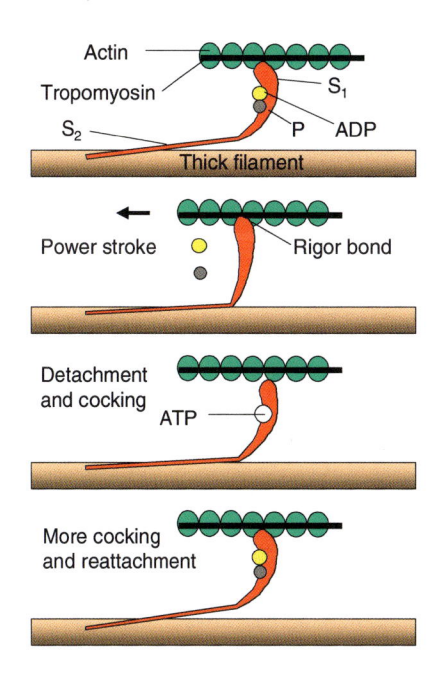

Figure 15. The S_1 ATPase cycle during contraction. See text for description.

Topic 5: The Rigor Bond

Following the power stroke, S_1, depleted of ADP and P, is strongly attached to actin. This attachment is called the rigor bond. Almost immediately, a new molecule of ATP binds to S_1 and the rigor bond breaks. Loosening of the rigor bond requires ATP binding.

If the supply of ATP runs low, as it does after death, rigor bonds persist. Thick and thin filaments remain tightly connected by crossbridges. The rigidity of skeletal muscles that results from persistent rigor bonds after death is called rigor mortis.

Topic 6: Cocking S_1

As S_1 with bound ATP detaches from actin, it bends a little and rotates with respect to S_2. ATP is quickly split to ADP and P and S_1 bends a little more. It is now primed and ready to attach to another binding site on actin.

Topic 7: The Crossbridge Cycle – A Reiteration

Animation: Crossbridge Cycle
[Available in the electronic edition of this textbook]

- A bent S_1, with bound ADP and P, stiffly attaches to two adjacent actin subunits.
- Immediately, the ADP and P are released and, simultaneously, S_1 forcefully unbends (power stroke).
- The power stroke drives the thin filament about 5.5 nm toward the other half of the sarcomere.
- A molecule of ATP binds to S_1; this greatly weakens the bond between S_1 and actin and they separate.
- As S_1 detaches from actin, it bends a little.
- The ATP that is bound to S_1 is now hydrolyzed to ADP and P, which remain attached to S_1.
- As ATP is split, S_1 bends further. It is now cocked and ready to attach to the next actin binding site.

This cycle continues until tropomyosin moves to cover the actin binding sites. As long as these sites are available, the cycle can repeat several hundred times per second per crossbridge.

Notice that actin activates the ATPase activity of S_1 by increasing the rate of product release (ADP and P). The turnover number of the S_1 ATPase is increased several orders of magnitude.

Topic 8: Asynchrony of Crossbridge Action

There are about 150 myosin molecules on each half of each thick filament. Each of these has two S_1 heads. They do not all tug together on the surrounding thin filaments but operate asynchronously, presumably in random fashion, on the available actin sites. The total force generated between thick and thin filaments, and the rate of sarcomere shortening, depend on the number of crossbridges cycling at any instant. It has been suggested that the two S_1 heads on each myosin molecule might act alternately, as one would tug on a rope hand-over-hand; however, this has not been proved.

Selected References for Chapter 2:

- M.S. Forbes and N. Sperelakis, Ultrastructure of Mammalian Cardiac Muscle. In N. Sperelakis (Ed.), *Physiology and Pathophysiology of the Heart, 3rd Edition*, Chapter 1, Kluwer Academic Publishers, 1995.
- A.J. Brady, Contractile and Mechanical Properties of the Myocardium. In N. Sperelakis (Ed.), *Physiology and Pathophysiology of the Heart, 3rd Edition*, Chapter 19, Kluwer Academic Publishers, 1995.
- C. Lynch III, The Biochemical and Cellular Basis of Myocardial Contractility. In D.C. Warltier (Ed.), *Ventricular Function*, Chapter 1, Williams & Wilkins, 1995.
- K.P. Roos, Mechanics and Force Production. In G.A. Langer (Ed.), *The Myocardium, 2nd Edition*, Chapter 6, Academic Press, 1997.
- I. Rayment, The Structural Basis of the Myosin ATPase Activity, *J. Biol. Chem.* 271:15850-15853, 1996.
- R. Cooke, The Sliding Filament Model: 1972–2004, J. Gen. Physiol. 123: 643-656, 2004.
- J. M. Ervasti, Costamers: the Achilles' Heel of Herculean Muscle, J. Biol. Chem. 278: 13591-13594, 2003.
- The Dystrophin-Associated Glycoprotein Complex (DGC), Leiden Muscular Dystrophy pages, http://www.dmd.nl/DGC.html.

Chapter 3

Cardiac Muscle: Excitation

This chapter treats the mechanisms of excitation in cardiac muscle.
Part 1 describes the excitatory system of the heart.
Part 2 describes excitation-contraction coupling in cardiac muscle - it is similar, but not identical, to excitation-contraction coupling in skeletal muscle.
Part 3 presents the ionic mechanisms responsible for action potentials in working myocytes.
Part 4 presents the ionic mechanisms responsible for rhythmicity and determination of heart rate.

Part 1: Excitatory System of the Heart

Topic 1: Introduction

The heart does not require nerves to make it beat - it is not neurogenic. Its autonomic innervation is responsible for important changes in frequency and strength, but does not initiate the beat. Instead, the working myocardium is activated by action potentials that originate in special cardiac myocytes. Thus, the heartbeat is myogenic rather than neurogenic. Transplanted hearts with no extrinsic innervation beat rhythmically.

Figure 1
Excitation of the heartbeat consists of the following stages:

- Rhythmic generation of action potentials in the sinus node (often called the sinoatrial node or SA node).
- Conduction of action potentials throughout the atrium and to the atrioventricular node (AV node).
- Conduction of action potentials through the AV node to the bundle of His.
- Conduction of action potentials through the His-Purkinje system to working myocytes of the ventricles.
- Conduction of action potentials through working ventricular myocytes.

Topic 2: Shapes of Cardiac Action Potentials

Figure 2
Action potentials from the SA node and AV node have a slower rise than those from atrial and ventricular myocardium and from the His-Purkinje system. They also have less overshoot (the portion above zero mV), and they start from a less polarized membrane potential (about -60 mV compared to about -85 mV). In addition, action potentials from the nodes do not have stable resting potentials but show pacemaker potentials (diastolic depolarization). Pacemaker potentials are the basis of automaticity.

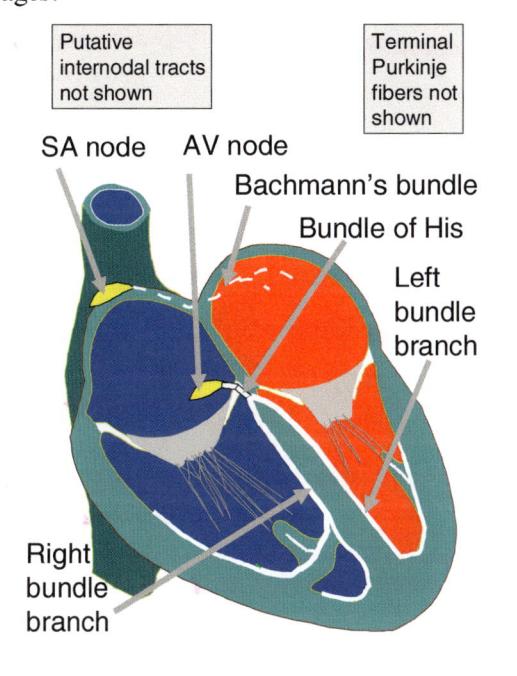

Figure 1. The excitatory system of the heart.

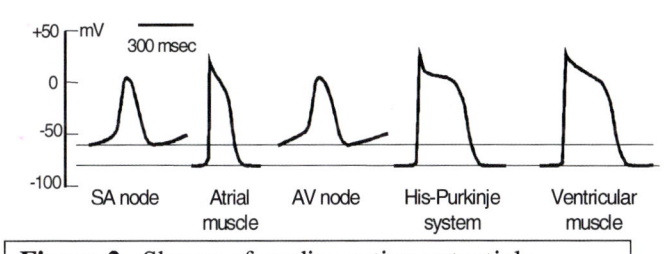

Figure 2. Shapes of cardiac action potentials.

Topic 3: Rhythmic Generation of Action Potentials in the SA Node

The SA node is an elongated oval mass of cells and connective tissue about 10-20 mm long. It is located subepicardially along the anterio-lateral junction of the superior vena cava and the right atrium. The SA node contains two different types of myocytes called P cells (pale, pacemaking), and T cells (transitional).

P cells are very small and nearly spherical. They are embedded in a connective tissue matrix that surrounds a large central artery. Groups of P cells are electrically connected to each other by gap junctions. P cells generate action potentials. They do so spontaneously and rhythmically. This behavior is called automaticity.

The frequency of action potentials generated by P cells in the SA node normally sets the pace for the entire heart (*i.e.* determines the heart rate). When this is true, the heart is said to be on a sinus rhythm.

T cells are more elongated and are located near the periphery of the SA node. Their appearance is intermediate between P cells and ordinary atrial myocytes. T cells are connected to P cells and to each other by gap junctions. T cells near the margin of the node connect to ordinary atrial cells at intercalated disks. T cells relay the action potentials generated in P cells to the surrounding atrial myocardium.

Topic 4: Conduction through the Atrium

From the SA node, the impulse is rapidly conducted as a wave of depolarization to the AV node and throughout both atria along ordinary atrial myocytes. The velocity of atrial conduction is about 1 m/sec. The impulse reaches the AV node in about 40 msec and depolarizes the entire atrial myocardium in about 90 msec. The duration of the atrial action potential (roughly 200 msec) is considerably longer than its conduction time. Consequently, during most of the atrial activation period most of the atrial myocytes are contracting. The result is an atrial beat that is more synchronous than it is peristaltic. Repolarization is not propagated as a regular wave through the atria.

There is a large bundle of atrial fibers that runs from the SA node behind the aorta to the left atrium. This structure is called Bachmann's bundle. It is presumed that action potentials traveling from the SA node through Bachmann's bundle assist in left atrial depolarization.

Tracts of atrial myocytes that look histologically different from ordinary atrial fibers and run from SA node to AV node have been described. They are called internodal tracts. It has been suggested that internodal tracts facilitate impulse conduction to the AV node. There is no compelling evidence for this function. In fact, even the existence of internodal tracts is in doubt. [Some textbooks depict internodal tracts as prominent bundles - they are not.]

Topic 5: Conduction through the AV Node

The AV node is a mass of cells located subepicardially in the posterior wall of the right atrium. It lies near the interatrial septum just above the base of the heart where the septal leaflet of the tricuspid valve is attached. Its longest dimension is roughly 20 mm. The cells in the core of the AV node are mainly P cells. Most of the periphery contains T cells intermixed with ordinary atrial myocytes. The distal part of the node makes a transition into the bundle of His, which penetrates the base of the heart through the central fibrous body (right fibrous trigone).

P cells in the AV node possess latent automaticity. If left to their own devices they would generate action potentials spontaneously and rhythmically. However, their frequency of spontaneous firing is less than that of P cells in the SA node. Consequently, AV nodal action potentials are normally driven at the frequency of P cells in the SA node. If the SA node fails, the AV node can take up the duty of pacing the ventricles, but at a lower than normal frequency.

Conduction through the AV node is very slow (only about 0.1 m/sec) and requires over 100 msec. Consequently, activation of the His-Purkinje system (ventricular conduction system) is delayed, giving the atria a chance to complete their contraction before the ventricles begin theirs.

Action potentials can be conducted in either direction through the AV node, but conduction in the retrograde direction is considerably slower than in the normal direction.

Topic 6: Conduction through the His-Purkinje System

The His-Purkinje system consists of:
- The bundle of His (also called the His bundle)
- The left and right bundle branches
- The terminal Purkinje fibers

The predominant and most important type of cell in the His-Purkinje system is the Purkinje cell. Purkinje cells have very large diameters. They have a poorly developed system of myofibrils and, therefore, have a pale appearance. They are specialized for rapid conduction of the impulse

The distal part of the AV node blends into the bundle of His, which penetrates the central fibrous body and runs along the membranous part of the interventricular septum. Its length is about 20 mm and its diameter about 4 mm.

As the muscular part of the interventricular septum is reached, the bundle of His branches into the left and right bundle branches. The left bundle branch continues distally along the left side of the interventricular septum. It branches a variable number of times along the septum. The right bundle branch continues unbranched along the right side of the interventricular septum to the apex of the right ventricle, finally sending branches to papillary muscles and along the moderator band. More and more branching occurs on both left and right sides as the bundles pass through the apex and then travel up along the endocardial surfaces of the ventricular free walls.

Along the apex and the left and right free walls, and along the left side of the interventricular septum, the conduction system branches profusely into terminal Purkinje fibers. These fibers form a dense interweaving network on the endocardial surface and some of them penetrate into the myocardium for as much as a third of its thickness.

Purkinje cells in the His-Purkinje system are electrically connected to each other with gap junctions at intercalated disks. Impulse conduction along each Purkinje cell and from cell to cell is very rapid. The conduction velocity is about 1-4 m/sec. The wave of depolarization reaches nearly the entire endocardial surface of both ventricles within about 30 msec after leaving the AV node. Rapid conduction of action potentials through the His-Purkinje system is essential to assure that all parts of the ventricular myocardium contract nearly simultaneously rather than piece-by-piece.

Purkinje cells in the His-Purkinje system are latent pacemakers; *i.e.* they have the potential for automaticity. The spontaneous firing frequency of Purkinje cells is less than that of either the SA node or AV node. Therefore, they do not normally get a chance to express their own intrinsic rhythm, but are driven at nodal frequency. If anything happens to prevent supraventricular impulses from reaching the ventricles, Purkinje cells, usually in the His bundle or main bundle branches, start pacing. Most commonly, this problem is caused by conduction failure in the AV node (AV block). Purkinje cell automaticity is important for keeping the beat going (albeit at a low rate) when AV conduction fails.

Topic 7: Conduction through Working Ventricular Myocytes

The His-Purkinje system promptly gets the wave of depolarization to the vicinity of the working myocardium. However, the final stage in excitation involves conduction of action potentials cell-to-cell through the working myocardium itself. Conduction velocity in the working myocardium is much slower than through the Purkinje system. In the ventricular free walls, a wave of depolarization passes from endocardial to epicardial surfaces at a velocity of about 0.4 m/sec, and requires roughly another 30 msec to depolarize all the working myocytes. In the interventricular septum, the wave of depolarization passes from left to right since the septum is supplied by terminal Purkinje fibers only from the divisions of the left bundle branch, not the right.

The duration of action potentials in epicardial myocytes is considerably less than in endocardial myocytes. This disparity has an important consequence. Although the epicardial myocytes are the last to depolarize, they are the first to repolarize. Consequently, in the ventricular free walls, a wave of repolarization passes from epicardial to endocardial surfaces, in the opposite direction to the wave of depolarization.

Topic 8: Each Atrial or Ventricular Contraction is a Synchronous Twitch of All Its Fibers

You should recall that during a sustained contraction of skeletal muscle, motor units fire asynchronously. The contraction can be smooth rather than jerky because twitches in many motor units are out of phase with each other. Increased force of contraction in skeletal muscle is caused by recruitment of more motor units and by increased excitation frequency of individual motor units. If excitation frequency increases sufficiently, summation of contractions and even complete tetanus can occur.

The situation is quite different in cardiac muscle. Action potentials in cardiac muscle, unlike those in skeletal muscle, propagate from cell to cell through gap junctions. An impulse starting in the SA node progressively excites all atrial fibers and they contract synchronously. An impulse relayed through the AV node progressively excites all ventricular fibers and they contract synchronously.

In addition, cardiac muscle fibers, unlike skeletal muscle fibers, can only contract in individual twitches; summation of contractions is absent. Therefore, cardiac muscle cannot be tetanized. The explanation for lack of summation lies in the duration of the cardiac action potential; it lasts so long that the membrane remains practically inexcitable until after the relaxation phase of the twitch is over.

In cardiac muscle, changes in the force and velocity of contraction are not caused by recruitment of more muscle fibers or by summation of twitches. Rather, they are caused by changes in sarcomere length and contractility as explained in Chapter 4.

Part 2: Excitation-Contraction Coupling

Topic 1: Introduction

The trigger for contraction is the movement of tropomyosin on thin filaments in a way that uncovers the sites on actin to which S_1 heads of myosin can bind. Contraction is terminated when tropomyosin moves back to cover these sites again. The position of tropomyosin is determined by the concentration of free Ca^{++} around thin filaments. The Ca^{++} concentration around thin filaments responds to action potentials traveling over the sarcolemma and T tubules. The process by which action potentials initiate contraction is called excitation-contraction (EC) coupling.

Topic 2: Temporal Relationship among the Action Potential, Ca^{++} Concentration, and Contraction

Figure 3
This figure shows the timing between the action potential and the resulting contraction. The ionic mechanism of the action potential in working myocardium will be described in Part 3 of this chapter. For now, notice that the action potential is very long and has about the same duration as the contraction. This figure also shows the change in cytoplasmic free Ca^{++} concentration. Notice that contraction closely tracks Ca^{++} concentration, but lags appreciably behind. The phase lag between cytoplasmic free Ca^{++} and contraction is due to series elasticity as it is in skeletal muscle.

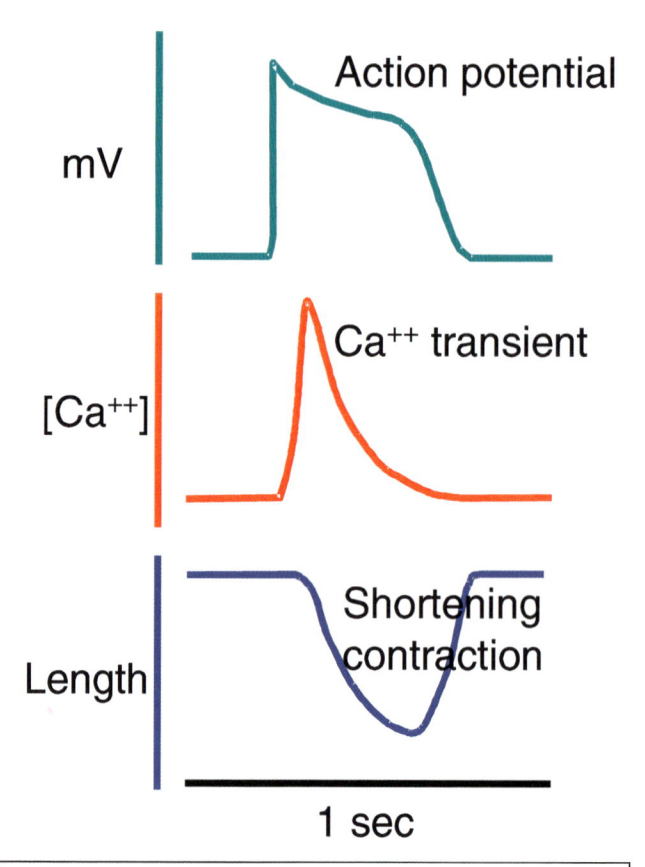

Figure 3. Temporal relationship among the action potential, cytoplasmic free Ca^{++} concentration, and a shortening contraction in cardiac muscle. Constant-length contractions (isometric) last somewhat longer than the shortening contraction shown here.

Cardiac Muscle: Excitation

Topic 3: Ca^{++} Entry into the Myocyte and Ca^{++}-Induced Ca^{++} Release from the SR

Figure 4

This figure is repeated here to remind you of the anatomical relationships among sarcolemma, T tubules, junctional SR, network SR, and sarcomeres. These are the structural elements involved in EC coupling.

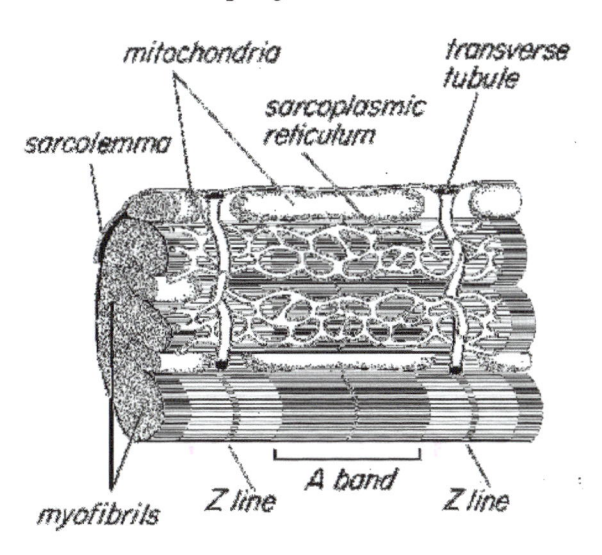

Figure 4. General relationships among myofibrils, sarcolemma, T tubules, sarcoplasmic reticulum, and mitochondria in cardiac muscle. Drawing by Dr. Donald Stubbs.

Figure 5

Here we zoom in on the region of close approximation between T tubule membrane and junctional SR membrane. These membranes are separated by a narrow cleft about 12 nm wide. We add two types of Ca^{++} channels.

- In T tubule membrane we have L-type Ca^{++} channels. These are also called dihydropyridine (DHP) receptors, since drugs in the dihydropyridine class, such as nifedipine, block them. The dihydropyridines are a major class of Ca^{++} channel blockers that are important in the treatment of angina, hypertension, and heart failure. DHP receptors are present all along the sarcolemma and T tubules. They are particularly concentrated at the sites of close contact with junctional SR. Their probability of opening is greatly increased by membrane depolarization; in other words, they are voltage-gated channels.

- In junctional SR membrane we have Ca^{++}-release channels (CRCs). These are also called ryanodine receptors. Ryanodine is a drug that influences CRCs and is important in experimental work but currently has no clinical use. CRCs open in response to Ca^{++} that enters the cell through DHP receptors during the action potential. Thus, CRCs are Ca^{++}-gated Ca^{++} channels. CRCs are spatially related to the DHP receptors of the T tubules.

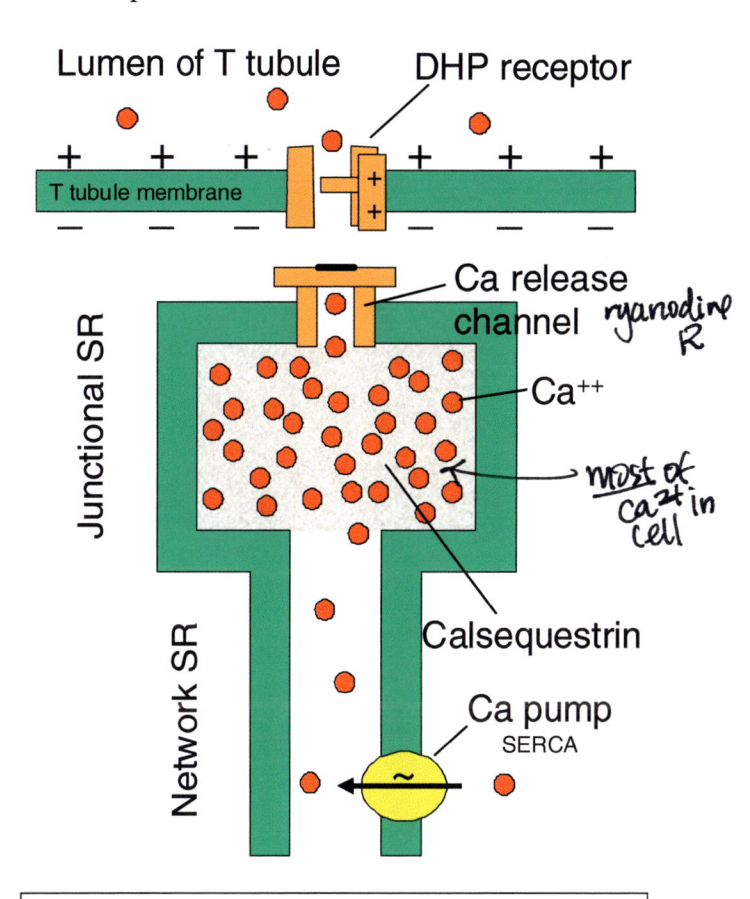

Figure 5. The players involved in the excitation-contraction coupling process in cardiac muscle. Resting state.

In Figure 5, the system is at rest (diastole). There is no action potential. The resting membrane potential is about -85 mV. Both types of Ca^{++} channels are closed. The Ca^{++} concentration in the lumen of the T tubule is about 2-3 mM. A huge amount of Ca^{++} is sequestered within the junctional SR, most of which is loosely bound to calsequestrin. Primary Ca^{++} pumps in the network SR and sarcolemma, and Na$^+$-Ca^{++} exchangers in the sarcolemma and T tubules, keep the concentration of Ca^{++} in the cytoplasm exceedingly low (about 0.1 µM).

Entry of Ca^{++} during the Action Potential
Figure 6

The initial excitatory event is an action potential traveling along the sarcolemma. It continues along the T tubules into the interior of the cardiomyocyte. Membrane depolarization during the action potential causes the DHP receptors to open. Consequently, a little Ca^{++} enters the cell.

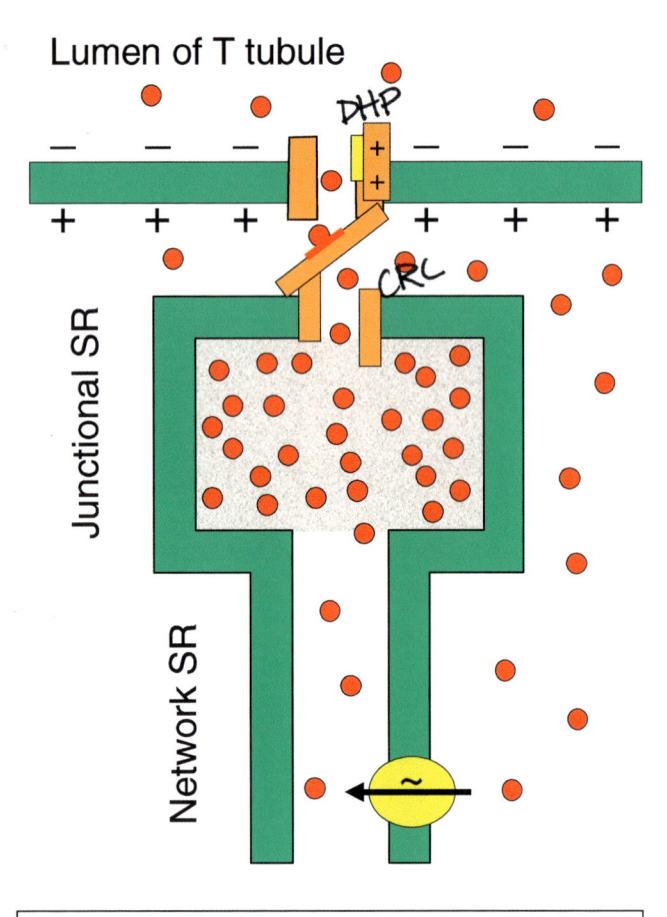

Figure 6. Excitation-contraction coupling. The active state.

Ca^{++}-Induced Ca^{++} Release from the Junctional SR

When just a little Ca^{++} enters through the DHP receptors, its concentration increases markedly in the tiny space between the two membranes. Ca^{++} binds to CRCs. When Ca^{++} binds to a CRC its probability of being open is vastly increased. Consequently, Ca^{++} rapidly diffuses out of the junctional SR through the CRCs. This process is called Ca^{++}-induced Ca^{++} release. The Ca^{++} initially released by this process probably induces more Ca^{++} release, thereby amplifying the response. Much more Ca^{++} is released from the junctional SR through CRCs than enters the cell through DHP receptors. The released Ca^{++} then diffuses through the cytoplasm along the myofilaments, reaching a concentration of roughly 2 μM (a 20-fold increase). When Ca^{++} encounters a troponin complex, it binds to TnC.

CRCs open only briefly upon being activated by Ca^{++}. A burst of Ca^{++} release occurs and then, in spite of an elevated Ca^{++} concentration around them, the CRCs close. Theories to explain this apparent inactivation of CRCs are currently not established sufficiently to be included here.

[Note: In skeletal muscle, the mechanism for inducing Ca^{++} release from CRCs is different than it is in cardiac muscle. In skeletal muscle, a conformational change in the DHP receptor in response to a membrane voltage change is thought to be more important in signaling the underlying CRC than is Ca^{++} influx. The signal apparently involves a direct mechanical interaction between the DHP receptor and the CRC.]

[Animations for EC-coupling are available in the electronic edition.]

These animations depict:
- the action potential along the T tubule membrane
- opening of L-type Ca^{++} channels (DHP receptors)
- Ca^{++}-induced Ca^{++} release from junctional SR
- diffusion of Ca^{++} to the myofilaments
- activation of the troponin-tropomyosin complex by Ca^{++}
- the crossbridge cycle
- removal of Ca^{++} from the sarcoplasm by the Na$^+$-K$^+$ pump and Na$^+$-Ca^{++} exchanger in the sarcolemma, and by SERCA in the sarcoplasmic reticulum.

Topic 4: The Troponin-Tropomyosin Trigger

Figure 7

Prior to excitation, when the concentration of Ca^{++} in the cytoplasm is about 0.1 μM, TnC is devoid of Ca^{++} and is weakly attached to TnI. In turn, TnI is attached to actin and to TnT. TnT is a rod that spans about three actin subunits, but is not attached to them. However, TnT is attached to tropomyosin. In other words, TnT links TnI to tropomyosin. Tropomyosin is an even longer rod (about 42 nm) that spans about 7.5 actin subunits. This arrangement holds tropomyosin rather loosely over seven actin sites that otherwise could bind S$_1$ heads.

Cardiac Muscle: Excitation

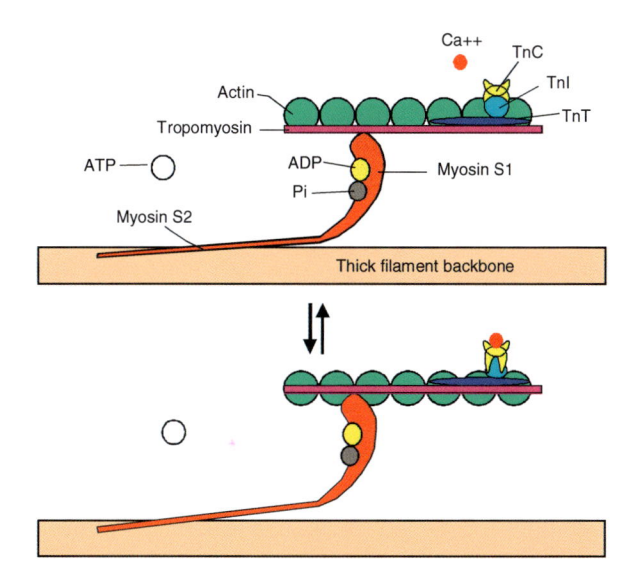

Figure 7. Ca^{++}-induced transition of the troponin-tropomyosin complex. When the available Ca^{++}-binding site on TN-C is empty, tropomyosin covers the sites on actin that could otherwise bind to myosin S$_1$. When Ca^{++} binds to the available site on TN-C, the troponin-tropomyosin complex moves out of the way.

Response of the Troponin-Tropomyosin Complex to Ca^{++} Binding

When a single Ca^{++} ion binds to TnC, a cascade of conformational changes is induced in the troponin-tropomyosin complex, which results in uncovering the sites on actin that can bind S$_1$ heads. [Note: In skeletal muscle, two Ca^{++} ions must bind to TnC, but in cardiac muscle there is only one available Ca^{++} binding site on TnC.] *more sensitive to Ca^{2+}?*

Upon excitation, the Ca^{++} concentration rises about 20-fold and some of the Ca^{++} ions bind to TnC. This induces a conformational change in TnC such that its attachment to TnI gets stronger. This, in turn, induces a conformational change in TnI, which causes it to detach from actin. Then the entire complex shifts. Tropomyosin moves further into the actin double helix groove and the S$_1$ binding sites on actin are exposed. Now, as shown in the following animation, the crossbridge cycle proceeds. Tension is generated. Shortening and thickening occur.

Binding of Ca^{++} to TnC is a reversible process - it remains attached for only a few crossbridge cycles before spontaneously unbinding. Therefore, troponin-tropomyosin complexes trigger and then reset repetitively as long as cytoplasmic free Ca^{++} is sufficiently elevated.

Topic 5: The Dose-Response Relationship for Ca^{++}

Figure 8

The amount of Ca^{++} released during a single excitatory event is much less than that required for a maximal response. Only a fraction of the troponin-tropomyosin complexes is triggered at any instant. If the amount of Ca^{++} released from the SR during an excitatory event increases, then a greater fraction of the troponin-tropomyosin complexes will be triggered and the contraction will be stronger. In fact, the amount of Ca^{++} released from the SR during an excitatory event is one of the most important determinants of the force and speed of contraction. This behavior contrasts to that in skeletal muscle where nearly maximal thin filament activation is produced with each excitatory event.

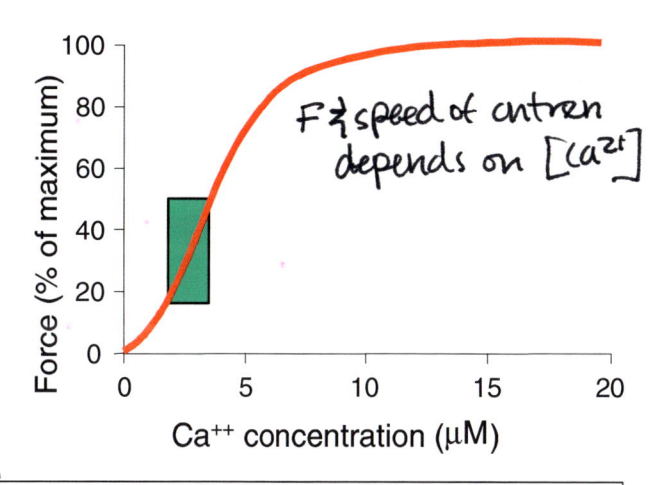

F & speed of contren depends on [Ca^{2+}]

Figure 8. The dose-response relationship for Ca^{++}. Isometric force is plotted as a function of cytoplasmic free Ca^{++} concentration. This type of relationship is sometimes called an activation curve. The rectangle shows the range of Ca^{++} concentration and relative force production for a normal heartbeat in an individual at rest.

The steepness of the curve is much greater than expected for simple binding of one Ca^{++} ion to TnC. This characteristic implies positive cooperativity in the triggering process. The mechanisms for cooperativity are somewhat speculative, but can be tentatively described as follows:

- When a Ca^{++} binding event activates a troponin-tropomyosin complex, crossbridges start cycling, and tension is exerted on actin. The resulting distortion of actin subunits increases the stability of the troponin-tropomyosin complex in its triggered state. This effect can be measured as an increase in the affinity of

TnC for Ca^{++}. The greater the number of crossbridges cycling, the greater is this effect.
- Triggering of one troponin-tropomyosin complex by a Ca^{++} ion makes it easier for other Ca^{++} ions to trigger adjacent troponin-tropomyosin complexes. This effect might be related to the fact that tropomyosin molecules overlap each other a little.

Regardless of the mechanism, cooperativity markedly increases the sensitivity of the response to small changes in Ca^{++} concentration.

Topic 6: Removal of Ca^{++} and Relaxation

See Figure 3 again
The concentration of Ca^{++} around the myofilaments rises quickly during the beginning of an excitatory event, and then gradually decreases during the remainder of the action potential. The decrease results from operation of the following three Ca^{++} transporters (in order of quantitative importance):
- The primary Ca^{++} pump in the tubular SR (SERCA), which pumps Ca^{++} back into the tubular SR.
- The Na^+-Ca^{++} exchange carrier in the sarcolemma and T tubules, which pumps Ca^{++} out of the cell.
- The primary Ca^{++} pump in the sarcolemma, which pumps Ca^{++} out of the cell (quantitatively much less important than the Na^+-Ca^{++} exchanger).

These transporters are in operation continuously. During the early part of excitation, when cytoplasmic Ca^{++} concentration is rising, Ca^{++} is released from the junctional SR through CRCs faster than the transporters remove it from the cytoplasm. Later during excitation, as pointed out above, the CRCs shut down, allowing the transporters to clear the cytoplasm of previously released Ca^{++}.

As the concentration of cytoplasmic Ca^{++} goes down, crossbridge activity diminishes and eventually ceases.

In the following animation, the three transporters that remove Ca^{++} from the cytoplasm are added to the earlier animation, which showed only the processes responsible for increasing cytoplasmic Ca^{++}.

Topic 7: Myocyte Ca^{++} Balance and Effect of Heart Rate

As long as the heart rate remains constant, the amount of Ca^{++} pumped back into the tubular SR exactly equals the amount released from the junctional SR during each contraction-relaxation cycle. The average amount of Ca^{++} in the SR remains constant. In addition, the amount of Ca^{++} pumped out of the myocyte by the Na^+-Ca^{++} exchanger and the primary Ca^{++} pump equals the amount entering the cell via Ca^{++} channels. Thus, total cell Ca^{++} remains constant.

There is a complication. Between action potentials, CRCs occasionally open spontaneously. The frequency of spontaneous opening is far less than it is during excitation, but whenever it occurs, a little Ca^{++} is released (this is called a Ca^{++} spark). Some of the Ca^{++} released between action potentials is simply pumped back into the SR. However, some of it is pumped out of the cell, resulting in a gradual decline of Ca^{++} in the SR. Spontaneous Ca^{++} sparks do not release enough Ca^{++} to cause contraction, but they do release enough to result in an appreciable loss of Ca^{++} from the SR between action potentials. The amount lost depends on the amount of time between action potentials.

Figure 9
If the heart rate decreases, more Ca^{++} is lost from the SR due to Ca^{++} sparks. Consequently, less Ca^{++} is available for release during each excitatory event, and over the next several beats the force of contraction gradually goes down. If the frequency of excitation increases, the SR retains more Ca^{++} and the force of contraction gradually goes up. The stepwise change in force of contraction with changes in heart rate is called the staircase phenomenon (it also called treppe and sometimes the Bowditch effect).

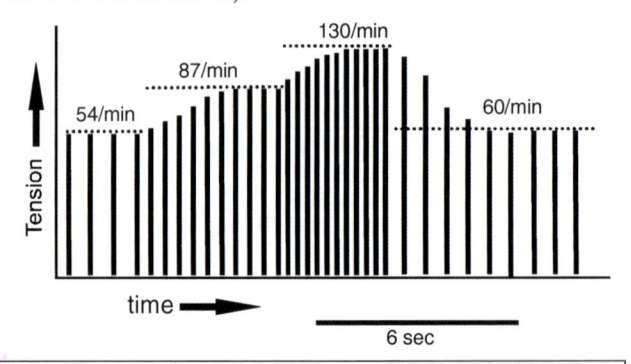

Figure 9. The staircase phenomenon (treppe). Isometric tension is influenced by heart rate.

Cardiac Muscle: Excitation

Part 3: Action Potentials of Working Myocytes

Topic 1: General Features of Myocardial Action Potentials

Figure 10
This figure illustrates the shape and nomenclature of action potentials in working myocardium and Purkinje fibers. The most obvious and most important feature of the cardiac action potential is its duration. It lasts a long time, normally about 200-350 msec in ventricular myocytes. Action potentials in skeletal muscle last only a few msec. The duration of ventricular action potentials is greatest in endocardial myocytes and progressively decreases toward the epicardial surface. The duration of atrial action potentials is less than that of ventricular action potentials.

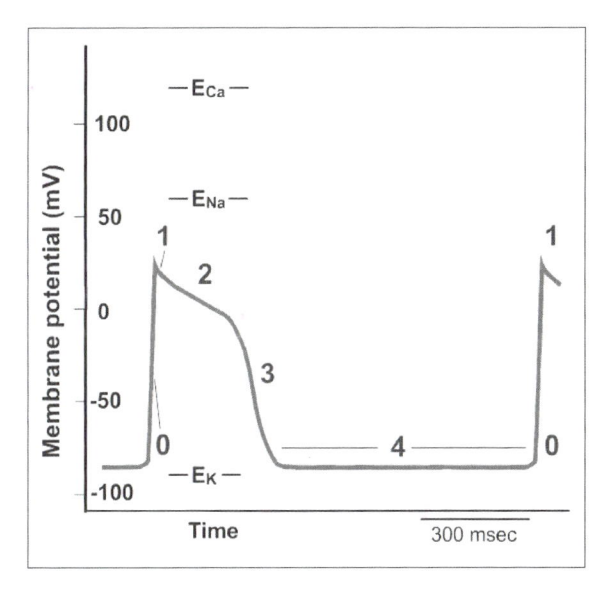

Figure 10. The nomenclature for action potentials in working myocardium and Purkinje cells. The phases (0-4) are described in the text. The equilibrium potentials for K^+, Na^+, and Ca^{++} are shown for reference during the discussion of ionic mechanisms.

A long action potential is required in cardiac muscle to provide a long refractory period. Consider a wave of depolarization passing over the ventricular conduction system and working myocardium. At any given location the refractory period must last until the entire ventricular myocardium is depolarized and the excitatory impulse dies out. Otherwise, it might not die out at all. It might re-excite regions that have already regained excitability resulting in reverberating circuits of depolarization that continue endlessly. This kind of abnormal electrical activity is called reentry and is responsible for many kinds of arrhythmias. Action potential duration can be less in myocytes near the epicardial surface since these are the last myocytes to be excited.

Topic 2: A Few Rules Necessary for Understanding Action Potentials

You should recall the following principles of membrane excitability:
- When an ion channel opens, specific types of ions can move through it across the membrane. They move from the side having the higher electrochemical potential for the ion, to the side having the lower electrochemical potential. This means that at normal resting potentials, Na^+ and Ca^{++} ions will move inward when their channels open, but K^+ ions will move outward when their channels open.
- Ionic currents resulting from channel opening cause depolarization when the current is in the inward direction, and cause hyperpolarization (or repolarization) when the current is in the outward direction.
- If the permeability to one type of ion increases as a result of channel opening, the membrane potential (V_M) moves toward the equilibrium potential for that ion (E_{ion}).

[Tutorial: Membrane Potentials]
[Available in electronic edition]

Topic 3: Ionic Mechanisms

Phase 0: Rapid Depolarization
Rapid depolarization is caused by inward current through voltage-gated fast Na^+ channels. This current is called the fast inward Na^+ current or I_{Na}. It lasts only an instant since the Na^+ channels rapidly inactivate.

Rapid depolarization is essential to produce rapid conduction of the impulse along each cell and, especially, from cell to cell. Action potentials at any site are triggered by passive depolarization spreading ahead from upstream active sites. When passive depolarization at a downstream site reaches threshold, an action potential fires. The time required to reach threshold is determined largely by the abruptness and amplitude of upstream depolarization (also by intracellular conductance and, therefore, cell diameter). Thus, I_{Na} causes rapid conduction of the impulse along the network of myocardial cells. The pacemaking cells in the SA node (P cells) do not have significant I_{Na}. Therefore, they do not have a rapid depolarization phase and they conduct very slowly. This is also true of P cells in the AV node. Slow conduction in the AV node is essential to assure that the ventricles do not start contracting before the atria are finished contracting.

Phase 1: Transient Repolarization
This phase is caused by outward current through channels called transient outward channels (these are mainly K^+ channels but Cl^- channels may also be involved). Transient outward current is designated I_{to}. It is initiated by the depolarization produced by I_{Na} and by the rise in cytoplasmic Ca^{++} concentration that begins about this time. Most transient outward channels inactivate quickly. The function of phase 1 is not entirely clear. It seems to have something to do with action potential duration but the mechanism is not understood.

Phase 2: Slow Repolarization or Plateau
This is the most interesting and complex phase of the myocardial action potential. The membrane remains depolarized during phase 2 mainly because of inward current through L-type Ca^{++} channels (dihydropyridine receptors). This current is called $I_{Ca(L)}$. It is also called the slow inward current, I_{si}. It is initiated by the depolarization produced by I_{Na}. L-type Ca^{++} channels inactivate slowly during the plateau. Inward $I_{Ca(L)}$ provides the Ca^{++} required for triggering Ca^{++}-induced Ca^{++} release from the junctional SR (see Part 2 of this chapter).

Two other kinds of channels are important in maintaining the plateau, K_1 channels and background channels. The K_1 channels (also called inwardly rectifying K^+ channels) are open during phase 4 and are important in setting the resting potential. The outward current through K_1 channels is called I_{K1}. K_1 channels have a very important property; they instantly close as the membrane depolarizes. $I_{Ca(L)}$ is small in magnitude and would be ineffective in maintaining the plateau if the K_1 channels remained open. Inhibition of I_{K1} by depolarization allows $I_{Ca(L)}$ to keep V_M far from the equilibrium potential for K^+ (E_K).

There are background channels for Na^+ and Ca^{++}. The inward current through these channels, I_{bkg}, is very small but occurs all the time. Background channels are not voltage gated. After the K_1 channels are turned off by depolarization, I_{bkg} contributes appreciably to maintaining membrane depolarization during the plateau.

Thus, the long duration of the plateau and refractory period results from:
- Activation of slowly inactivating $I_{Ca(L)}$ by the depolarization produced by I_{Na}.
- Inhibition of I_{K1} by depolarization.
- Continuous I_{bkg}.

During phase 2 another type of K^+ channel, the delayed K^+ channel, gradually opens and carries an outward current called I_K. Inward $I_{Ca(L)}$ and outward I_K fight each other, attempting to drive V_M in opposite directions. As $I_{Ca(L)}$ gradually declines (due to inactivation) and I_K gradually increases, the membrane slowly repolarizes.

Phase 3: Rapid Repolarization
This phase is caused mainly by outward I_K. Delayed K^+ channels open with ever increasing frequency as phase 2 progresses. At the same time, L-type Ca^{++} channels gradually inactivate. Eventually, the K^+ channels win overwhelmingly, and outward I_K repolarizes the membrane. During phase 3, delayed K^+ channels slowly begin to close and K_1 channels open again. Outward I_{K1} contributes to final repolarization and then holds V_M at resting potential during phase 4.

Phase 4: Resting Potential
The resting potential is set mainly by outward current through K_1 channels. Between action potentials, so many K_1 channels are open that V_M is held near E_K.

The background channels are much less abundant than K_1 channels. The small inward current through these background channels, I_{bkg}, causes some depolarization and accounts for the fact that resting potential is depolarized a few mV compared to E_K.

During phase 4 (and final part of phase 3) the voltage-gated Na^+ channels reactivate. They cannot reactivate until the membrane repolarizes. This is the reason that the refractory period lasts about as long as the action potential.

If you would like to step through each component of the action potential in more detail click here
[Tutorial: Ventricular Action Potential]
[Available in electronic edition]

Topic 4: A Summary of the Ionic Currents in Working Myocytes

- **I_{Na}:** Responsible for rapid depolarization (phase 0). Rapid depolarization activates L-type Ca^{++} channels and is necessary for rapid conduction.
- **I_{to}:** Responsible for transient repolarization (phase 1).
- **$I_{Ca(L)}$:** Partly responsible for the plateau (phase 2) and the long duration of the refractory period. Provides the Ca^{++} that triggers Ca^{++}-induced Ca^{++}-release from the SR.
- **I_K:** Responsible for rapid repolarization (phase 3).
- **I_{K1}:** Largely responsible for setting the resting potential (phase 4). Depolarization turns off this outward current, thereby allowing inward $I_{Ca(L)}$ and I_{bkg} to maintain the plateau.
- **I_{bkg}:** Contributes, along with $I_{Ca(L)}$, to the plateau. Responsible for the fact that resting potential is depolarized a few mV compared to E_K.

Part 4: Action Potentials of Pacemaking Cells and Automaticity

Topic 1: Introduction

The pacemaking cells (P cells) in the SA node generate action potentials spontaneously and rhythmically. This property is called <u>automaticity</u>. The normal range of frequencies in the SA node is roughly 52-90 cycles/min. These impulses spread into the surrounding transitional cells (T cells) and then into the working atrial myocardium, as described in Part 1 of this chapter.

P cells in the AV node also have the property of automaticity. They can make action potentials at a frequency of about 40-60 cycles/min. They normally don't get the chance to do so since they are driven by the higher frequency impulses from the SA node.

Purkinje cells in the His-Purkinje system can also pace when left to their own devices, but at very slow rates (20-40 cycles/min). If impulse conduction through the AV node fails (AV block) Purkinje cells, usually in the His bundle or main bundle branches, take over the function of pacing the ventricles, but the heart rate is very low. When pacing originates from a site other than the SA node, that site is called an <u>ectopic focus</u>.

In some abnormal circumstances, even ordinary working myocytes can begin pacing and become ectopic foci.

The essential feature for automaticity is that there is no stable resting potential during phase 4. Instead, the membrane gradually depolarizes toward threshold for firing an action potential. Such a drift in membrane potential during phase 4 is called <u>diastolic depolarization</u> or the <u>pacemaker potential</u>.

The rate of diastolic depolarization and the amount of depolarization necessary to reach threshold determine the frequency of pacing, *i.e.* the heart rate.

Topic 2: General Features of P Cell Action Potentials

Action potentials from P cells in the SA node and AV node are similar to each other in shape and ionic mechanism except that phase 4 lasts longer in the AV node.

Figure 11
Notice the following differences from the action potentials of working myocytes described in Part 3:

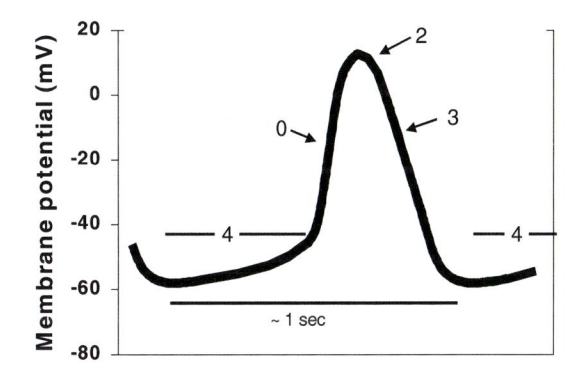

Figure 11. The nomenclature for action potentials in P cells.

- There is no resting potential. Instead, during phase 4, there is diastolic depolarization.
- The maximum amount of hyperpolarization at the beginning of phase 4 is about -60 mV. Compare this to the resting potential during phase 4 in working myocytes of about -85 mV.

- The upstroke of the action potential (phase 0) is not abrupt as it is in working myocytes. It is much more gradual. In addition, the overshoot is not as great.
- The threshold for triggering an action potential is about -40 mV, compared to about -70 mV in working myocytes.
- There is no phase 1.
- The plateau (phase 2) is hardly noticeable.

Topic 3: Determination of Heart Rate

Figure 12

The rate of diastolic depolarization (normally in the SA node) and the amount of depolarization necessary to reach threshold determine the frequency of pacing, *i.e.* the heart rate. This is illustrated in the figure. The steeper the rate of diastolic depolarization, the sooner threshold is reached for firing the next action potential and heart rate is increased.

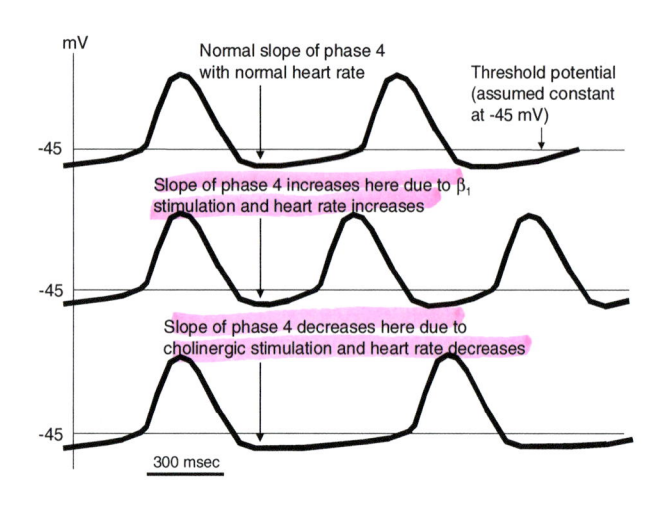

Figure 12. Effect of changes in the slope of the SA node pacemaker potential (phase 4) on heart rate.

Topic 4: Ionic Mechanism of P Cell Action Potentials

Certain channel types that are present in working myocytes are absent (or greatly reduced) in P cells. These are:
- **K₁ channels.** Their absence eliminates I_{K1}. Consequently, the membrane potential is not clamped near E_K during phase 4. This is the fundamental reason that P cells show diastolic depolarization and spontaneous action potentials while working myocytes normally do not.
- **Voltage-gated, fast Na⁺ channels.** Their absence eliminates I_{Na}. Consequently, depolarization during phase 0 depends on inward $I_{Ca(L)}$ and is much more gradual than in working myocytes or Purkinje cells. Absence of I_{Na} also causes the overshoot to be less. These effects cause conduction velocity to be much slower. The small diameter of P cells also contributes to slow conduction velocity.
- **Transient outward channels.** Their absence eliminates I_{to} and phase 1.

On the other hand, certain channel types are important in P cells that are not important in working myocytes. These are:
- **f channels.** f channels are voltage-gated, but they open in response to repolarization rather than to depolarization. They start opening during phase 3 after the membrane has repolarized to about -50 mV. More and more of them open as repolarization continues. They conduct both Na⁺ and K⁺ ions. There is, at this time, a much stronger driving force on Na⁺ than there is on K⁺. Consequently, when f channels open, an inward Na⁺ current results. This current is called I_f. It retards further repolarization and begins the process of diastolic depolarization. [For reasons that are no longer important, f originally stood for funny. Perhaps f could now imply an effect on frequency.]
- **T-type Ca⁺⁺ channels.** T-type Ca⁺⁺ channels are voltage-gated. They open when the membrane depolarizes to roughly -55 mV (compared to about -50 mV for L-type Ca⁺⁺ channels). They carry an inward Ca⁺⁺ current called $I_{Ca(T)}$.

Phase 0: The upstroke. When diastolic depolarization during phase 4 reaches threshold a Ca⁺⁺ action potential is triggered. The inward current, $I_{Ca(L)}$, is carried by L-type Ca⁺⁺ channels. $I_{Ca(L)}$ is small in magnitude, but slow to inactivate. The result is a gradual and prolonged depolarization.

Phase 1: Transient repolarization. Absent.

Phase 2: Slow repolarization or plateau. There is no actual plateau and no definite distinction between phase 2 and phase 3. The rate of repolarization gets progressively faster during phase 2 and the beginning of phase 3.

Phase 3: Rapid repolarization. Delayed K⁺

channels gradually open while L-type Ca^{++} channels gradually close. Outward I_K eventually overwhelms inward $I_{Ca(L)}$ and the membrane repolarizes. As it repolarizes, the delayed K^+ channels begin closing. The membrane only repolarizes to about -60 mV. There are at least two reasons for this:
- There are no K_1 channels and, therefore, no outward I_{K1} to assist repolarization and to hold V_M near E_K.
- f channels start opening at around -50 mV. They carry inward I_f which not only helps prevent further repolarization, but begins to cause depolarization.

Phase 4: Diastolic depolarization, or pacesetter potential. As delayed K^+ channels continue closing, the background Na^+ and Ca^{++} channels remain open and carry inward I_{bkg}. This inward current, although very small, is capable of slowly depolarizing the membrane since there is no offsetting outward I_{K1}. However, if this were the only mechanism for diastolic depolarization, it would be a very slow process and the heart rate would be very low. The rate of diastolic depolarization is greatly increased by I_f, $I_{Ca(T)}$, and $I_{Ca(L)}$.

Diastolic depolarization is started by inward I_f and then supplemented, first by $I_{Ca(T)}$ and then by $I_{Ca(L)}$. Depolarization continues until the threshold for firing the next Ca^{++} action potential is reached (about -40 mV).

Topic 5: A Summary of the Ionic Currents in P Cells

Figure 13
- I_f contributes to diastolic depolarization (especially the early portion).
- $I_{Ca(T)}$ contributes to diastolic depolarization (especially the middle portion).
- $I_{Ca(L)}$ contributes to diastolic depolarization (especially the last portion) and is responsible for the upstroke of the action potential (phase 0).
- I_K is responsible for repolarization (phases 2 and 3).
- I_{bkg} would cause a very slow diastolic depolarization as I_K inactivates if not obscured by the more rapid depolarization caused by I_f, $I_{Ca(T)}$, and $I_{Ca(L)}$.

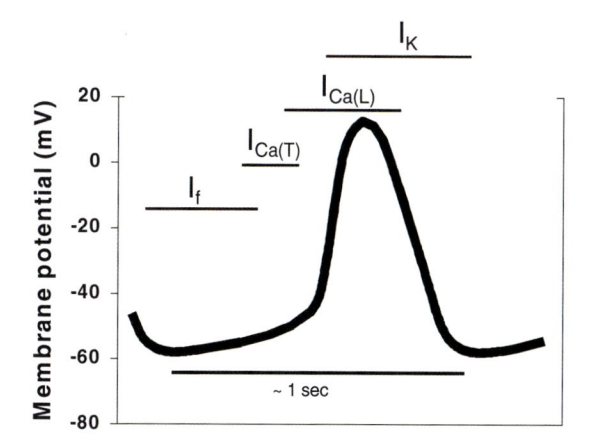

Figure 13. Approximate timing of the important ionic currents involved in P cell action potentials. Of course, the currents do not stop abruptly as might be implied in this figure. Inactivation is a gradual process.

Topic 6: T Cell Action Potentials

T cells possess fast Na^+ channels and K_1 channels but not as many as do working myocytes. Their action potentials are intermediate between those of P cells and working myocytes. In the SA node, conduction velocity progressively increases as the wave of depolarization travels to the atrial myocardium. In the AV node, conduction velocity gradually decreases as the impulse travels from atrial myocardium to P cells.

Topic 7: Pacing by Purkinje Cells

Purkinje cells have all the same channels possessed by working myocytes. In addition, they have f channels and, in certain circumstances, show diastolic depolarization and automaticity. Ordinarily, however, Purkinje cells are driven at nodal frequency and do not have a chance to express their own slower rhythm. Moreover, when driven at nodal frequency diastolic depolarization due to I_f is suppressed and the membrane potential remains stable at about -85 mV during phase 4. This effect is called <u>overdrive suppression</u>.

Remember that f channels are opened by repolarization. At -85 mV, most of them are open and there is an appreciable inward I_f. There is also some inward I_{bkg}. Why don't these inward currents cause diastolic depolarization? The explanation is that at -85 mV outward I_{K1} is so large that it keeps the membrane potential clamped near E_K.

If overdrive from a higher frequency pacemaker is suddenly stopped, Purkinje cells in the His-Purkinje system begin to depolarize. After a few seconds, depolarization somewhere in the system (usually in the His bundle or main bundle branches) reaches threshold (about -70 mV) and a Na$^+$ action potential fires, which results in a ventricular beat. After the first beat, the site that fired the action potential shows diastolic depolarization and automaticity, *i.e.* it continues firing action potentials and sets the pace for the ventricles. In other words, it becomes an ectopic focus.

How does relief from overdrive result in depolarization?

One explanation relates to the Na$^+$-K$^+$ pump. With each action potential, a little Na$^+$ enters the cell and a little K$^+$ leaves. The Na$^+$-K$^+$ pump must continuously pump Na$^+$ out and K$^+$ in to maintain their normal intracellular concentrations. When a cell stops making action potentials, the Na$^+$-K$^+$ pump slows since not as much Na$^+$ and K$^+$ need to be pumped. The Na$^+$-K$^+$ pump is electrogenic. In Purkinje cells, it can contribute significantly to the membrane potential. Therefore, when the Na$^+$-K$^+$ pump slows, the membrane depolarizes by a few mV.

How does depolarization of Purkinje cells by a few mV lead to rhythmic diastolic depolarization and automaticity?

One explanation is that the depolarization (perhaps caused by reduced Na$^+$-K$^+$ pump activity) closes some of the K$_1$ channels and decreases I$_{K1}$ enough that it no longer prevents the membrane potential from responding to inward I$_f$ and I$_{bkg}$.

Topic 8: Pacing by Working Myocardial Cells

Working cardiac myocytes do not have f channels or T-type Ca^{++} channels. They normally do not have pacemaker potentials. Unlike Purkinje cells, they do not show automaticity even when left to their own devices. However, during periods of hypoxia (as in myocardial ischemia) ectopic foci can appear in the working myocardium. Hypoxia can cause considerable membrane depolarization. The depolarization can lead to development of phase 4 pacesetter potentials and automaticity, a phenomenon called depolarization-induced automaticity. The mechanism of depolarization-induced automaticity is not clear but probably involves activation of L-type Ca^{++} channels and perhaps Na$^+$ channels.

How does hypoxia cause depolarization of myocytes?

There exits in many cells, including cardiomyocytes, a type of K$^+$ channel that is sensitive to ATP. Its probability of opening increases as the concentration of ATP decreases. This channel is called the K$_{ATP}$ channel. During hypoxia, the concentration of ATP declines. The result is inhibition of the Na$^+$-K$^+$ pump and opening of K$_{ATP}$ channels. At first, outward I$_{K(ATP)}$ tends to hyperpolarize the membrane. However, with time, the concentration of K$^+$ decreases in the cells and increases in the extracellular spaces around the cells. These concentration changes cause E$_K$ to change to a depolarized value. The open K$_{ATP}$ channels keep the membrane potential clamped near E$_K$. Therefore, the membrane depolarizes. The rise in extracellular K$^+$ concentration can be quite large since, during ischemia, there is little blood flow to rinse out the interstitial spaces.

Chapter 4

Cardiac Muscle: Regulation of Contraction

This chapter discusses the mechanisms by which force, velocity, and frequency of cardiac muscle contraction are adjusted.
Part 1 deals with intrinsic, automatic responses to changes in preload and afterload.
Part 2 treats the mechanisms involved in regulation of force, velocity, and frequency by extrinsic agents, especially autonomic neurotransmitters.

Part 1: Intrinsic Regulation of Contraction

Topic 1: Preliminaries

Passive tension is experimentally determined by stretching a muscle while it is not contracting. The curve relating passive tension to muscle length closely resembles the behavior of a rubber band.

Active tension is experimentally determined at the peak of an isometric contraction. The tension actually measured is called the total tension. To get active tension, the previously measured passive tension is subtracted from total tension. This process is repeated at various lengths to construct length-tension curves.

Preload is the passive tension in a muscle just before it begins to contract. Preload increases as the muscle is stretched beyond its slack length. For any cardiac chamber, preload is determined by the volume of blood that it contains just before it contracts.

Afterload is the active tension a muscle must generate in order to shorten. For any cardiac chamber, afterload is determined by the pressure that must be generated in order to eject blood. For example, aortic pressure is normally the main determinant of left ventricular afterload. Failure of an outflow valve to open properly increases resistance to blood flow out of the chamber and, therefore, increases afterload. Aortic stenosis is an important example.

We describe here certain automatic responses to changes in preload and afterload. These responses are due to intrinsic mechanisms. They do not depend on extrinsic input from neural or humoral agents.

Topic 2: The Active Length-Tension Curve
Figure 1

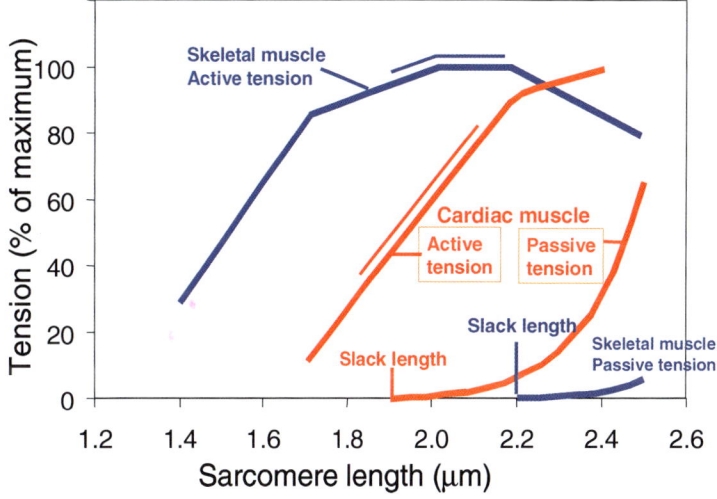

Figure 1. Length-tension relationships for cardiac and skeletal muscle. The normal operating ranges are indicated by secondary lines just above the main active tension curves. In cardiac muscle, the operating range can extend to longer sarcomere lengths (as much as 2.4 μm) with increases in diastolic filling.

[The normal operating range for skeletal muscle varies with different muscles. The range shown here is probably the most common; however, some skeletal muscles operate at much longer lengths. For example, a certain wrist extensor muscle has been carefully studied and apparently operates at sarcomere lengths of about 2.6-3.4 μm (R.L. Lieber et al., J. Neurophysiol. 71:874-881, 1994).]

[Note: It should be understood that sarcomere length shorter than slack length can be achieved only by active shortening. If the ends of a muscle fiber or single myofibril are passively brought closer to each other than the slack length, the thick and thin filaments do not slide over each other and the sarcomeres do not shorten. Instead, the fibers and fibrils buckle and get wavy. Then when the muscle actively contracts, this slack must be taken up by myofilament sliding driven by crossbridge power strokes before any active tension can be generated.]

In cardiac muscle, the useful range of sarcomere lengths is about 1.8-2.4 µm. Over this range, active isometric force increases as sarcomere length increases. The length-tension relationship over the normal working range is much steeper in cardiac muscle than it is in skeletal muscle.

Use the following interactive program to cement your understanding of the length-tension relationship for cardiac muscle and to compare it to that for skeletal muscle. At each sarcomere length, note the amount of overlap between thick and thin filaments and between thin filaments from opposite Z lines.
[Special: Length-Tension Relationship]
[Available in electronic edition of this textbook]

Topic 3: Mechanism of the Active Length-Tension Relationship

How can we account for the fact that cardiac muscle contracts much more forcefully as its sarcomeres get longer? We will describe three mechanisms.

Increasing Sarcomere Length Brings the Thick and Thin Filaments Closer to Each Other

As a sarcomere is stretched, it gets thinner, and all the filaments get slightly closer to each other. The decrease in separation between thick and thin filaments is only a few tenths of a nanometer, but this is apparently enough to make crossbridges more likely to connect. In addition, those crossbridges that do connect might be stronger because of a better mechanical advantage. In addition, it has recently been found that as the filament spacing becomes more compact, the myosin heads tend to reorient at angles that are presumably more favorable for attaching to actin.

This explanation also accounts for the modest effect of sarcomere length on active tension in skeletal muscle at sarcomere lengths between about 1.75 and 2.05 µm. The next two mechanisms operate only in cardiac muscle.

Increasing Sarcomere Length Causes an Immediate Increase in the Sensitivity to Ca^{++}
Figure 2
As sarcomere length increases, the triggering mechanism (troponin-tropomyosin) becomes more sensitive to Ca^{++}. The explanation for this effect again relates to the fact that as sarcomeres get longer, they get thinner. Decreasing inter-filament spacing results in more (and perhaps stronger) crossbridges. Perhaps you recall the discussion of cooperativity in Chapter 2. The force exerted on actin by crossbridges results in stabilization of the troponin-tropomyosin complex in its triggered conformation, and increases the affinity of TnC for Ca^{++}. In addition, triggering of a troponin-tropomyosin complex increases the probability that Ca^{++} will trigger adjacent complexes. With decreased spacing between thick and thin filaments, the above cooperative processes are augmented and sensitivity to Ca^{++} is increased.

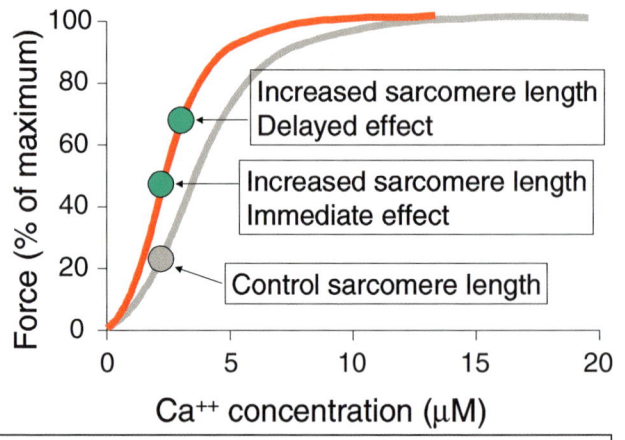

Figure 2. The dose-response relationship for Ca^{++} at two different sarcomere lengths. The circles indicate cytoplasmic Ca^{++} concentration at the peak of the Ca^{++} transient. The immediate effect of increasing sarcomere length is an increase in sensitivity to Ca^{++}. The delayed effect is increased Ca^{++} release from the SR.

This effect is not important in skeletal muscle because enough Ca^{++} is released from the SR during each excitatory event to produce nearly maximal thin filament activation. Thus, an increase in sensitivity to Ca^{++} has little or no consequence.

Increasing Sarcomere Length Causes a Gradual Increase in Ca^{++} Release from the SR
See Figure 2 again
Ca^{++}-induced Ca^{++} release from the junctional SR increases as sarcomere length increases. This effect develops gradually over a period of a few minutes following a change in sarcomere length and leads to a gradual increase in contractile force, which contributes importantly to the steepness of the length-tension relationship in cardiac muscle.

Note that in cardiac muscle, as sarcomere length increases from 2.2 µm to 2.4 µm, active tension continues to increase even though the maximum number of crossbridges decreases. This apparent anomaly is due to increased Ca^{++} release and increased sensitivity to Ca^{++}. These effects override the effect of having fewer crossbridges.

Increasing Sarcomere Length Does Not Cause Increased Force of Contraction by Producing Greater Overlap between Thick and Thin Filaments

A common misconception is that the increased contractile force resulting from increased sarcomere length is caused by greater overlap between thick and thin filaments. This is not true, as can readily be seen in Special: Length-Tension Relationship.

Topic 4: The Passive Length-Tension Relationship

See Figure 1 again

Passive tension is zero at a sarcomere length of about 1.9 μm. This is slack length. Sarcomeres automatically go to their slack length when they are neither contracting nor being stretched. As a myofibril is stretched, its sarcomeres become longer and develop passive tension.

This kind of elastic behavior is not attributable to any interaction between thick and thin filaments or to any structure directly connected in series to thick or thin filaments such as Z lines. It is often called parallel elasticity since the elastic elements responsible for it behave as though they are arranged in parallel with the contractile elements. We now know that parallel elasticity over the working range of fiber lengths is mainly due to the giant protein titin. [Remember that titin molecules connect Z lines to M lines and hold the thick filaments in the center of the sarcomere.]

Note that the passive tension curve for cardiac muscle is much steeper than for skeletal muscle. In other words, passive stiffness is greater in cardiac muscle. In addition, the slack length is less. These differences are due mainly to differences in titin. Cardiac titin is stiffer than skeletal muscle titin.

If skeletal muscle fibers are passively stretched beyond their optimal length, active isometric tension decreases owing to less overlap between thick and thin filaments, and eventually reaches zero when there is no longer any overlap. On the other hand, when cardiac myocytes are stretched beyond optimal sarcomere length (about 2.3-2.4 μm) further elongation of sarcomeres becomes nearly impossible. This large increase in stiffness at abnormally long sarcomere lengths results partly from titin, but extracellular collagen fibers also play a role and help protect against overfilling of the cardiac chambers.

As a cardiac chamber fills during diastole, its walls are passively stretched. The sarcomeres become longer and skinnier, and passive tension develops. As wall tension increases, the pressure in the chamber increases. Increased chamber pressure resists further diastolic filling. Thus, passive stiffness is an important determinant of diastolic filling. One type of congestive heart failure is due primarily to increased stiffness of the ventricular wall. This so-called diastolic dysfunction impairs ventricular filling during diastole.

Restoring Forces

During the relaxation phase of a twitch, myocytes spring back to their slack length. Recoil is forceful and fast. In cardiac muscle, recoil can be even faster that the shortening phase of the twitch. Recoil does not depend on an external load to pull the fiber back to slack length (although this might contribute), but can result entirely from internal restoring forces.

The principal restoring force is titin. In the I bands, titin molecules are very springy. They not only resist passive stretch, but also resist compression. Titin determines the slack length of sarcomeres.

Topic 5: The Effect of Sarcomere Length on Shortening Velocity

In the normal operating range of sarcomere length, there is a steep positive relationship between sarcomere length and the initial velocity of shortening – the greater the sarcomere length, the faster the shortening. This relationship is quite similar to that for active isometric tension *vs.* length.

The effect of sarcomere length on shortening velocity and, to a lesser degree, on isometric force underlie Starlings Law of the Heart (see Chapter 7), without which there could not be a stable, closed circulatory system.

Topic 6: The Effect of Afterload on Shortening Velocity

Figure 3

Increasing the afterload to any striated muscle

reduces the speed of shortening; it also reduces the distance of shortening. These effects are not surprising since they are commonly observed for skeletal muscle in our ordinary movements – the greater the resistance, the slower the movement. Cardiac muscle obeys the same rule. The effect of afterload on initial speed of shortening is called the force-velocity relationship.

If the afterload is increased just to the point that shortening velocity is zero, the contraction is isometric. In this case, the afterload is equal to the isometric tension generated by the muscle. If the afterload is zero, shortening velocity is maximum.

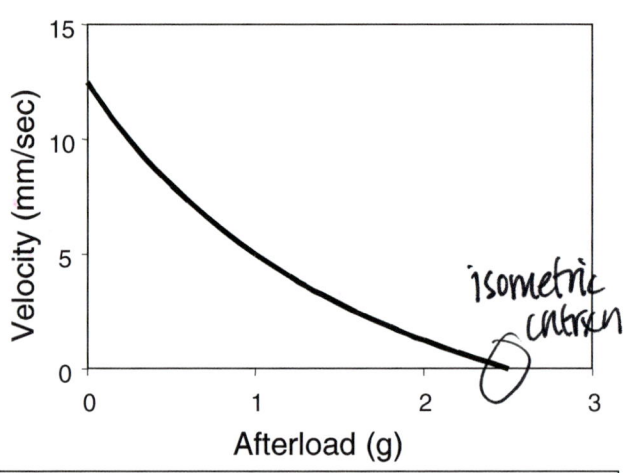

Figure 3. The force-velocity relationship for cardiac muscle. This graph merely indicates that increasing the load decreases the speed that the load can be lifted.

Part 2: Effects of Extrinsic Agents on Contraction

Topic 1: Introduction

Changes in sarcomere length automatically influence the force and velocity of contraction by mechanisms that are intrinsic to the myocyte, as discussed in Part 1 of this chapter. These responses do not require changes in neural or hormonal input. Here in Part 2 we discuss regulation of contraction by extrinsic agents, especially neurotransmitters.

Definition of Contractility:
The term contractility refers to the ability of a muscle to generate force and speed. Contractility can be increased or decreased by a variety of extrinsic agents. These effects are called inotropic effects. Thus, we speak of positive and negative inotropic agents. For example, epinephrine (adrenalin) is a positive inotropic agent since it increases the ability of cardiomyocytes to generate force and increases their velocity of shortening.

Certain intrinsic responses are also considered changes in contractility. These are:
- The increased force and speed that result from a gradual increase in Ca^{++} release from the SR following an increase in sarcomere length.
- The increased force and speed that result from increased heart rate.

The increases in force and speed that result directly and immediately from increased sarcomere length are not considered increases in contractility. This distinction can be confusing.

Topic 2: Actions of the Autonomic Nervous System on the Heart

The autonomic nervous system does not initiate or conduct the rhythmic waves of depolarization responsible for the heartbeat. However, it importantly modifies contractility, heart rate, conduction velocity, action potential duration, contraction duration, and the speed of relaxation.

Sympathetic fibers to the heart are postganglionic and parasympathetic fibers are preganglionic. Both divisions of the autonomic nervous system form plexuses on the epicardial surface of the heart. The parasympathetic preganglionic fibers synapse with postganglionic fibers on the epicardial surface or within the myocardium. The postganglionic neurons of both divisions penetrate the myocardium and terminate as thin axons that run parallel to the myocytes. There are no elaborate junctions between nerve terminals and myocytes as there are in skeletal muscle. Instead, the neurotransmitters are released by exocytosis from a series of swellings along the terminal portions of the axons known as varicosities. The transmitters then diffuse in the general extracellular space to nearby membranes where they act on specific membrane receptors.

Sympathetic Effects

Sympathetic neurons supply the SA node, AV node, atrial myocardium, ventricular myocardium, and coronary blood vessels. Their neurotransmitter is norepinephrine (noradrenalin). Norepinephrine activates adrenergic receptors on P cells, T cells, working myocytes, and smooth muscle cells of coronary vessels. The most important type of adrenergic receptor on myocytes is the β_1 receptor, although β_2 and α_1 receptors are also present and can be involved in some circumstances.

Increased sympathetic activity to the heart causes:
- Increased contractility of atria and ventricles (positive inotropic effect).
- Increased heart rate (positive chronotropic effect).
- Increased conduction velocity, most notably in the AV node (positive dromotropic effect).
- Decreased duration of action potentials in working myocardium with earlier and faster relaxation (positive lusitropic effect). This effect is necessary to achieve high heart rates.
- Increased coronary blood flow, which is a secondary consequence of the positive inotropic and chronotropic effects. Coronary blood flow is discussed in Chapter 16, Part 4.

Decreased sympathetic activity, of course, has the opposite effects.

It is important to realize that the normal heart of a resting individual is constantly under the influence of sympathetic nerve activity. Either increases or decreases from this background level of activity can have effects. The background level of activity is called sympathetic tone.

Parasympathetic Effects

The SA node and AV node are both richly supplied with parasympathetic postganglionic fibers. The working atrial myocardium is also parasympathetically innervated, but to a lesser degree. The ventricles are hardly innervated at all by parasympathetics. The neurotransmitter released from postganglionic parasympathetic fibers is acetylcholine. Acetylcholine activates muscarinic receptors on P cells, T cells, and working atrial myocardium.

Increased parasympathetic activity to the heart causes :
- Decreased heart rate (negative chronotropic effect).
- Decreased conduction velocity in SA node, atrial myocardium, and AV node (negative dromotropic effect). Very strong parasympathetic stimulation can completely block impulse conduction through the AV node.
- Decreased atrial contractility (negative inotropic effect) and decreased duration of atrial action potentials (yes, decreased AP duration). These effects are probably not very important.

There is normally at rest a considerable degree of parasympathetic tone to the heart, which keeps the heart rate well below what it would be otherwise. In a resting person, there is more parasympathetic tone to the heart than sympathetic tone. Consequently, if muscarinic receptors are pharmacologically blocked (e.g. with atropine), the heart rate increases considerably. If β_1 receptors are blocked (e.g. with propranolol), the heart rate decreases only moderately.

The mechanisms of these sympathetic and parasympathetic effects are discussed in the following topics.

Topic 3: Stimulation of β_1 Adrenergic Receptors: Effects on Contractility and Duration of Contraction

---

Figure 4

Norepinephrine is the neurotransmitter released from postganglionic sympathetic neurons. Epinephrine is the hormone secreted from the adrenal medulla. They both activate β_1 adrenergic receptors on atrial and ventricular working myocardium. The result is increased contractility and faster relaxation. The degree of β_1 adrenergic receptor stimulation is the most important determinant of cardiac contractility and duration of contraction!

The mechanism of the response is complex. It is outlined in Figure 4 and described below. The following animation might help [best to run it one frame at a time].

Animation: Beta1 Adrenergic Stimulation
[Electronic edition only]

Activation of Protein Kinase A

Binding of norepinephrine or epinephrine to a β_1 receptor initiates a G-protein cascade that results in activation of protein kinase A (PKA). The intermediates in this process include a G-protein called G_s, adenylyl cyclase, and cyclic AMP (cAMP) as shown in Figure 4.

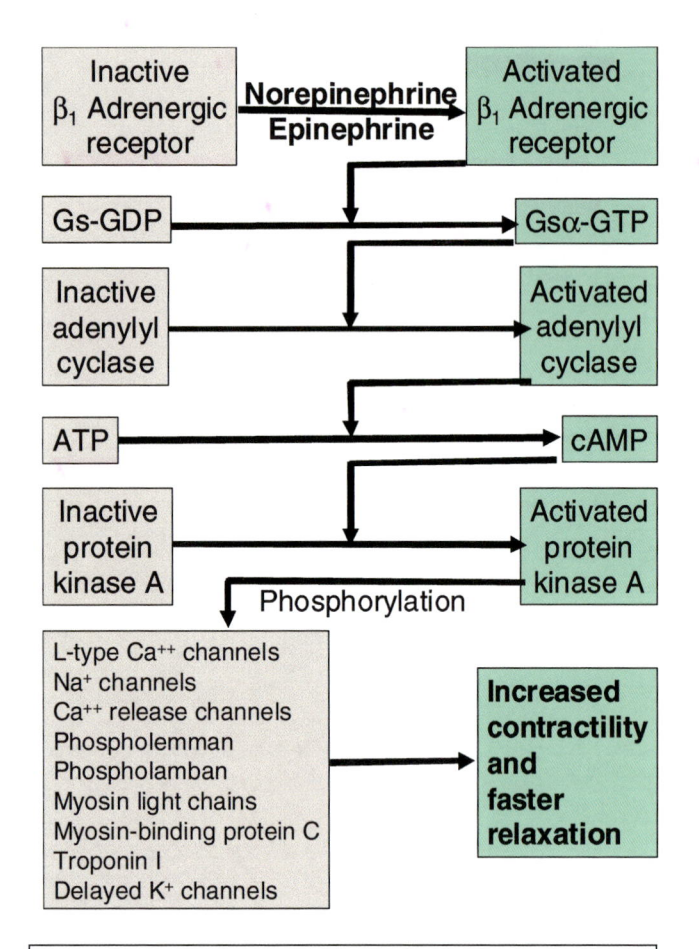

Figure 4. Summary of the processes by which stimulation of β₁ adrenergic receptors leads to increased cardiac contractility and faster relaxation.

Effects of Phosphorylation by Protein Kinase A

PKA phosphorylates several proteins involved in the action potential, EC-coupling, contraction, and relaxation, thereby altering their properties. The first set of phosphorylations listed here results in increased Ca^{++} entry into the cell and release from the junctional SR. The amount of Ca^{++} diffusing along the myofilaments and activating the troponin-tropomyosin triggers is thereby increased.

- **L-Type Ca^{++} Channels (DHP Receptors)**: When DHP receptors are phosphorylated by PKA, they tend to stay open longer upon being activated by membrane depolarization. The amount of Ca^{++} that enters the cell with each action potential is increased, and the stimulus for Ca^{++}-induced Ca^{++} release from the SR is increased.
- **Voltage-Gated Na$^+$ Channels**: Inward Na$^+$ current through these channels is responsible for the fast depolarization phase of the myocardial action potential. When these channels are phosphorylated by PKA, they start conducting Ca^{++} as readily as Na$^+$. The resulting inward Ca^{++} current contributes an additional stimulus for Ca^{++}-induced Ca^{++} release from junctional SR.
- **Ca^{++} Release Channels (CRCs, Ryanodine Receptors)**: When CRCs are phosphorylated they become more sensitive to Ca^{++}.
- **Phospholemman**: When phospholemman is phosphorylated by PKA it inhibits the Na$^+$-Ca^{++} exchanger in the sarcolemma. This leads to a slight increase in sarcoplasmic Ca^{++} concentration.
- **Phospholamban**: When phospholamban is phosphorylated its inhibitory effect on the Ca^{++} pump in the tubular SR (SERCA) is diminished. In other words, the activity of SERCA increases. Phosphorylated phospholemman and phospholamban work in concert to increase contractility: decreased activity of the Na$^+$Ca^{++} exchanger slightly elevates sarcoplasmic Ca^{++} while increased activity of SERCA pumps this excess Ca^{++} into the SR. The amount of Ca^{++} in the SR builds up and, therefore, more can be released through CRCs with each excitatory event.

The next set of phosphorylations affects crossbridge action.

- **Myosin Regulatory Light Chains**: When myosin regulatory light chains are phosphorylated, they stiffen the stem of S$_1$ heads, making crossbridges stronger.
- **Myosin-Binding Protein C**: When myosin-binding protein C is phosphorylated, it causes a slight lateral movement of S$_1$ heads so that they get closer to thin filaments, thereby increasing the probability of making crossbridges.

The final set of phosphorylations influences duration of contraction and speed of relaxation.

- **Phospholamban (again)**: Increased activity of SERCA hastens relaxation by removing Ca^{++} from the cytoplasm faster. Whenever contractility is increased because of β₁ adrenergic stimulation, heart rate is also increased. At faster heart rates, it is important for relaxation to proceed faster.
- **Troponin I (TnI)**: When TnI is phosphorylated, the affinity of TnC for Ca^{++} decreases. This effect in itself would tend to reduce activation of crossbridges, but it is obscured by the great increase in cytoplasmic Ca^{++} concentration. The importance of this effect is that it aids in hastening relaxation by allowing Ca^{++} to come

off TnC faster.
- **Delayed K⁺ Channels**: These channels are important in the repolarization phase of cardiac action potentials. Phosphorylation of delayed K⁺ channels causes earlier repolarization and, therefore, briefer action potentials. Again, this effect contributes to earlier and faster relaxation, which is important at higher heart rates.

The overall effect of β_1 adrenergic stimulation in working myocardium is a stronger, faster, and briefer contraction.

Summary of β_1 adrenergic effects:
- Increased contractility due to increased Ca^{++} release from SR.
  - Increased inward Ca^{++} current during the action potential.
  - Increased sensitivity of Ca^{++}-induced Ca^{++}-release from SR.
  - Decreased activity of sarcomemmal Na^+Ca^{++} exchanger (due to phosphorylated phospholemman)
  - Increased activity of SERCA (due to phosphorylated phospholamban).
- Increased contractility due to effects on crossbridges.
  - Increased strength of crossbridges.
  - Increased number of crossbridges.
- Decreased duration of contraction and increased speed of relaxation.
  - Decreased duration of the action potential
  - Increased activity of SR Ca^{++} pump.
  - Decreased affinity of TnC for Ca^{++}.

Topic 4: Stimulation of β_1 Adrenergic Receptors: Effects on Heart Rate

The SA and AV nodes are richly supplied by both divisions of the autonomic nervous system and are under continuous sympathetic and parasympathetic tone.
Animation: Beta1 Adrenergic Stimulation of P Cells

The plasma membrane of P cells has β_1 adrenergic receptors that are activated by norepinephrine (released during sympathetic nerve activity) or epinephrine (circulating from the adrenal medulla). The result is a G_s-protein cascade that leads to activation of protein kinase A (PKA). PKA phosphorylates L-type Ca^{++} channels, which causes $I_{Ca(L)}$ to be larger during the late stages of the pacemaker potential.

In addition to the above effect of phosphorylation, G_s subunits (probably the $\beta\gamma$ subunits) have a direct effect on f channels to increase I_f. cAMP also has a direct effect to increase I_f.

These effects of β_1 adrenergic stimulation result in a steeper slope of the pacemaker potential so that it reaches threshold for firing a Ca^{++} action potential sooner. In the SA node, steeper diastolic depolarization increases the heart rate. Decreased sympathetic activity has the opposite effects and heart rate decreases.

Topic 5: Stimulation of β_2 Adrenergic Receptors

There are β_2 receptors on atrial and ventricular myocytes. Stimulation of β_2 adrenergic receptors by epinephrine results in increased contractility but this effect is much less important than stimulation of β_1 adrenergic receptors. For a little more information click here. [Beta2 adrenergic receptors on cardiomyocytes]

Topic 6: Stimulation of α_1 Adrenergic Receptors

Atrial and ventricular myocytes also possess α_1 adrenergic receptors that can be activated by epinephrine and norepinephrine. The result is increased contractility and increased duration of the action potential. These effects are far less important than the effects of β_1 adrenergic stimulation, and are noticeable only after β_1 receptors are pharmacologically blocked. Ordinarily the effect of sympathetic nerve stimulation or circulating epinephrine is a decrease in the action potential duration, the response to α_1 activation being overridden by that of β_1 activation. For a little more information about mechanism, click here. [Alpha1 adrenergic receptors on cardiomyocytes]

Topic 7: Stimulation of Muscarinic Acetylcholine Receptors: Effects on Contractility and Action Potential Duration

Atrial and ventricular myocytes also have muscarinic acetylcholine receptors. These receptors can be activated by acetylcholine released from postganglionic parasympathetic nerve endings. The result is reduced contractility and reduced action potential duration. For the mechanism of these effects, click here. [Effects of acetylcholine on contractility and action potential duration]

The importance of these effects in working myocardium is questionable. In fact, parasympathetic nerves very poorly innervate the ventricles (if at all). The real importance of muscarinic acetylcholine receptors is in pacemaking tissue (SA node and AV node) where their activation leads to lower frequency of action potential generation.

Topic 8: Stimulation of Muscarinic Acetylcholine Receptors: Effects on Heart Rate

Increased parasympathetic activity to the SA node causes increased release of acetylcholine, which activates muscarinic receptors on P cells. The result is a G_i-protein cascade that leads to inhibition of adenylyl cyclase. Consequently, cAMP concentration and PKA activity are reduced. The result is less phosphorylation of L-type Ca^{++} channels and less direct activation of f channels by cAMP. Diastolic depolarization becomes flatter and takes longer to reach threshold. The heart rate decreases. Decreased parasympathetic activity has the opposite effects and heart rate increases.

Animation: Parasympathetic Stimulation of P Cells

Parasympathetic activity can reduce heart rate by another mechanism involving a type of K^+ channel called the K_{ACh} channel. K_{ACh} channels are activated by the βγ subunit of G_i. They carry an outward K^+ current called $I_{K(Ach)}$. Parasympathetic stimulation of the SA node results in an outward $I_{K(Ach)}$ that hyperpolarizes the membrane of P cells. When diastolic depolarization begins from a hyperpolarized level (i.e. more negative than -60 mV), it takes longer to reach threshold and the heart rate decreases. Under normal circumstances, this mechanism is probably not as important as those involving I_f and $I_{Ca(L)}$. However, when parasympathetic activity is very intense, this mechanism can produce a profound drop in heart rate. It probably accounts for the very slow heart rates seen in vasovagal syncope. Hyperpolarization of P cells and T cells in the AV node by $I_{K(Ach)}$ probably contributes to the AV nodal block that can be produced by strong vagal stimulation.

Topic 9: Cardiac Glycosides

Cardiac glycosides can increase the contractility of cardiac muscle and have been used to treat failing hearts for centuries [described to the medical profession in 1785 by Withering, but known in folk medicine much earlier]. The most commonly used cardiac glycoside for treating heart failure is digoxin, which is one of the glycosides that can be obtained from digitalis (which is the dried leaf of the foxglove plant). For experimental work, we often employ another plant cardiac glycoside called ouabain since it is more water-soluble than digoxin.

Figure 5
Cardiac glycosides act by inhibiting the Na^+-K^+ pump. The sequence of events is described Figure 5

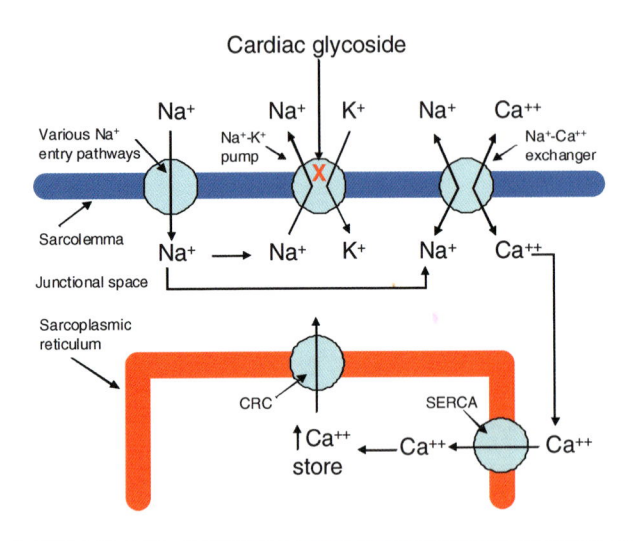

Figure 5. Mechanism for positive inotropic effect of cardiac glycosides. Na^+ continuously leaks into cardiac myocytes through various channels and carriers and is normally pumped out at the same rate by the Na^+-K^+ pump. When this pump is inhibited by a cardiac glycoside, Na^+ concentration rises in the narrow space between the sarcolemma and the junctional SR. Some of this Na^+ is ejected by the Na^+-Ca^{++} exchanger, which can operate in either direction depending on relative concentrations. This raises intracellular Ca^{++} concentration – not enough to trigger Ca^{++}-induced Ca^{++} release through the calcium release channels (CRCs), but enough for the SR Ca^{++} pump (SERCA) to gradually load the SR with a little more Ca^{++}. Then when excitatory events occur, more Ca^{++} is released through the CRCs and contractility is increased.

Endogenous Ouabain

The adrenal cortex secretes a hormone having a chemical structure that is apparently identical to that of ouabain. This hormone is called endogenous ouabain (EO). It normally circulates in the blood in detectable amounts and presumably exerts a slight, but continuous, inhibitory effect on Na^+-K^+ pumps everywhere. Secretion of EO from the adrenal cortex (and also from the hypothalamus) increases in response to elevated plasma and cerebrospinal fluid Na^+ concentrations, and one of its normal roles may be to promote natriuresis (renal Na^+ loss), thereby helping to restore plasma and CSF Na^+ concentrations to normal. EO can promote natriuresis by inhibiting Na^+-K^+ pumps in renal tubules and in vascular smooth muscle. The latter effect induces constriction of precapillary resistance vessels, leading to increased MAP and pressure diuresis (described in Chapter 15). The vasoconstricting effect of EO involves the Na^+-Ca^{++} exchanger as described above for cardiac muscle.

Excessive dietary salt induces hypertension in many people. A major theory for the mechanism of this connection has recently been presented by M.P. Blaustein *et al.* (*Am. J. Physiology*, 302: H1031-H1049, 2012). Endogenous ouabain plays a central role in this very interesting theory.

Chapter 5

The Cardiac Cycle

Here we treat the mechanical features of the heartbeat and associated events.
Part 1 describes the motions of the heart during the cardiac cycle, and explains how these motions eject blood from the ventricles during systole and draw blood back into the ventricles during diastole.
Part 2 defines the various phases or periods of the cardiac cycle.
Part 3 describes the major events associated with the cardiac cycle and their relationships to each other.
Part 4 explains the concept of ventricular pressure-volume loops.

Part 1: The Motions of the Heart

Topic 1: The Fibrous Skeleton of the Heart

Figure 1
The rims of all four valves (tricuspid, mitral, pulmonic, and aortic) are attached to fibrous rings that are embedded in a connective tissue sheet that separates the atria from the ventricles. These fibrous structures form the base of the heart (or cardiac skeleton) as shown in Figure 1. The atrial and ventricular muscles are also attached to the fibrous rings. Understanding the motions of the heart is aided by appreciating that all the moving parts are attached to the fibrous skeleton.

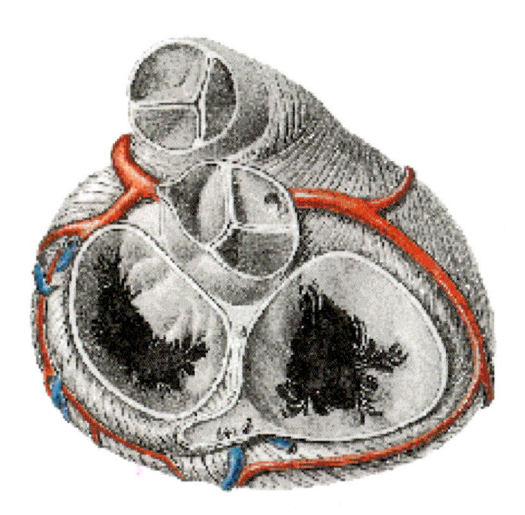

Figure 1. The fibrous skeleton of the heart (base of the heart) and the heart valves, looking down. Top of figure is anterior edge of heart. Make sure you can identify the valves and the coronary arteries.

From the *Medical Illustration Library*, Sobotta Cardiology/Pulmonology Anatomy Collection, 1996, Williams & Wilkins.

Topic 2: Movements of the Valves

Inflow and outflow valves allow the ventricles to pump blood in a preferred direction, into the aorta and pulmonary artery. The atrioventricular (AV) inflow valves, mitral and tricuspid, close whenever ventricular pressures exceed atrial pressures, and open when these pressure gradients reverse. The outflow valves, aortic and pulmonic, open whenever ventricular pressures exceed aortic or pulmonary arterial pressures respectively, and close when these pressure gradients reverse. Valve openings and closings are abrupt, essentially all-or-none, events.

The free edges of the AV valve cusps are tethered to the ventricular walls by *chordae tendineae* and papillary muscles. At the onset of ventricular systole the papillary muscles contract, thereby preventing eversion of the valves into the atria, a condition called mitral or tricuspid prolapse.

Click here [Movie: MitralValveMotion] for an echocardiogram movie showing the action of a mitral valve. In this movie, the left atrium is below the left ventricle. Left atrial and ventricular motions are also shown. [The author thanks Dr. Paul Boor, Dept. of Pathology, UTMB for this movie.]

Topic 3: Movements of the Atria

When the atria contract, their internal volume is decreased, internal pressure is increased, and blood is propelled into the ventricles. The atria only have outflow valves, mitral and tricuspid, no true inflow valves. Nevertheless, the atria pump mainly into the ventricles. This is possible because during atrial contraction the orifices of the venae cavae and pulmonary veins constrict, thereby providing an appreciable resistance against retrograde flow. It is useful (though not really accurate) to visualize atrial ejection of blood as simply the result of a decrease in the radius of curvature of the atria. Ventricular ejection of blood is more interesting, as you shall see.

Atrial contraction is the final event of the ventricular diastolic period. Most ventricular filling occurs early during ventricular diastole. Atrial contraction accounts for only about 15-20% of total diastolic ventricular filling in a resting individual. This final burst of ventricular filling, though quantitatively small, puts some extra stretch on the ventricular muscle fibers, which is thought to prime them for their contraction. This extra stretch is called the atrial kick.

The main function of the atria is to serve as blood reservoirs. The atrial walls are very distensible. Blood returning from the systemic circuit expands them during ventricular systole with nearly enough blood to refill the ventricles during ventricular diastole. The atrial blood reservoirs allow for very rapid ventricular filling as soon as the AV valves open. Here are some more details on atrial filling in case you are interested [Atrial filling].

Topic 4: Movements of the Ventricles

The ventricles are pressure pumps; they drive blood through the pulmonary and systemic circuits principally by generating positive pressure during systole. Ventricular suction plays a lesser, but important, role, as we shall see. Click here for more on the forces that drive blood around the circuit [Forces from behind and in front].

During systole the base of the heart is pulled toward the apex, with the apex itself remaining relatively stationary. Initially, shortening of the ventricles is accompanied by a small increase in transverse circumference. However, as soon as the outflow valves open and blood begins to be ejected, ventricular circumference decreases.

As systole proceeds, the ventricular myocytes not only shorten; they also thicken. Consequently, the ventricular wall gets thicker and internal dimensions decrease more than do external dimensions. The increase in wall thickness begins in the interventricular septum, continues into the apex, and then on up the free walls. There is also an important twisting motion of the ventricles during systole, especially the base of the heart with respect to the relatively stationary apex.

These systolic motions, especially twisting, cause the ventricles to become less spherical. For a given surface area, a sphere contains more volume than any other shape. Therefore, the change in shape contributes to systolic ejection of blood, especially from the left ventricle.

During diastole, the ventricles untwist, get longer, and increase in external circumference. They increase even more in internal circumference as the walls get thinner. These diastolic motions draw blood into the ventricles from the atria and intrathoracic veins.

Ejection of blood by the ventricles is accomplished by (in decreasing order of importance):

- Decreased external circumference
- Shape change, largely due to twisting.
- Decreased external length due to the base of the heart being pulled down toward the apex.
- Increased wall thickness, including apex and interventricular septum.

Topic 5: An Animated Cartoon of the Heartbeat

[Animation: Heartbeat]
This animation shows a more or less frontal view of a heart. To make it move, click the start button. This cartoon is obviously not anatomically correct, nor does it illustrate all of the features of cardiac motion described above. For example, it does not illustrate systolic twisting and diastolic untwisting of the ventricles. The animation attempts to illustrate three important features of ventricular systole:

- Base to apex shortening (accompanied by a downward stretch of the atria and all attached large blood vessels).
- Decrease in external circumference.
- Increase in wall thickness with a large decrease in internal circumference and length. The increase in wall thickness begins in the interventricular septum, continues into the apex, and then on up the free walls.

The animation also shows that the atria undergo two filling/emptying cycles for each heartbeat. This behavior will be explained in Part 3.

Topic 6: Special Features of Right Ventricular Ejection

Figure 2
The right ventricular free wall is much thinner and weaker than is the left ventricular free wall, consistent with the fact that the right ventricle normally must generate less than 20% of the pressure generated by the left ventricle.

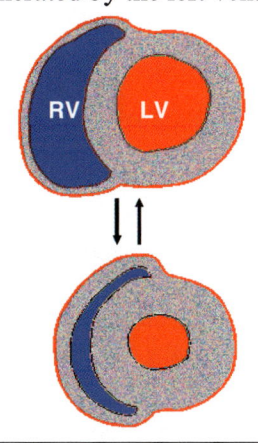

Figure 2. A diagrammatic cross-section through the ventricles showing that the thin right ventricular free wall moves close to the interventricular septum during systole (down arrow).

The right ventricular free wall can be considered a large pocket attached to the side of the left ventricle as shown in Figure 2. It ejects blood largely by its free wall coming closer to the interventricular septum; a motion often likened to the action of a bellows. The bellows motion is an effective way to move large volumes of fluid against low pressures without much effort. In addition, as the left ventricle contracts it pulls on the right ventricle, wrapping it more tightly around the interventricular septum, which at the same time bulges into the right ventricle.

Topic 7: Diastolic Suction

As mentioned, during diastole the ventricles untwist. This motion occurs mainly during the first phase of diastole, the isovolumetric relaxation period (see *Part 2* of this chapter). The sudden forceful untwisting of the ventricles causes an abrupt decrease of intraventricular pressure, and as soon as the AV valves open, blood is sucked into the ventricles from the atria. This phenomenon is called diastolic suction. Click here for a deeper look at the timing and importance of left ventricular untwisting [Left ventricular untwisting].

untwisting of vent ⇒ diastolic suction ⇒ vent fill

A second contributor to diastolic suction is the tendency of all striated muscle fibers to spring back to their slack length following a shortening contraction. This phenomenon is probably due to the elastic properties of the giant protein, titin.

Topic 8: Systolic Suction

The base-to-apex shortening of the ventricles during the early part of systole stretches the atria and attached veins in a downward direction, expanding them like accordions. The resulting drop in atrial pressure sucks blood from the *venae cavae* and pulmonary veins.

Topic 9: Relationship between Wall Tension and Chamber Pressure

The wall tension (**T**) that must be generated to produce a given amount of pressure (**P**) within a heart chamber depends upon the radius of curvature of the chamber wall (**r**). Roughly

$$T = P \cdot r / 2$$

$P = \dfrac{2T}{r}$ $\downarrow r \Rightarrow \uparrow P$

This relationship, known as the Laplace equation, will be discussed more thoroughly in Chapter 9.

A variety of cardiac dysfunctions, including valvular defects, eventually lead to abnormally dilated ventricular chambers, causing **r** to increase. In these cases, the ventricular walls must contract more forcefully than they normally do in order to develop adequate intraventricular pressures.

↑r ⇒ ↑T (F of cntrxn) to maintain P
problem w/ ventricular dilation

46   Chapter 5

Part 2: The Phases of the Cardiac Cycle

Topic 1: Introduction

Figure 3

The cardiac cycle is divided into two major phases – systole and diastole. These, in turn, are divided into briefer periods. Since we are dealing with a cycle the starting point is arbitrary. We will start with the beginning of ventricular systole. The ventricles have already filled with blood during diastole while the atrioventricular (AV) valves were open and the aortic and pulmonic valves were closed.

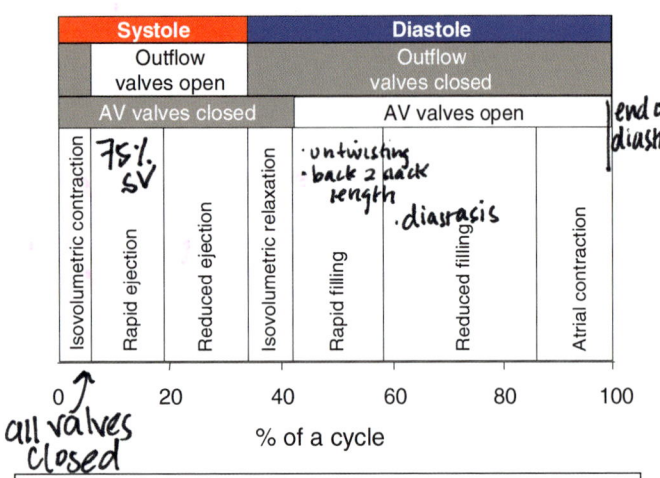

Figure 3. The phases of the cardiac cycle.

Topic 2: Ventricular Systole

The Isovolumetric Contraction Period

When the ventricles begin to contract, pressure is rapidly generated in the ventricular chambers and, consequently, the AV valves immediately close. This event (AV valve closure) marks the beginning of ventricular systole. Enough pressure is soon generated to open the aortic and pulmonic valves, but until these outflow valves actually open the ventricles are closed chambers containing constant volumes of blood - ventricular pressures rise, while volumes remain constant. Thus, the period between closure of the inflow valves and opening of the outflow valves is called the isovolumetric contraction period. [At normal heart rates in a person at rest (60-80 beats per min) this period lasts for about 6% of the total cardiac cycle.]

The Ejection Period

As soon as ventricular pressures just exceed outflow pressures the outflow valves open and blood is ejected into the root of the aorta from the left ventricle, and into the pulmonary artery from the right ventricle. The ejection period is divided into two sub-phases.

The Rapid Ejection Period: The initial propulsion of blood from the ventricles, especially the left ventricle, has been described as an impulse akin to striking a golf ball with a golf club. Ejection is sudden and forceful. Considerable momentum is imparted to the blood. [The rapid ejection period normally lasts for about 13% of the total cycle, and accounts for roughly 75% of total stroke volume.]

The Reduced Ejection Period: The ventricles begin to relax. Systolic ejection continues, but at a reduced rate. As the ventricles relax, ventricular pressures decline and soon the aortic and pulmonic valves snap shut. This event (outflow valve closure) marks the end of ventricular systole. [The reduced ejection period normally takes about 15% of the total cycle. Systole, therefore, takes roughly 35% of the total cardiac cycle.]

Topic 3: Ventricular Diastole

The Isovolumetric Relaxation Period

At the instant the aortic and pulmonic valves snap shut, the ventricles once again become closed chambers. As the ventricular muscle finishes relaxing ventricular pressures rapidly drop, but until the AV valves open, ventricular volumes remain constant. [The isovolumetric relaxation period lasts for about 8% of the total cycle.]

The Filling Period

When ventricular pressures drop just below atrial pressures, the AV valves open and blood flows into the ventricles from the atria and great veins. The filling period is divided into three sub-phases.

The Rapid Filling Period: When the AV valves first open, blood rapidly flows into the ventricles from the distended atria. Rapid ventricular filling is partly driven by atrial pressure, but is greatly augmented by ventricular suction. As mentioned in Part 1, ventricular suction is the result of 1) ventricular untwisting and 2) forceful return of each muscle fiber to its slack length (probably caused by the elastic properties of titin). [The rapid filling period lasts for about 16% of the total cardiac cycle, and accounts for about 65% of total diastolic filling of the ventricles.]

The Cardiac Cycle

The Reduced Filling Period: Blood continues to return to the right ventricle from the periphery *via* the *venae cavae* and right atrium, and to the left ventricle from the pulmonary bed *via* the pulmonary veins and left atrium. As the ventricles fill with blood, ventricular pressures gradually increase, thus opposing further filling. At resting heart rates, blood flow into the ventricles nearly drops to zero toward the end of the reduced filling period. For this reason, the reduced filling period is sometimes called the period of diastasis. [The reduced filling period lasts for about 28% of the total cycle in a resting person.]

The Atrial Contraction Period: Finally, near the end of ventricular diastole, the atria contract, and a little more blood is squirted into the ventricles, priming the ventricular pump. [The atrial contraction period lasts for about 14% of the total cycle and accounts for roughly 15-20% of ventricular filling.]

Topic 4: Changes in Heart Rate Affect the Duration of Diastole More than Systole

When heart rate increases (*e.g.* during exercise), all phases of the cardiac cycle decrease in duration. However, the duration of diastole is affected by changes in heart rate more than is the duration of systole. The phase of diastole affected the most by changes in heart rate is, of course, the reduced filling period.

Part 3: The Events of the Cardiac Cycle

Topic 1: Introduction

Figure 4
The names of the phases are mainly based on ventricular volume changes and on valve actions. There are, however, several other processes associated with the cardiac cycle, including pressure changes (ventricular, aortic, and atrial), heart sounds, and the electrocardiogram. All these processes together are known as the events of the cardiac cycle. Understanding how the heart works requires understanding these events and their temporal relationships with respect to each other.

Figure 4 shows idealized tracings of the events of the cardiac cycle for a person at rest. Only data pertaining to the left heart are shown. Data for the right heart are similar in time course, but the pressures are lower. An interactive, dynamic chart of the events is available [Special: Events].

Topic 2: Left Ventricular Volume

During the isovolumetric contraction and relaxation periods, ventricular volume remains constant. During the ejection period, ventricular volume decreases (more rapidly during the rapid ejection period than during the reduced ejection period). During the filling period, ventricular volume increases (more rapidly during the rapid filling period than during the reduced filling period). During the atrial contraction period (which is the final part of ventricular filling), ventricular volume increases further. Note the following:

- The volume of blood in the left ventricle at the end of diastole (following atrial contraction) is called the left ventricular end-diastolic volume.
- The volume of blood in the left ventricle at the end of systole is called the left ventricular end-systolic volume.
- The end-systolic volume is always appreciable and serves as a reserve that can be dipped into when contractility increases during exercise.
- The difference between end-diastolic volume and end-systolic volume (*i.e.* the volume that is ejected during systole) is called the stroke volume.
- The stroke volume divided by the end-diastolic volume is called the ejection fraction and is normally about 60-70%. An abnormally low ejection fraction is a very important clinical sign of a failing heart; it can be estimated non-invasively using echocardiography.
- During the final part of the reduced filling period (just before atrial contraction) essentially no more ventricular filling occurs (at resting heart rate). Clearly, the duration of the reduced filling period can be decreased somewhat without interfering with diastolic filling of the ventricles.
- The initial rate of ventricular filling is comparable to the initial rate of ventricular ejection. This surprising behavior results from forceful diastolic suction as discussed in Part 1.

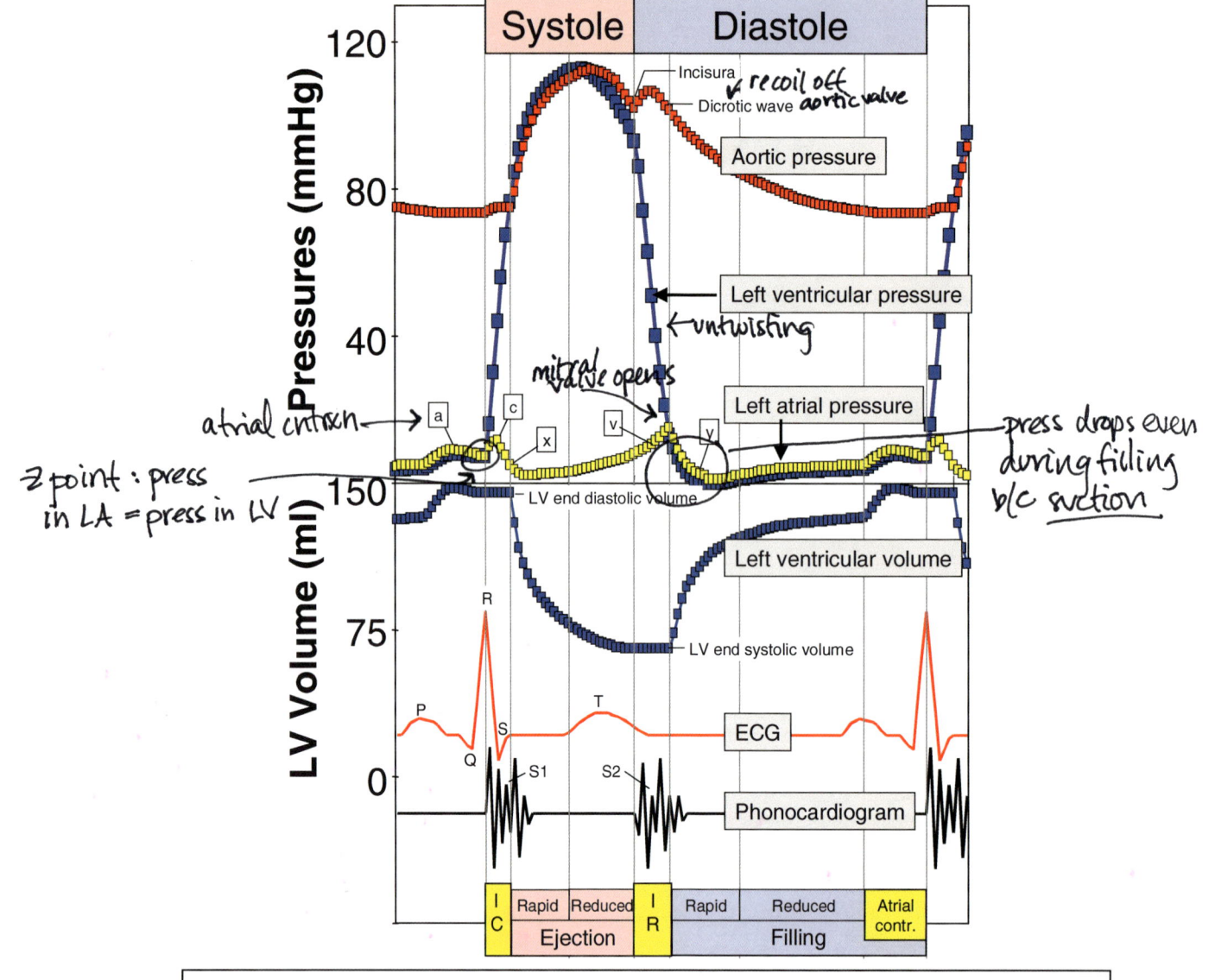

Figure 4. The events of the cardiac cycle. These are idealized traces representing the events at a normal, resting heart rate. The points along the pressure and volume curves are spaced one hundredth of a cycle apart (10 msec apart if the heart rate is 60/min). IC = isovolumetric contraction period, IR = isovolumetric relaxation period.

Topic 3: Left Ventricular Pressure

Ventricular pressure shoots up very steeply during the isovolumetric contraction period. After the aortic valve opens, ventricular pressure continues rising, but not as steeply; the energy of ventricular contraction is now used more to eject blood than to develop pressure. Pressure continues to rise, however, until a little past the end of the rapid ejection period. Then, during the reduced ejection period, left ventricular pressure declines.

During isovolumetric relaxation, ventricular pressure drops precipitously, largely because of ventricular untwisting [Left ventricular untwisting]. Ventricular pressure then continues to drop through part of the rapid filling period because of elastic recoil of the ventricular muscle fibers. Note that ventricular pressure drops during this time even as rapid ventricular filling proceeds. This is clearly a suction phenomenon. Soon, however, ventricular pressure starts rising and continues to rise gradually for the duration of the reduced filling period. This gradual rise in ventricular pressure results from the fact that as the ventricle fills with blood its walls become stretched and passive wall tension is generated.

Finally, during atrial contraction, a little hump in ventricular pressure is seen which reflects the relatively small additional ventricular filling caused by atrial contraction.

The pressure in the left ventricle at the end of systole is called the left ventricular end-systolic pressure. The pressure at the end of diastole is called the left ventricular end-diastolic pressure.

Topic 4: Aortic Pressure

Aortic pressure gradually rises and then gradually falls during the ejection period as the volume of blood in the arterial tree rises and falls. During the rapid ejection period, blood is forced into the arterial tree faster than it runs out through the microcirculation to the veins. Thus, during the rapid ejection period the volume of blood contained in the arterial tree, and consequently the pressure in the arterial tree, increase. The diameter of the aorta increases by roughly 30%. During most of the reduced ejection period, blood runs out of the arterial tree across the microcirculation faster than it is forced in from the left ventricle, and consequently, arterial blood volume and pressure decrease. This cyclic pressure change begins in the root of the aorta and rapidly travels as a wave (the pulse wave) out the arterial tree. The arterial pulse wave will be treated in more detail in Chapter 13.

As the arterial tree swells with blood during the rapid ejection period, tension in the arterial walls increases. Throughout the remainder of the cardiac cycle, elastic recoil resulting from this wall tension squeezes blood out of the arterial tree through the microcirculation. As the aortic valve closes, however, there is a very brief period of retrograde flow in the root of the aorta. A small amount of blood is actually squeezed backward toward the closing aortic valve. This retrograde flow is thought to assist aortic valve closure by banging into the closing valve. As the valve snaps shut, blood bounces off of it creating a secondary pressure wave that travels away from the heart along the arterial tree, riding piggy-back on the primary pressure wave. This reflected wave is called the dicrotic wave. The sharp indentation between the primary wave and the dicrotic wave is called the incisura.

Except for superposition of the dicrotic wave, aortic pressure simply declines gradually throughout diastole and the next isovolumetric contraction period, until the next ejection period. During this time, blood continues to flow through the microcirculation, powered by elastic recoil of the arterial walls.

The maximum pressure achieved in the arteries during systole is called the arterial systolic pressure. The minimum pressure reached in the arteries at the end of diastole is called the arterial diastolic pressure. The difference between arterial systolic and diastolic pressures is called the pulse pressure.

Topic 5: Left Atrial Pressure

The pressure fluctuations in the left atrium are characterized by three crests, called the *a*, *c*, and *v* waves, and by two troughs, called the *x* and *y* waves.

- The *c* wave begins with the onset of ventricular systole and peaks roughly midway through the isovolumetric contraction period. It is caused by a small amount of blood propelled back into the left atrium before the mitral valve is fully closed. Bulging of the closed mitral valve back into the left atrium probably contributes to the *c* wave.
- The *x* wave (or *x* descent) is caused by movement of the base of the heart toward the apex during the rapid ejection period. This movement expands the atria like accordions with a consequent drop in pressure that sucks blood into the atria from the thoracic veins. The *x* wave would begin at the start of the isovolumetric contraction period if it were not obscured by the *c* wave.
- The *v* wave is caused by atrial filling as blood circulates back to the heart during ventricular systole and the isovolumetric relaxation period. At the instant the mitral valve opens, blood is sucked into the left ventricle from the left atrium and left atrial pressure drops very quickly. Thus, the peak of the *v* wave marks the instant of mitral valve opening.
- The *y* wave (or *y* descent) results from the fact that during the rapid filling period blood is sucked out of the left atrium by the recoiling left ventricle faster than it passively flows into the left atrium from the pulmonary veins. As atrial filling continues during the reduced filling period of the ventricle, atrial pressure gradually rises, thus completing the *y* wave.
- The *a* wave, of course, results from atrial contraction and is completed just prior to the onset of ventricular systole.
- Immediately preceding ventricular systole, left atrial and left ventricular pressures are essentially equal; this pressure is sometimes called the *z* point.

It is not traditional to present tracings for atrial

volume changes during the cardiac cycle and none is provided here. However, it should be clear from the atrial pressure trace that there are two cycles of atrial volume change for each ventricular cycle. First, atrial volume continuously increases from the beginning of ventricular systole until the peak of the *v* wave, and then decreases immediately after the AV valves open. Atrial volume increases again during the reduced filling period of the ventricles, and then abruptly decreases during atrial contraction. Thus, there are two atrial volume cycles for each beat of the ventricles as illustrated in [Animation: Heartbeat].

Topic 6: Pressure Crossovers and Valve Action

Valves open or close when there are pressure crossovers. For example, at the beginning of systole, just as left ventricular pressure becomes greater than left atrial pressure, the mitral valve closes. At the instant left ventricular pressure becomes greater than the pressure in the root of the aorta, the aortic valve opens. During the early part of diastole, just as left ventricular pressure falls below left atrial pressure, the mitral valve opens. Analogous relationships take place in the right heart.

There is one curious exception to the above rule. Shortly after the end of the rapid ejection period, left ventricular pressure falls slightly below aortic pressure, but the aortic valve remains open. Blood continues to move from left ventricle to aorta during the reduced ejection period, against a slight pressure difference. This curiosity results from the fact that the momentum imparted to blood as it is ejected during the rapid ejection period keeps it moving into the aorta even after the pressures reverse. The aortic valve is able to close under the influence of the pressure gradient only after the momentum of the ejecting blood has sufficiently subsided.

A normal aortic valve, when open, provides almost no resistance to ejection of blood from the left ventricle to the root of the aorta. Consequently, there is almost no pressure drop from the left ventricle to the aorta during the ejection period. Thus, while the aortic valve is open, left ventricular pressure closely follows aortic pressure, rising during the rapid ejection period and then falling during the reduced ejection period.

Topic 7: The Heart Sounds

In normal, young adults, only two heart sounds, named S_1 and S_2, can be routinely auscultated (heard) using a stethoscope. Two additional heart sounds can sometimes be heard in apparently healthy people (S_3 in children and S_4 in old people) but these sounds are usually a sign of some abnormality in young or middle-aged adults. S_1 and S_2 are caused mainly by vibrations of the valves following their abrupt closure.

Abnormal sounds from the heart include murmurs and clicks that usually result from valvular diseases; they will not be discussed here.

The first heart sound, S_1, is produced mainly by closure of the AV valves at the beginning of systole. In fact, the beginning of S_1 is generally taken to mark the beginning of systole. S_1 has two major components: M_1 followed closely by T_1. M_1 is related to mitral valve closure and T_1 is related to tricuspid valve closure. Ordinarily these components fuse into a single audible sound by stethoscopic examination, but can be resolved by phonocardiography.

The second heart sound, S_2, is produced mainly by closure of the semilunar valves. It marks the beginning of diastole. S_2 has two major components: A_2 followed by P_2. A_2 is related to aortic valve closure and P_2 is related to pulmonic valve closure. During inspiration, the interval between A_2 and P_2 is large enough (>30 msec) that two separate sounds (a split heart sound) can usually be distinguished using the stethoscope. During expiration, P_2 moves closer to A_2 and usually only a single sound can be heard. The occurrence of a split S_2 in normal people decreases with age.

The third heart sound, S_3, occurs toward the end of the rapid filling period. Traditionally it has been ascribed to vibrations of the ventricular walls as they begin to expand. More recently, it has been determined that S_3 as heard with a stethoscope results from impact of the heart with the chest wall during rapid ventricular filling. S_3 is normally audible in children but tends to disappear with age. When present beyond age 35-40, S_3 is considered pathologic. When S_3 is auscultated, the sounds are said to be a ventricular diastolic gallop.

The fourth heart sound, S_4, occurs during atrial contraction, and as auscultated with the stethoscope is probably due to impact of the heart with the chest wall. It is almost never auscultated in normal young adults, but is often heard in apparently healthy old people. An audible S_4 results in a so-called atrial diastolic gallop (or presystolic gallop).

Topic 8: The Electrocardiogram

Cardiac cellular electrophysiology and the excitatory pathway in the heart were described in Chapter 3. As the excitatory wave of depolarization sweeps over the atrial muscle fibers and then the ventricular muscle fibers, electrical currents flow in the extracellular spaces around the heart. When the ventricular muscle fibers repolarize, electrical currents again flow in the extracellular spaces around the heart. These extracellular currents spread throughout the entire body since the extracellular spaces provide a conducting medium. Voltage differences exist along the lines of current flow. If the currents are intense enough, a cycle of voltage differences associated with each heartbeat can be recorded from electrodes connected to the skin. Such a recording is called an electro-cardiogram, ECG. The extracellular currents due to activity in the conduction system of the heart are too weak to be detected on the body surface; only currents due to activity in the working myocardial fibers are seen in surface ECGs.

An introduction to electrocardiography will be presented in Chapter 6. For now you need only be familiar with a few prominent features of a typical ECG trace obtained from electrodes connected to any two limbs, for example the right arm and the left leg (this set of electrode placements is called lead II). The following table lists the sources of the extracellular currents underlying each of these major features:

P wave	Depolarization of the atria
Q wave	Depolarization of most of the interventricular septum
R wave	Depolarization of the apex and most of the ventricular free walls
S wave	Depolarization of small portions of the interventricular septum and ventricular free walls just under the base of the heart
T wave	Repolarization of the ventricles

The Q, R, and S waves together are the QRS complex, which represents ventricular depolarization.

Topic 9: An Interactive, Dynamic Chart Showing the Events of the Cardiac Cycle

[Special: Events]
Use this special to confirm your knowledge of the phases and the events, and especially to examine the temporal relationships among the features of the events. The events can be run singly, all at once, or in any combination.

Part 4: Left Ventricular Pressure-Volume Loops

Topic 1: The Basics

Figure 5
Graphing left ventricular pressure against left ventricular volume during each heart beat results in a cyclic plot known as a left ventricular pressure-volume loop. The width of the loop is the stroke volume. The loop runs counterclockwise. To describe the left ventricular PV loop we will start at its lower right corner, which is the point just at the end of diastole (or beginning of systole).

Isovolumetric contraction period: With both valves closed, pressure rises perpendicularly at constant end-diastolic volume until it just exceeds aortic pressure and the aortic valve opens (upper right corner of loop).

Ejection periods: After the aortic valve opens, blood is ejected from the left ventricle into the aorta and left ventricular volume decreases. During the rapid and reduced ejection periods the pressure in the left ventricle rises and then falls, paralleling the pressure changes in the aorta. When left ventricular pressure falls just below aortic pressure, the aortic valve closes (upper left corner).

Isovolumetric relaxation period: With both valves now closed, pressure falls perpendicularly at end-systolic volume until it becomes just less than left atrial pressure and the mitral valve opens (lower left corner).

Filling periods: After the mitral valve opens, blood is rapidly sucked into the ventricle; volume increases, and pressure decreases during most of the rapid filling period. Subsequently, blood continues to flow passively from left atrium to left ventricle resulting in a gradual rise in left ventricular pressure. This rise in pressure continues as ventricular volume is further increased by atrial contraction just before the next systole begins (lower right corner).

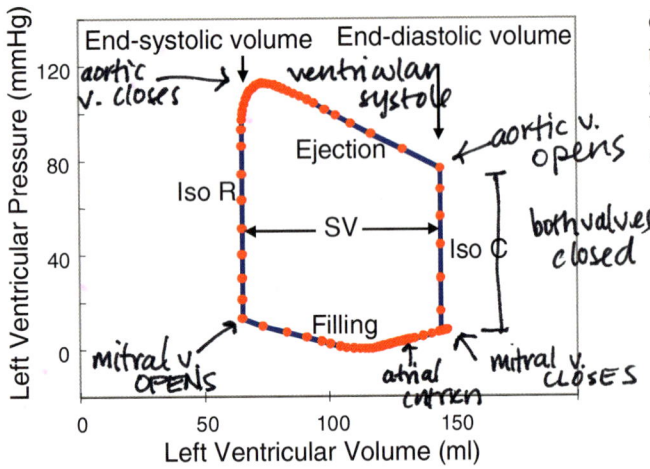

[Figure 5 annotations: aortic v. closes; ventricular systole; aortic v. opens; both valves closed; mitral v. opens; atrial contract; mitral v. closes]

Figure 5. Left ventricular pressure-volume loop. The points along the curve are spaced one hundredth of a cycle apart (10 msec apart if the heart rate is 60/min)
SV = Stroke volume ← so how does Δ press & vol Δ SV?
Iso C = Isovolumetric contraction
Iso R = Isovolumetric relaxation

It is important to note that during the ejection and filling periods, most ejection occurs while pressure is rising, and most filling occurs while pressure is falling. The latter fact is often unappreciated.

Topic 2: An Interactive, Dynamic Chart of Left Ventricular Pressure-Volume Data

[Special: PV Loop]
Static illustrations of left ventricular pressure-volume loops, such as the one shown in Figure 5, give no insight into the dynamics of the process. The PV loop special provided here should give you a feeling for the timing of the pressure-volume relationship. Clicking on any of the phase buttons brings up a rectangle on the chart. You can try to identify each phase in advance and then click up a rectangle for confirmation. The width of each rectangle (except for the isovolumetric periods) represents the volume change associated with each phase, and the height represents the pressure change. Note how little actually happens during the reduced filling period, although it takes a lot of time.

Topic 3: Control of Stroke Volume

Understanding the control of stroke volume is best done with reference to ventricular PV loops, and this is the focus of Chapter 7. At this point, in anticipation, we will make two important observations that have clinical relevance.

- Cardiac contractility determines how far to the left ejection proceeds before the aortic valve shuts. For example, a decrease in contractility shifts the end-systolic pressure-volume point (upper left corner) to the right, thereby increasing end-systolic volume and reducing stroke volume. An increase in contractility has the opposite effect; the end-systolic pressure-volume point shifts to the left and stroke volume increases. Reduced ventricular contractility is a common cause of congestive heart failure.

- The steepness of the PV curve during the reduced filling period and the atrial contraction period is a measure of the resistance to passive filling of the ventricle. If the slope of this curve increases (indicating reduced ventricular compliance), the end-diastolic pressure-volume point (lower right corner) tends to shift to the left, thereby reducing end-diastolic volume and stroke volume. An abnormally hypertrophied ventricular myocardium or myocardial hypoxia can result in reduced ventricular compliance. Reduced ventricular compliance is another important cause of congestive heart failure.

Topic 4: Valvular Defects

Normally, the segments of the PV loop representing the isovolumetric periods are vertical. However, if either the mitral valve or the aortic valve leaks (is incompetent) these segments are not vertical. The subject of valvular defects is beyond the scope of this chapter.

Topic 5: Stroke Work

The work performed by the left ventricle during each beat is equal to the area within a PV loop.

Chapter 6

Electrocardiography

This chapter introduces electrocardiography.
Part 1 discusses the flow of extracellular electrical currents around an advancing wave of depolarization.
Part 2 describes the principles and conventions of frontal-plane electrocardiography.
Part 3 describes the chest leads and the standard 12 lead electrocardiogram.
Part 4 discusses cardiac arrhythmias and illustrates the use of electrocardiography in their diagnosis. Other clinical uses of electrocardiography, for example in diagnosing and evaluating myocardial ischemia and infarction, are beyond the scope of this chapter.

Part 1: Basic Principles

Topic 1: Electrical Fields in a Volume Conductor

Figure 1

If a dipolar source of electrical current (*e.g.* a flashlight battery) is immersed in a tub of salt solution, an electrical field is set up in the conducting medium with current flowing from positive to negative poles. If the strength and orientation of the dipole and the properties of the medium are known, the structure of the electrical field can be deduced. For example, it is possible to predict the voltage difference between any two points in the field. Conversely, if the voltage differences among various points in the field are known, it is possible to predict the magnitude and direction of the dipole. If the magnitude and direction of the dipole change, then the voltage differences in the medium will change, providing information about the changes in the dipole.

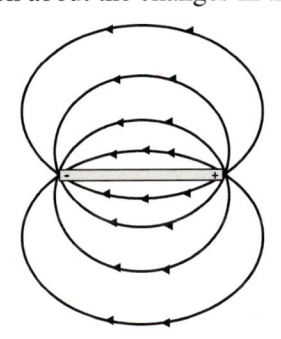

Figure 1. Electrical current from a dipolar source in a volume conductor (two-dimensional representation). The current that flows from positive terminal to negative terminal spreads out through the whole conductor. The density of electrical current decreases with distance from the source.

Topic 2: Extracellular Electrical Currents Caused by a Wave of Depolarization

Figure 2

Consider a strip of cardiac muscle immersed in a volume conductor. The muscle strip is in the process of depolarizing from left to right. We can think of this strip as being a single cell since gap junctions electrically connect all the cells.

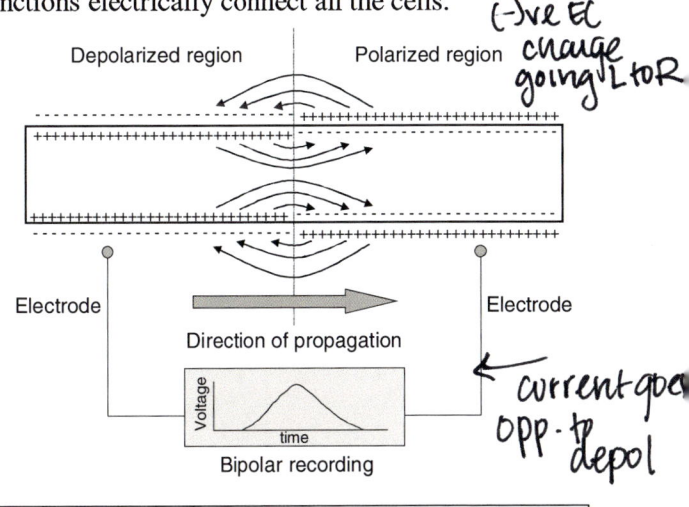

Figure 2. Electrical currents from a strip of cardiac muscle in a volume conductor. Extracellular current flows from regions that are not yet depolarized to regions that are already depolarized, opposite to the direction of propagation. In electrocardiography, the direction of the vector describing the resultant extracellular electrical field is, by convention, in the direction of propagation rather than in the direction of extracellular current flow. Electrodes placed anywhere along the lines of current flow detect a simple monotonic wave of voltage difference as propagation occurs from one end to the other of the muscle strip.

The outer surfaces of the cells ahead of the wave of depolarization are electrically positive with respect to the outer surfaces of the cells behind the wave of depolarization. Therefore, an electrical current flows in the extracellular space from right to left (*i.e.* from the cells that have not yet depolarized back to the cells that have already depolarized). The circuit is completed by current flowing through the cells as shown in the figure. This process is the same as the local currents that flow around the wave front of an action potential in any nerve or muscle fiber. The extracellular currents spread throughout the entire conducting medium, and if they are strong enough (*i.e.*, involve enough muscle mass), the electrical potential differences associated with these currents can be detected by electrode pairs located anywhere in the volume conductor. The extracellular record of a wave of depolarization along a linear strip of cardiac tissue is quite simple. Prior to depolarization, there is no voltage difference between two extracellular electrodes. During the wave of depolarization, the voltage difference rises and then falls. When the tissue is all depolarized, there is again no voltage difference because there is no flow of extracellular current.

Now consider the entire heart *in situ*. The wave of electrical activity that passes through the myocardium and initiates each beat of the heart causes electrical currents to flow in the extracellular spaces surrounding the heart. Since the extracellular spaces are continuous throughout the body, the electrical activity generated by the heart can be detected anywhere in the body or on the body surface. A recording of such electrical activity is called an electrocardiogram (ECG). In Holland, where clinical electrocardiography began, cardio is spelled with a K, so traditionally we say EKG.

The EKG as recorded from body surface electrodes is important in clinical diagnosis and evaluation. It is also useful in physiology for relating the various mechanical events of the cardiac cycle to the electrical events. This chapter will describe the features of the EKG as recorded from standard electrodes, and will explain the fundamentals of how cardiac electrical activity results in these features. The use of electrocardiography in examining arrhythmias will be introduced.

Topic 3: The Extracellular Electrical Vector during a Wave of Depolarization

The extracellular current that flows during a wave of depolarization is a vector quantity having both magnitude and direction. An arrow whose length is proportional to the magnitude of the extracellular current represents this vector. By tradition, the direction of the vector is opposite to the direction of extracellular current flow, designating the direction of the wave of depolarization. It is common jargon among electrocardiographers to refer to the direction of this vector as the direction in which the "electrical forces" are traveling.

Topic 4: Sequence of Events

Extracellular electrical fields from the whole heart are complex because of the tortuous path taken by the wave of depolarization. This path is determined by the conducting system as described in Chapter 3. Depolarization of the conducting system itself contributes little or nothing to the EKG because of its small mass compared to working myocardium.

The wave of depolarization passes over all the atrial muscle while traveling from SA node to AV node. In the ventricles, the working myocardium of the interventricular septum is the earliest to depolarize; depolarization begins roughly a third of the way down the septum on its left side and quickly spreads to the right. Then the free walls of the left and right ventricles depolarize; first at the apex, and then up toward the base of the heart. Depolarization of the apex and free walls begins at the endocardial surface and progresses to the epicardial surface. The free walls and septum just under the base of the heart are the last regions to depolarize. Repolarization of the ventricles occurs in a direction that is roughly opposite to that of depolarization.

Thus, the resultant vector representing the extracellular electrical field around the heart continuously changes in magnitude and direction as depolarization and repolarization proceed. This changing vector can be followed accurately by electrical measurements from skin electrodes. There have been many attempts to make predictions of the electrical measurements from knowledge of cardiac depolarization pathways. These attempts are not especially useful and are out of the scope of this chapter. Therefore, from here on, the subject becomes almost entirely empirical.

Electrocardiography

Part 2: Frontal-Plane Electrocardiography

Topic 1: The Einthoven Limb Leads

British physiologist Augustus Waller in 1887 made the first electrocardiogram from surface electrodes in humans. In 1901 a Dutch physiologist, Willem Einthoven, invented an improved version of a recording device called the string galvanometer with which he made extensive electrocardiographic studies and established conventions in clinical electrocardiography that are still in use today.

Figure 3
Electrodes are attached to all four limbs. The electrode attached to the right leg is only used to ground the subject. The following three voltage differences are recorded.

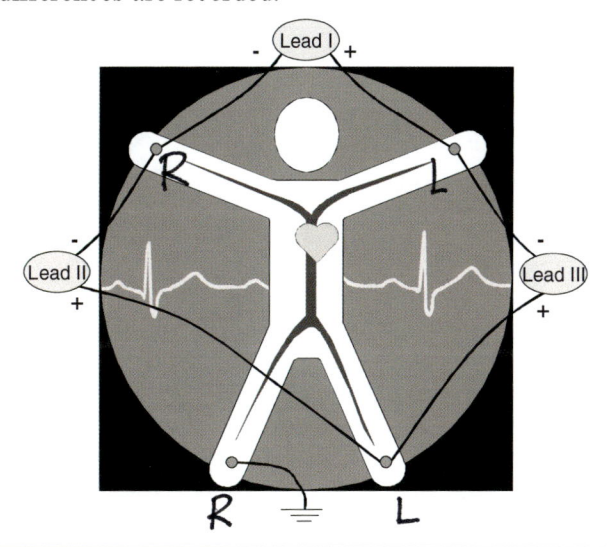

Figure 3. Electrode placements for the Einthoven limb leads.

Lead 1:
- Left arm *vs.* right arm.
- Polarity: The connections are arranged so that when the left arm is positive with respect to the right arm, an upward deflection is recorded (chart recorder, oscilloscope, computer).

Lead 2:
- Left leg *vs.* right arm.
- Polarity: The connections are arranged so that when the left leg is positive with respect to the right arm, an upward deflection is recorded.

Lead 3:
- Left leg *vs.* left arm.
- Polarity: The connections are arranged so that when the left leg is positive with respect to the left arm, an upward deflection is recorded.

Einthoven selected these polarities so that all of the major deflections of the EKG (the P, R, and T waves) usually go up.

Since the limbs conduct electricity, they serve as extensions of the electrodes. The same EKG patterns would be obtained if the electrodes were placed closer to the heart in a triangular arrangement, but wrists and ankles are convenient.

Topic 2: Unipolar Limb Leads

In a unipolar lead, the voltage difference between a so-called exploring electrode and an indifferent electrode (*i.e.*, one not influenced by cardiac electrical activity) is recorded. For the unipolar limb leads, the exploring electrode is one of the standard limb electrodes. The indifferent electrode can simply be the three limb electrodes connected to each other *via* resistors. However, in practice the indifferent electrode usually consists of only two of the limb electrodes connected to each other, with the third used as the exploring electrode. The neutrality of the indifferent electrode is not as good this way, but the signal is greatly augmented. Thus, these leads are called the augmented unipolar limb leads.

There are three standard augmented unipolar limb leads ("a" stands for augmented and "V" stands for voltage).
- Lead aVL = left arm *vs.* indifferent electrode.
- Lead aVR = right arm *vs.* indifferent electrode.
- Lead aVF = left leg (foot) *vs.* indifferent electrode.

In all cases, the polarities are arranged so that when the exploring electrode is positive with respect to the indifferent electrode, an upward deflection is recorded.

These three augmented unipolar limb leads together with the three Einthoven limb leads, provide information about electrical vectors in the frontal plane. Use of these six leads is called frontal-plane electrocardiography.

Topic 3: The Electrocardiogram from Einthoven's Standard Limb Leads

Figure 4
This is an idealized representation of an EKG recorded from lead 2.
- The P wave represents atrial depolarization.

- The QRS complex represents ventricular depolarization.
  - The Q wave occurs during depolarization of the interventricular septum.
  - The R wave occurs during depolarization of most of the ventricular myocardium.
  - The S wave occurs during depolarization of a small portion of the ventricular myocardium near the base of the heart (in the right ventricle, left ventricle, and septum).
- The T wave represents ventricular repolarization.

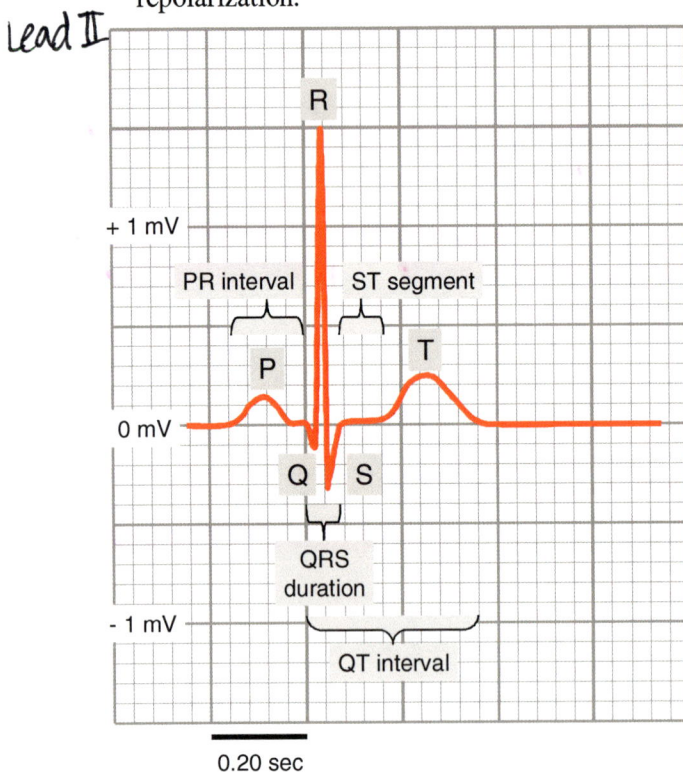

Lead II

Figure 4. The normal electrocardiogram recorded from lead 2. Conventional nomenclature is given.

Additional Nomenclature

Distances between two waves are called segments (*e.g.*, the ST segment). Distances that include at least one wave are called intervals (*e.g.*, the PQ interval and the QT interval). The PQ interval (from beginning of P wave to beginning of Q wave) is usually called the PR interval. Within the QRS complex, the first positive deflection is called the R wave. Subsequent positive deflections (abnormal) are called R', R'', etc. Negative deflections are called Q when they precede the R wave and S when they follow it.

Correlation between EKG Features and the Wave of Depolarization
Figure 5

Depolarization of the SA node, AV node, bundle of His, bundle branches, and the Purkinje fibers do not register on an EKG obtained from body surface electrodes. Figure 5 indicates their approximate timing.

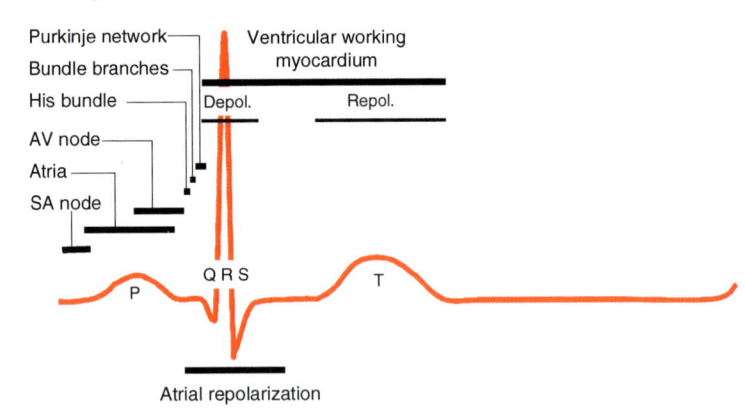

Figure 5. Correlation between the progress of the EKG and the progress of the excitatory process.

In addition to this figure, you might want to view [Animation: Correlation] [Some of the tweening is laughingly ragged, especially for ventricular depolarization and repolarization. Nevertheless, it should help for appreciating timing and synchrony.]

Repolarization

Repolarization of the ventricles does not travel the same path as depolarization and is probably not actually conducted from cell to cell. Nevertheless, there is an overall progression of repolarization from epicardial to endocardial surfaces – roughly the opposite direction to that of depolarization. The direction of the resultant vector for repolarization, therefore, normally approximates that for depolarization and the T wave is normally in the same direction as the R wave (up in the standard limb leads).

Repolarization of the atria is a different matter. It is not seen in EKGs. The reason often given is that atrial repolarization occurs during ventricular depolarization and the electrical signs of the former tend to be obscured by the much larger effects of the latter. However, this explanation cannot be correct since in complete block of the AV node, when atrial depolarization is not necessarily followed by ventricular depolarization, there is still no sign of atrial repolarization. It is possible that the small voltage vectors arising from repolarization of different parts of the atrial walls, simply cancel each other out.

Electrocardiography

Topic 4: The Electrical Axis of the Heart in the Frontal Plane

It is of frequent clinical value to estimate the direction of the resultant vector of the extracellular electrical field around the heart. The two dimensional direction in the frontal plane can be estimated from frontal-plane electrocardiography. There are two methods for doing this: graphical vector analysis using Einthoven's triangle and an approximation using the hexagonal lead system.

Einthoven's Triangle
Figure 6
Picture an equilateral triangle passing through the torso in the frontal plane. The center of the triangle is at the electrical center of the heart. Einthoven's standard limb leads detect approximately the same EKG patterns as would be obtained from electrodes placed at the apices of this triangle.

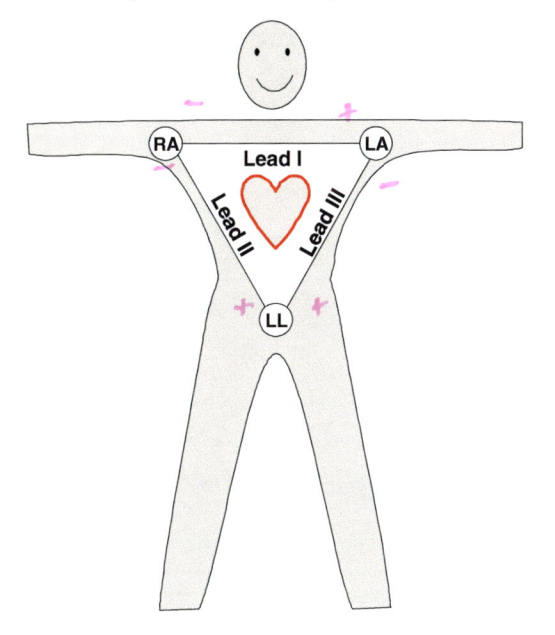

Figure 6. Einthoven's triangle.

Figure 7
Now, instead of the usual rectangular coordinate system for determining vectors, we do an analysis based on triangular coordinates. The method is described in the legend to Figure 7. The resultant electrical vector around the heart can be determined at any instant during the cycle. For example, we could determine the resultant vector at the peak of the P wave, R wave, or T wave. More commonly, however, the average vector during the entire QRS complex is determined rather than an instantaneous vector. The direction of this average vector is called the mean electrical axis of the QRS complex. It is determined using the net area enclosed by an entire QRS complex as the distance marked off along each lead axis, rather than the amplitude at any one instant. A simpler approximation that is sometimes used is to mark off the height of the R wave less the combined depths of the Q and S waves.

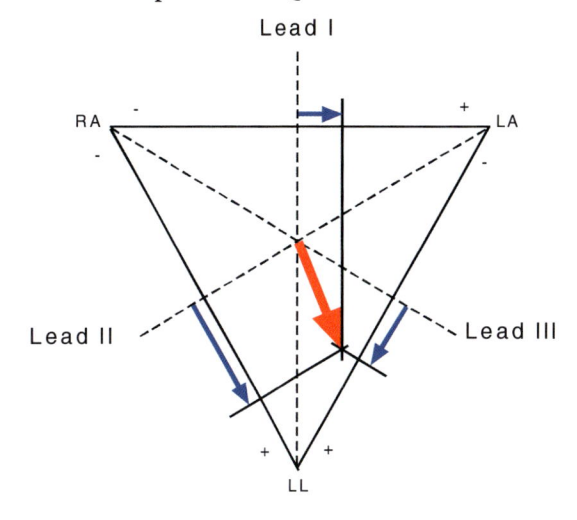

Figure 7. Frontal plane vector analysis using Einthoven's triangle. From the center of each lead axis, the voltage recorded by that lead is marked off (small arrows); toward the plus electrode if the deflection on the recording is up, and toward the minus electrode is the deflection is down. A line that is perpendicular to each lead axis is drawn from the end of each of these voltage marks. The three perpendicular lines intersect somewhere. An arrow drawn from the center of the triangle to this point of intersection (the big arrow) represents the vector in the frontal plane for this particular set of voltages. Any two of the three standard limb leads are sufficient to determine the electrical axis - the third is redundant. This procedure can be applied at any instant during the cycle, for example at the peak of the P wave, peak of the R wave, or peak of the T wave. More commonly, the average QRS vector is determined as described in the text.

The Hexaxial Lead System
Figure 8
Lead 1 reveals the component of the resultant vector in the horizontal axis. Lead 2 reveals the component in the +60 degree axis, etc. Altogether, the six limb leads register the vector components in six different axes separated from each other by 30°. An important rule is that the lead having the axis that is closest to the direction of the resultant extracellular electrical vector is the lead in which the EKG deflection is the biggest. This lead is perpendicular to the lead in which the EKG deflection is the smallest. The resultant electrical

axis of the R wave can be estimated (plus or minus 15 degrees) simply by determining in which of the six leads the R wave is biggest. The mean electrical axis of the QRS complex is given approximately by the lead axis that is perpendicular to the one having the smallest QRS signal.

Range of Normal
See Figure 8 again
The electrical axis is given in degrees. A vector pointing horizontally to the left of the person is 0 degrees and a vector pointing straight down is +90 degrees as shown in the figure. Anywhere within -10 degrees to +100 degrees is considered to be within the normal range. Between about -10 and -30 is borderline. Beyond these limits are left axis deviation and right axis deviation. Determination of the electrical axis of the heart has importance in diagnosing ventricular hypertrophies. For example, left ventricular hypertrophy tends to cause left axis deviation and right ventricular hypertrophy tends to cause right axis deviation.

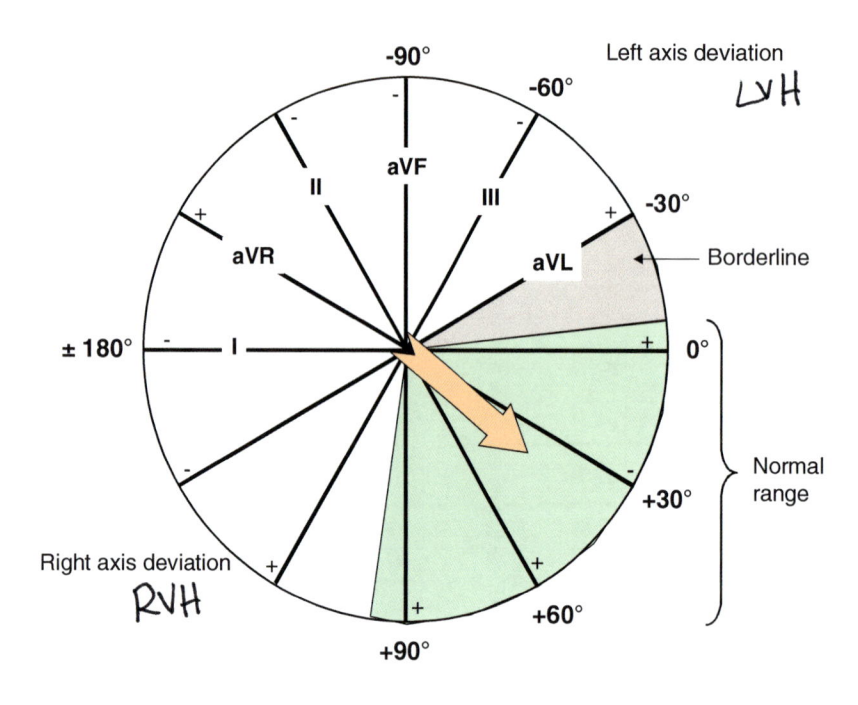

Figure 8. The lead axes for the hexaxial lead system and the normal range for the mean electrical axis of the QRS complex.

Part 3: The Chest Leads and the Standard Twelve Lead Electrocardiogram

Topic 1: The Chest Leads

Figure 9
There are six standard chest leads (also called precordial leads), as shown in the figure. They are unipolar leads, which means that the voltage difference recorded is between the chest electrode and an indifferent electrode, which in this case is the three limb leads connected to each other. The chest leads give vector information in the transverse plane as shown in the figure. For details about electrode placement, see EKG texts.

Topic 2: The Standard Twelve Lead Electrocardiogram

Clinically, it is customary to record brief segments of the three Einthoven limb leads, plus the three

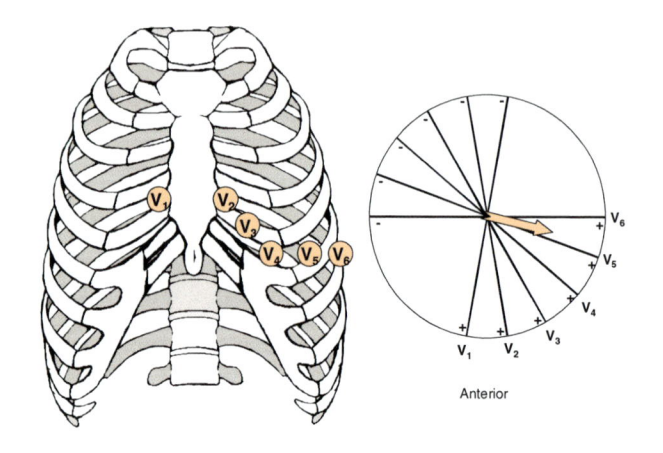

Figure 9. Locations of the six standard chest (precordial) leads, and the transverse axes that they represent.

unipolar limb leads, plus the six chest leads. Often a longer rhythm strip is also recorded, usually from lead 2.

Conventions are as follows:
- Horizontal
  o Chart speed is 25 mm/sec. Therefore, 1.0 cm horizontal represents 0.4 sec.
  o The chart is marked off with a light vertical line every mm and a heavy vertical line every 5 mm.
  o Therefore, each small square (box) horizontally is 0.04 sec and each large square is 0.2 sec (200 msec).
- Vertical
  o Standard voltage calibration is 1.0 mV/cm. One large square vertically is 0.5 cm and, therefore, represents 0.5 mV.
  o Sometimes, when a deflection is especially large, amplification is reduced. There should always be a voltage calibration mark visible on the record.

Sometimes reproducing the EKG strip may enlarge or reduce the squares, but 10 small horizontal divisions should always represent 0.4 seconds and 10 small vertical divisions usually represent 1.0 mV.

Figure 10

This is a somewhat idealized drawing of a strip from lead II showing a normal sinus rhythm. There are several rules of thumb for quickly calculating heart rate from a rhythm strip. The one I like the best is simply to divide 300 by the number of large squares between consecutive R waves. If rhythm is not regular, then a more laborious procedure must be used for determining average heart rate.

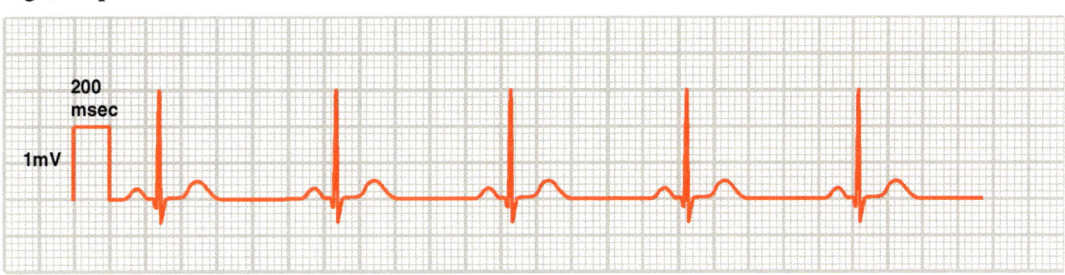

Figure 10. Normal sinus rhythm.

Part 4: Arrhythmias

Topic 1: Normal and Abnormal Sinus Rhythms

This is only a brief introduction to cardiac arrhythmias (which are also called dysrhythmias). Please consult pathophysiology and electrocardiography textbooks for more extensive study.

When the SA node is the pacemaker, the rhythm of the heart is called a sinus rhythm. Normal sinus rhythms range from about 52 to 90 beats/min. A sinus rhythm greater than 100 beats/min is called sinus tachycardia. A sinus rhythm less than 60 beats/min is sinus bradycardia.

In both sinus tachycardia and sinus bradycardia the EKG has a normal appearance except for the duration of its components. Endurance athletes often have a nonpathological sinus bradycardia resulting from increased parasympathetic tone. Rhythmic changes in heart rate associated with breathing are often observed – increased rate during inspiration, decreased rate during expiration. This phenomenon is called sinus arrhythmia. It is caused by rhythmic fluctuation in parasympathetic activity to the heart during the respiratory cycle. Sinus arrhythmia does not usually indicate any abnormality.

Topic 2: Depolarization Initiated from Abnormal Locations

Any site other than the SA node that initiates an excitatory wave of depolarization is called an ectopic focus. Mechanisms include reentry and ectopic pacemaker activity. Reentry occurs when some conduction defect results in a wave of depolarization that takes a path circling back on itself. If the returning wave finds a region of tissue that has regained excitability, a new, premature wave of depolarization can be triggered.

Ectopic pacing can result from regions of the conducting system or injured working myocardium that have abnormally high rates of spontaneous diastolic depolarization. In addition, if the SA node is depressed or conduction from it is blocked, a subsidiary pacemaker takes over and produces ectopic (escape) rhythms. These abnormalities may originate in either the atria (atrial dysrhythmias) or the ventricles (ventricular dysrhythmias). They may produce either single premature beats, or prolonged abnormal rhythms.

Atrial Dysrhythmias
Figure 11

Atrial Premature Contractions: Premature beats (extrasystoles) are contractions triggered from abnormal locations. A premature contraction of atrial origin is identified by a P wave that arrives early and is usually distorted, followed by a normal QRS complex. The next EKG cycle then follows with the previous rhythm (*i.e.* the SA node resets so that the time between the premature beat and the next beat is normal).

Atrial Tachycardia: In atrial tachycardia, the heart rate is often as high as 200 beats/min. It may be of SA node origin (sinus tachycardia) or of ectopic origin (usually by a reentry mechanism). When the ectopic site is in atrial tissue or when it is in the AV node or bundle of His, the condition is called supraventricular tachycardia. Commonly, in supraventricular tachycardias P waves cannot be clearly identified.

Atrial Flutter: In atrial flutter (250-350 atrial beats/min), impulses reach the AV node so frequently that not all can pass. Usually only one passes on to the bundle of His for every 2 or more that arrive at the AV node. The typical EKG in atrial flutter has a saw tooth pattern, with several P waves for each QRS complex. In atrial flutter and, to a lesser extent, in atrial tachycardia, increases in cardiac output during exercise that would normally be mediated partly by increased heart rate, are compromised.

Atrial Fibrillation: In atrial fibrillation the walls of the atria quiver rather than pump. They quiver in completely disordered motion apparently caused by multiple microreentry loops of depolarization that go on and on endlessly. Most impulses reaching the AV node fail to penetrate, and ventricular frequency, while irregular and usually high, may not be excessive.

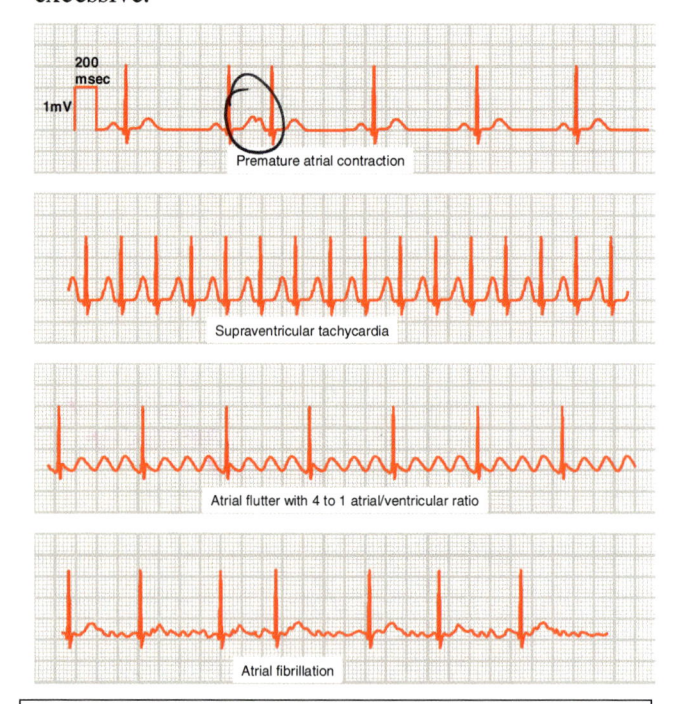

Figure 11. Atrial dysrhythmias (idealized drawings).

Ventricular Dysrhythmias
Figure 12

Ventricular Premature Contractions: An ectopic focus in the AV node or proximal His bundle sends waves of depolarization in both directions. The wave going up through the atria causes an abnormal P wave (which may be lost in the QRS complex), while the wave going to the ventricles follows its normal path and produces a relatively normal QRS complex. The resulting premature ventricular contraction is called a PVC.

Most ectopic foci are located below the His bundle (in the bundle branches, terminal Purkinje fibers, or damaged myocardium) and produce grossly abnormal QRS complexes. The retrograde waves of depolarization originating from these sites usually do not reach the SA node before it fires at its next regularly scheduled time. The normally timed impulse from the SA node, however, quickly dies out as it reaches tissue that has been made refractory by the premature ventricular impulse. Consequently, this SA node impulse is lost; it does not result in ventricular contraction. The ventricles must wait for the next regularly scheduled SA node event before they can contract again; this produces a so-called compensatory pause (*i.e.* the interval between the premature beat and the next beat is greater than usual). In a full compensatory pause, the normal R waves just before and just after the PVC are twice the normal R-R distance apart. The premature beat itself is generally not very forceful since the ventricles have not had time to fill during diastole with a normal amount of blood. However, the beat following the compensatory pause can be very forceful since, by then, the ventricles have filled with an abnormally large volume of blood. It is this hard beat following a PVC that often alerts the person. PVCs sometimes result from serious cardiac pathology, but they often afflict apparently normal hearts and are commonly the source of unnecessary anxiety.

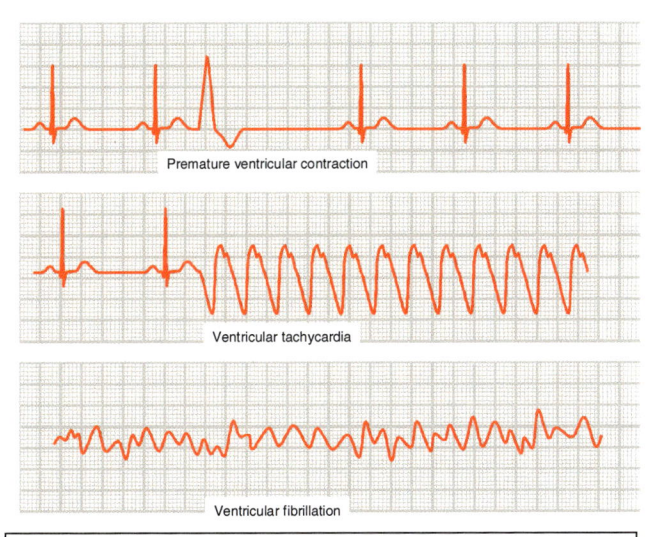

Figure 12. Ventricular dysrhythmias.

Ventricular Tachycardia and Flutter: Abnormally rapid heart rates driven by ectopic foci below the His bundle are called ventricular tachycardias. They can continue for long durations, but sometimes occur in short bursts of 10-20 beats called paroxysms. Their frequency ranges from about 100 to 250 beats /min and is generally regular. At rates so high that no clear ST segment can be detected, the arrhythmia is called ventricular flutter. As with ventricular extrasystoles, the QRS complexes are quite distorted. Ventricular flutter is often a transitional state leading to ventricular fibrillation.

Ventricular Fibrillation: Ventricular fibrillation is characterized by uncoordinated quivering, trembling, and twitching of the ventricular walls together with a chaotic EKG in which no semblance of QRS complexes is seen. No blood is pumped and the patient dies unless promptly defibrillated. The mechanism seems to involve reentry with complex, branching paths of depolarization returning upon themselves endlessly in what has been termed circus movement. Some investigators believe that repetitive firing of multiple ectopic pacemakers is also involved.

Topic 3: Atrio-Ventricular Conduction Defects

Figure 13

Various diseases and drugs can slow or even completely block conduction of impulses through the AV junctional tissue. There are three major categories of AV block.

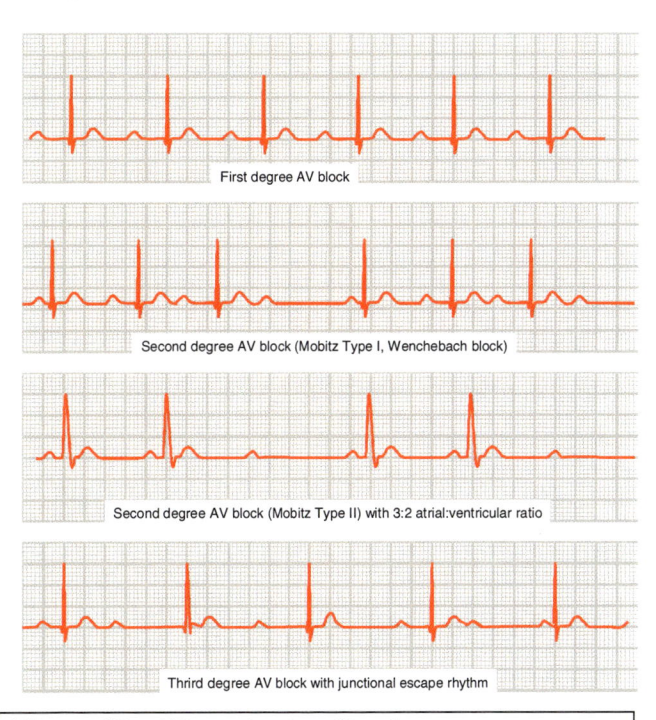

Figure 13. AV conduction disorders.

- **First Degree AV Block:** Conduction is slowed, but each impulse from the SA node eventually gets through and causes a QRS complex. The EKG is characterized by one P wave for each QRS complex, but the PR interval is prolonged (greater than 200 msec, one big square).
- **Second Degree AV Block:** Some, but not all, impulses from the SA node get through to the ventricles. Each QRS complex is preceded by a P wave, but there are more P waves than QRS complexes.
  o **Mobitz Type I** (also called Wenckebach block): The PR interval progressively increases in duration from beat to beat until, after a few beats, the impulse fails to get through the AV node.
  o **Mobitz Type II:** Here there is no gradual

lengthening of the PR interval, in fact it may not be prolonged at all. Instead, there is an occasional unexpected failure of AV conduction. This type of second degree heart block is much more serious than Wenckebach block.

- **Third Degree AV Block:** This is also called complete heart block. No impulses from the SA node get through the AV junction. The ventricles must depend on some ectopic focus for their rhythm, which, consequently, is quite slow. The EKG shows multiple P waves for each QRS complex with no evidence of coordination between atrial and ventricular electrical activity.

Chapter 7

Regulation of Stroke Volume

Afterload, preload, and contractility act together to determine stroke volume. This is accomplished by effects on the velocity at which cardiac muscle fibers shorten and thicken. There is also an effect of heart rate on stroke volume.

This chapter discusses:
- The effect of afterload on stroke volume
- The end-systolic pressure-volume relationship and end-systolic elastance
- The effect of preload on stroke volume
- The end-diastolic pressure-volume relationship and ventricular compliance
- Starling's Law of the Heart and the Starling effect
- Ventricular function curves (Starling curves)
- Ventricular afterload performance curves
- Hyper and hypo effectiveness of the heart
- The Anrep effect
- The effects of exercise on stroke volume
- The effect of high heart rates on stroke volume

Part 1: Effect of Afterload on Stroke Volume

Topic 1: Introduction

Stroke volume is determined by afterload, preload, and contractility. These effects will be explained by using left ventricular pressure-volume loops. If you need to refresh your knowledge of PV loops, click here [Special: PV Loop].

Afterload and preload are not primary adjustable parameters of the system; they are determined by heart rate, contractility, total peripheral resistance, venous capacity, and total blood volume as explained in subsequent chapters. Afterload, preload, and contractility determine stroke volume by their effects on the velocity of cardiac muscle fiber shortening (with a small contribution from fiber thickening). Velocity is increased by increased preload and by increased contractility. Velocity is decreased by increased afterload.

Parts 1-3 of this chapter discuss the effects of changing afterload, preload or contractility individually. In each case, the other two variables are experimentally held constant. The principal experimental arrangement for doing this is called the heart-lung preparation (see below).

Topic 2: Left Ventricular Intrinsic Reserve

Figure 1

The normal left ventricle (LV) has the potential to develop far more pressure than is ordinarily necessary to eject its stroke volume. This is true even without any increase in contractility or in preload. We will call this property intrinsic reserve to distinguish it from another property called inotropic reserve mentioned later in this chapter. Intrinsic reserve is illustrated in Figure 1.

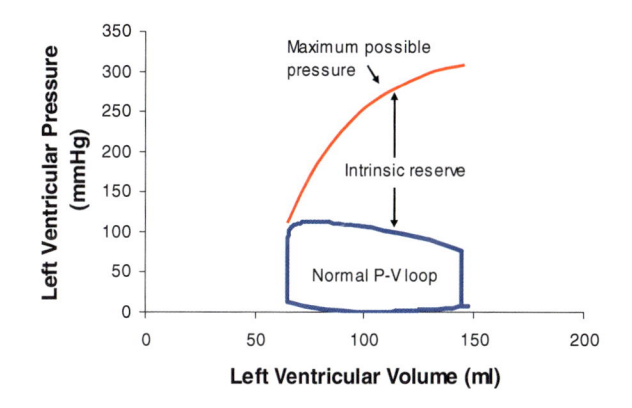

Figure 1. The property of left ventricular intrinsic reserve. The data for this figure are based on the author's, *A Working Simulation of Left Ventricular Performance* (unpublished).

[margin note: most reserve at beginning of systole]

At the beginning of systole, the aortic valve opens well before maximum LV pressure can be reached, so there remains considerable reserve. This reserve gradually diminishes during ejection and essentially disappears at the end of systole.

The maximum possible pressure declines during ejection for two reasons: 1) the sarcomeres get progressively shorter, and 2) the intensity of activation diminishes with time.

Note that at any degree of ejection, the ventricle can never generate more pressure than allowed by the maximum pressure curve at that degree of ejection.

[A famous experiment was to allow a heart to contract at various contained volumes after clamping the aorta. No blood could be ejected, *i.e.* the contraction was isovolumetric. The maximum isovolumetric pressure was recorded. The isovolumetric pressure-volume curve obtained was very much like the curve in Figure 1, called the maximum possible pressure curve. It showed that the more dilated the ventricle within normal limits, the more forcefully it could contract. This important finding is usually attributed to Otto Frank who published his work (on frogs) in 1895, although similar findings had been published previously by others. The maximum pressure curve of Figure 1 is not quite the same as the Frank curve since the latter does not account for the effect of time on the intensity of activation.]

Topic 3: Increased Afterload Reduces Stroke Volume by Reducing the Velocity of Shortening

Figure 2
This PV loop illustrates the consequences of increasing afterload (with preload and contractility held constant).

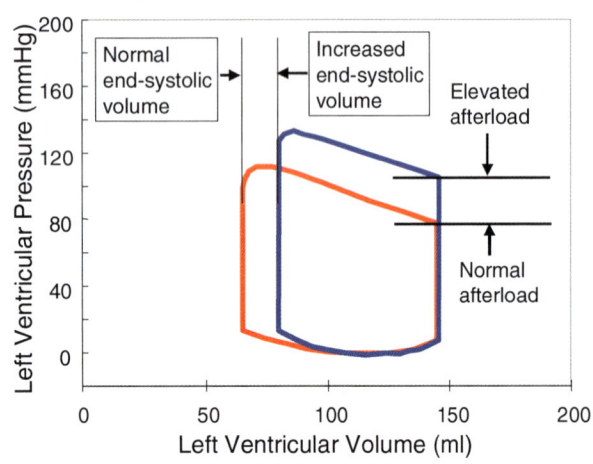

Figure 2. Effect of increased afterload on left ventricular pressure-volume loop.

Note the following:
- Ventricular pressure must rise to a higher level before the aortic valve opens and ejection starts.
- Ejection stops at an elevated end-systolic volume; therefore, stroke volume is reduced. The obvious explanation for this effect is that the shortening velocity of cardiac muscle fibers is reduced because of the increased afterload. Reduced shortening velocity leads to reduced ejection rate and, therefore, less ejection can take place before the fibers start to relax.
- The actual end-systolic pressure-volume point falls just a little short of the Frank curve.

Topic 4: What Determines the End of Systole and Closure of the Outflow Valves?

Any muscle fiber can shorten only when the tension it is capable of developing exceeds the load it is working against. As cardiac muscle fibers shorten during systole, the maximum tension they can generate subsides because of shortening and because of time. Eventually tension and, therefore, chamber pressure no longer exceed the load and no more ejection can take place. Systole is over. The aortic valve closes abruptly since the pressure difference (ventricular minus aortic) was already slightly reversed (Chapter 5, Part 3, Topic 6) and the only thing holding the valve open had been the momentum of ejecting blood.

Topic 5: The End-Systolic Pressure-Volume Relationship

Figure 3
Two more loops corresponding to different afterloads are added to Figure 2. A curve is drawn through the end-systolic pressure-volume points. This curve is called the end-systolic pressure-volume relationship (ESPVR) and is usually a fairly straight line; its slope is called the end-systolic elastance.

The ESPVR is a little to the right of the Otto Frank curve), and theoretically is very close to the maximum pressure curve.

Regulation of Stroke Volume 65

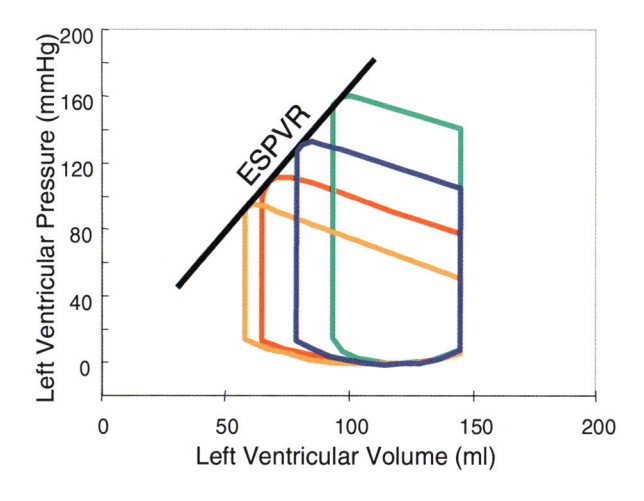

Figure 3. Effect of various afterloads to demonstrate the end-systolic pressure-volume relationship.

↑ afterload [inc press in aorta] ⟹
↓ SV
↑ ESV w/ no Δ in EDV
SV = EDV − ESV

Part 2: Effect of Preload on Stroke Volume

Topic 1: Left Ventricular Pressure-Volume Loop

Figure 4
A change in preload is represented on the PV loop as a change in end-diastolic volume. Since increased preload causes increased shortening and thickening velocity, it results in increased ejection velocity. Consequently, more ejection occurs prior to relaxation and stroke volume increases. The end-systolic volume remains the same as it was before the increase in preload.

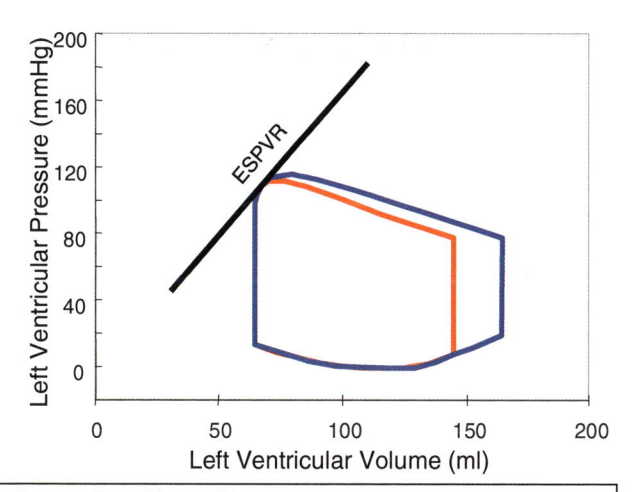

Figure 4. Effect of increased preload on the left ventricular pressure-volume loop.

Figure 5
More loops corresponding to different preloads are added. Regardless of the amount of preload (within the normal range shown here), end-systolic volume remains constant; this is an incredibly important property of the heart.

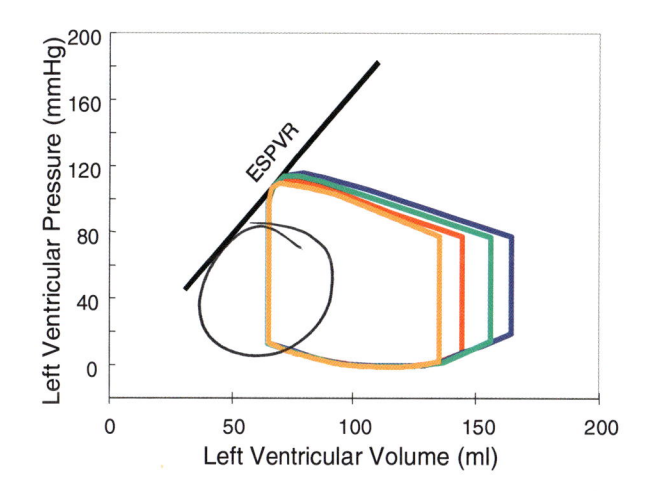

Figure 5. Left ventricular pressure-volume loops with various preloads..

Topic 2: Starling's Law of the Heart

We see from Figure 5 that increased preload leads to increased stroke volume. This crucial principle of cardiac function is known as Starling's Law of the Heart. The change in stroke volume exactly equals the change in end-diastolic volume over the normal range of preloads. The explanation for Starling's Law is, as we have seen, the increase in velocity of shortening and thickening of cardiac muscle fibers at increased preloads within the normal range of sarcomere lengths (up to 2.4 μm).

Figure 6
Ernest Starling *et al.* published this finding in 1914. They employed an experimental arrangement called the heart-lung preparation, which is diagrammed in Figure 6 (in case you are interested). Starling's Law is often called the Frank-Starling Law.

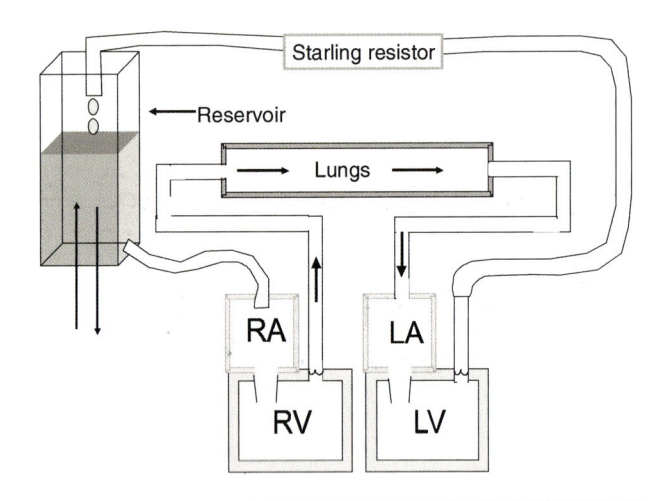

Figure 6. Diagram of the heart-lung preparation, an experimental arrangement usually applied to anesthetized dogs for studying the automatic responses of the heart to controlled changes in inflow pressure (preload) and outflow pressure (afterload). Various blood vessels are tied off or cannulated so that blood, after being ejected from the left ventricle, flows into an open reservoir instead of the systemic vascular system. It then flows from the reservoir into the right atrium, and is subsequently pumped by the right ventricle through the lungs and back to the left ventricle. The lungs are artificially ventilated to keep the blood oxygenated. The reservoir can be raised or lowered to adjust inflow pressure (right atrial pressure). A device called a Starling resistor is inserted into the outflow tubing in order to adjust outflow pressure. Pressures are monitored from the right atrium and the aorta. Flow rate into the reservoir is measured. [S.W. Patterson and E.H. Starling, *J. Physiol.* 48: 357, 1914.]

Topic 3: Ventricular Function Curves – Starling Curves

One of the important characteristics of any pump is how its output responds to changes in the inflow pressure. You might want to know this characteristic for some inanimate pump that you buy. You must know this characteristic for the heart.

Figure 7

This figure shows how left and right ventricular outputs respond to changes in mean left atrial pressure (MLAP) or mean right atrial pressure (MRAP) respectively. Again, afterload and contractility are held constant. Heart rate is also constant; therefore, the effects shown are entirely due to changes in stroke volume.

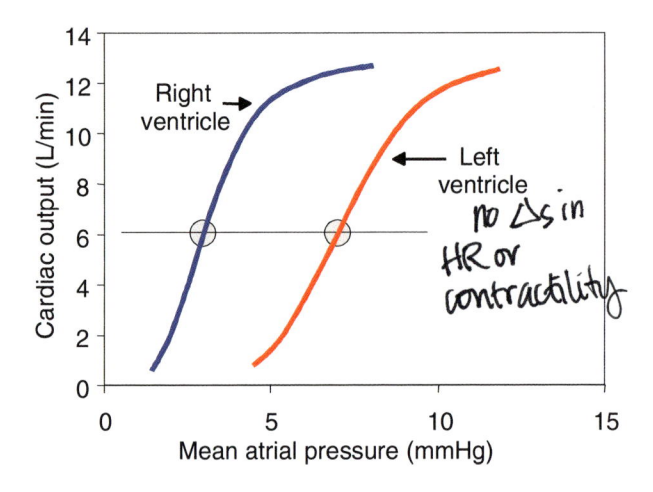

Figure 7. Left and right ventricular function curves. The circles represent the normal operating points.

The relationships shown in Figure 7 are called ventricular function curves. Sometimes they are called Starling curves. Notice the steep positive response of CO as inflow pressure increases within its normal range. This response is automatic; it does not require any changes in heart rate or contractility.

The effect of inflow pressure on CO is a corollary of Starling's Law of the Heart since it results from the fact that stroke volume increases as preload increases. Inflow pressure, together with ventricular compliance (see below), determines the amount of diastolic filling of the ventricle and, therefore, its preload.

The Starling effect accounts for the extremely important fact that the left heart always pumps blood onward at exactly the same rate as the right heart pumps blood to it. Left heart output, when averaged over a few beats, exactly equals right heart output.

[Note: Sometimes, instead of plotting CO as the dependent variable, stroke work is plotted, and the resulting curve is known as a Starling work curve. The amount of work done by the heart during each ejection period is best calculated as the area within a ventricular PV loop. However, simply multiplying stroke volume by mean arterial pressure gives a rough, but probably satisfactory, estimate of stroke work. There seems to be no advantage in Starling work curves over Starling output curves, but you probably should know about them.]

Regulation of Stroke Volume

Topic 4: Starling Curves for the Entire Heart

Figure 8
This figure shows Starling curves for the entire heart (including the lungs). Inflow pressure is either central venous pressure (CVP) or mean right atrial pressure (MRAP), which are essentially identical. [Note that Starling curves for the entire heart are the same as right ventricular function curves since the left ventricle must always keep up with the right ventricle.]

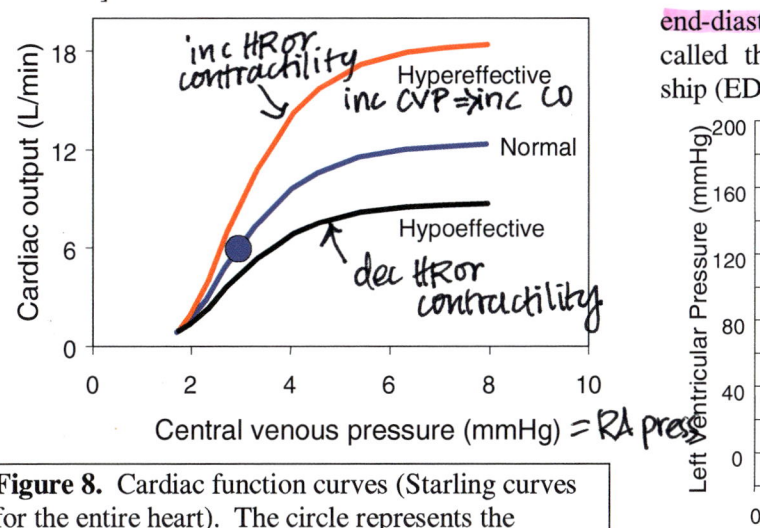

Figure 8. Cardiac function curves (Starling curves for the entire heart). The circle represents the normal operating point at rest. Effects on the Starling curve of making the heart hypereffective or hypoeffective are shown.

Pump output is very sensitive to inflow pressure. If inflow pressure increases even slightly, CO increases substantially. This response is automatic; it depends on the Starling effect rather than on changes in heart rate, contractility, or afterload. Thus, the Starling effect explains the fact that the heart automatically pumps blood onward at exactly the same rate that blood returns to it – cardiac output equals venous return.

MRAP, together with right ventricular compliance, determines right ventricular preload. As long as ventricular compliance remains constant, MRAP or CVP can be considered an index of preload to the entire pump.

Topic 5: Effects of Changing Heart Rate or Contractility on the Starling Curve

See Figure 8 again
If heart rate and/or contractility are changed then the Starling curve is shifted. A heart with an elevated ventricular function curve (due to increased heart rate and/or contractility) is said to be hypereffective, and one with a lowered ventricular function curve is called hypoeffective.

Topic 6: The End-Diastolic Pressure-Volume Relationship and Ventricular Compliance

Figure 9
This figure again illustrates left ventricular PV loops for various preloads. A curve is drawn through the end-diastolic pressure-volume points. This curve is called the end-diastolic pressure-volume relationship (EDPVR).

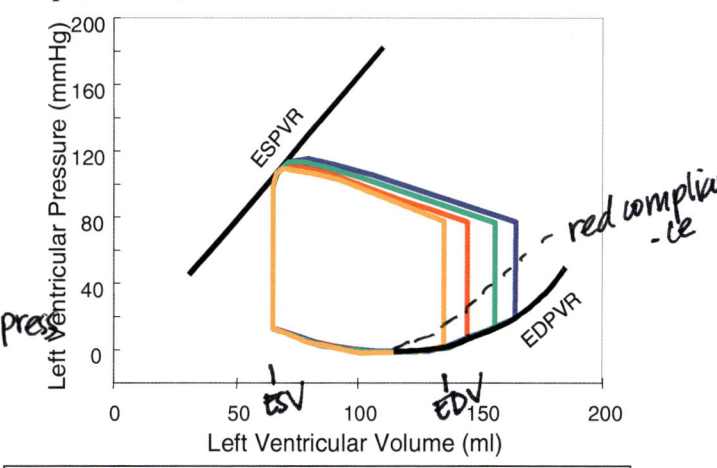

Figure 9. Left ventricular pressure-volume loops at various preloads, showing the normal end-diastolic pressure-volume relationship (EDPVR).

The EDPVR shows the pressure generated in the ventricle by the passive stretching of its walls as it fills with blood. The slope of the EDPVR is the reciprocal of ventricular compliance (the reciprocal of compliance is sometimes called elastance). Reduced ventricular compliance results in a steeper EDPVR.

Figure 10
We see in Figure 10 that if the EDPVR is abnormally steep (i.e. reduced compliance) but filling pressure remains normal, end-diastolic volume and, therefore, stroke volume are reduced. In order to maintain a normal stroke volume when ventricular compliance is abnormally low, the filling pressure must be abnormally high.

Changes in ventricular compliance are not important in regulating stroke volume under normal circumstances. However, various pathological conditions cause decreased ventricular compliance and can lead to congestive heart failure. This kind of heart failure is said to be caused by diastolic dysfunction.

Examples of pathological conditions that lead to reduced ventricular compliance are:
- Ventricular hypertrophy (a thicker ventricular wall is stiffer; *i.e.*, its distensibility is reduced).
- Myocardial ischemia (the myocardium does not fully relax during diastole because of inadequate pumping of Ca^{++} back into the sarcoplasmic reticulum).
- Pericardial diseases (cardiac tamponade and constrictive pericarditis).

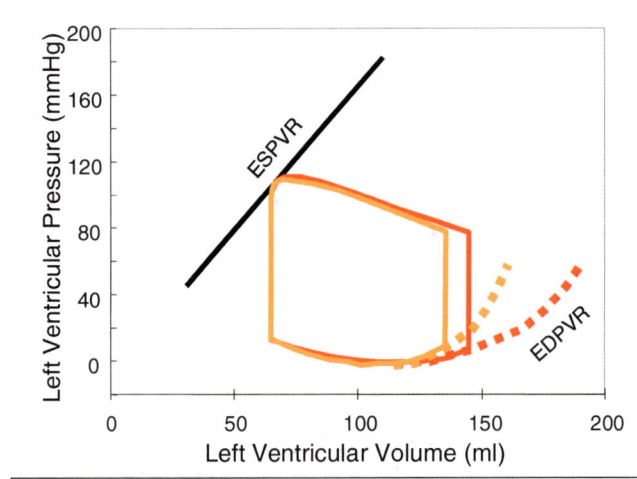

Figure 10. Decreased left ventricular compliance results in reduced end-diastolic volume and, therefore, decreased stroke volume.

Part 3: Effect of Contractility on Stroke Volume

Topic 1: Left Ventricular Pressure-Volume Loop

Figure 11

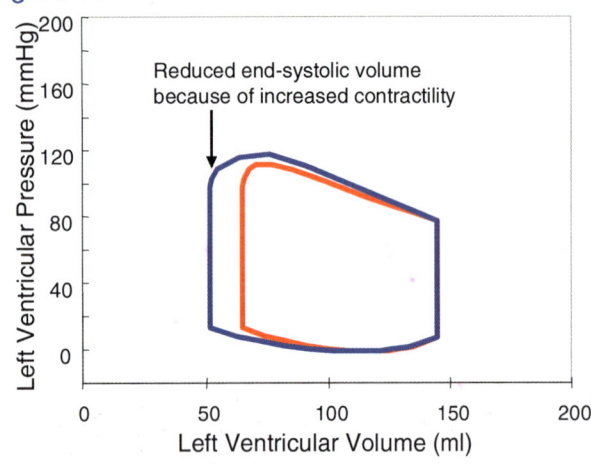

Figure 11. Effect of increased contractility on a left ventricular PV loop.

Since increased contractility causes increased rate of ejection, more ejection occurs prior to relaxation and stroke volume increases. The end-systolic volume becomes less than it was before the increase in contractility.

Figure 12
Figure 12 shows that increased contractility makes the ESPVR steeper.

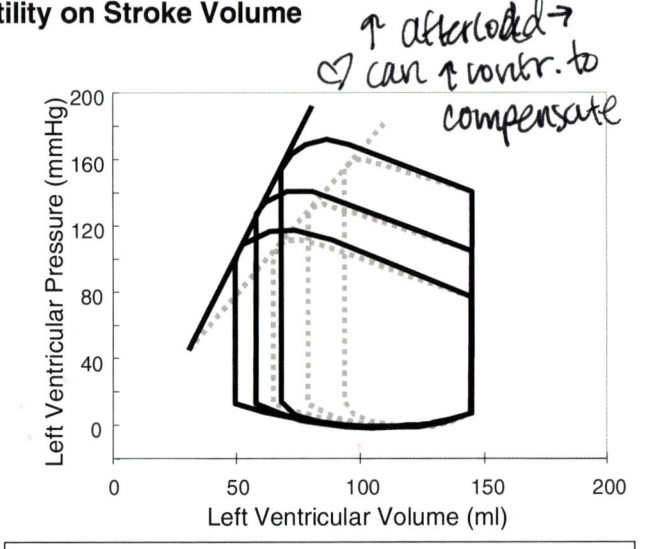

Figure 12. Effect of increased contractility on the ESPVR. Control PV loops at various afterloads are dotted gray. Solid black loops and ESPVR show the effect of increased contractility.

Increased contractility tends to cope with increases in afterload. On the other hand, if contractility is decreased for any reason, it becomes more difficult to cope with increases in afterload.

The slope of the ESPVR is called the end-systolic elastance and is an excellent index of contractility.

Topic 2: The Concept of Inotropic Cardiac Reserve

The degree to which contractility can be increased by extrinsic positive inotropic agents is called the

Regulation of Stroke Volume

inotropic cardiac reserve. It is often assessed by measuring stroke volume, stroke work, ejection fraction, *etc.* before and after administration of a positive inotropic drug. Inotropic reserve is often reduced in patients with heart failure, especially when associated with reduced contractility.

> **Topic 3: Pathological Conditions Often Associated with Decreased Ventricular Contractility**

This topic is outside the scope of this book; however, the following list might help to point you toward further study.

- Cardiomyopathies (primary diseases of cardiac muscle)
  - Idiopathic (*i.e.* cause not known)
  - Inflammatory
  - Metabolic
  - Infiltrative
  - Genetic
- Myocardial ischemia
- Myocardial infarction
- Myocarditis
- Cardiotoxic effects of drugs

[handwritten: dec vent contractility → systolic / diastolic dysfx]

Part 4: Automatic Compensations for Changes in Afterload

Now we will quit allowing only one variable to change at a time. We will examine how preload and contractility automatically respond to changes in afterload, and then explain how these responses result in a pump which can cope with a wide range of afterloads.

> **Topic 1: The Starling Effect**

Figure 13

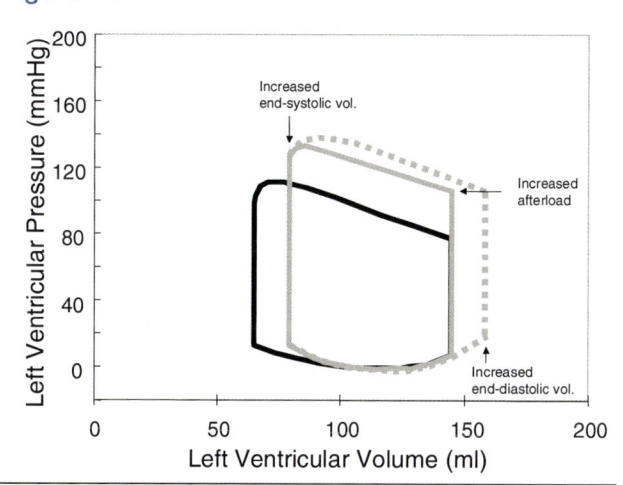

Figure 13. Within a few beats following an increase in afterload, the Starling effect returns stroke volume to normal.

Figure 13 shows the immediate effect of suddenly increasing the afterload (solid gray loop). Stroke volume is reduced. The next filling period, therefore, starts from an increased end-systolic volume and, since the usual amount of blood returns to the ventricle, end-diastolic volume increases (dotted gray loop). Because of the Starling effect, the next ejection is augmented and stroke volume

[handwritten left margin: b/c ↑ ESV]

returns to normal. [To be accurate, it should be noted that 2 or 3 beats following a change in afterload might be required before the original stroke volume is restored.]

> **Topic 2: The Anrep Effect**

Figure 14

During the subsequent 1-2 minutes following a change in afterload, a gradual change in ventricular contractility automatically occurs in a direction that compensates for the change in afterload. If afterload is increased, contractility gradually increases. Consequently, the end-systolic pressure-volume point and end-systolic volume gradually shift to the left. If several PV loops were shown, corresponding to various increases in afterload, you would see that the ESPVR becomes steeper; *i.e.* the end-systolic elastance increases.

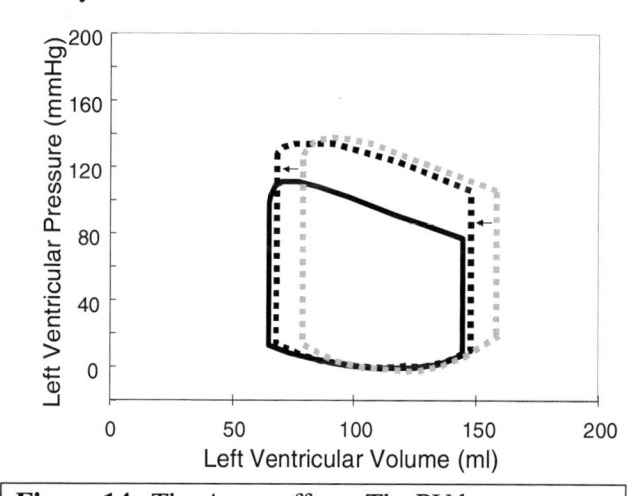

Figure 14. The Anrep effect. The PV loop gradually shifts to the left as contractility increases following increased afterload.

[handwritten bottom: Starling: ↑EDV → ↑CO (SV·HR=CO)]

As increased contractility causes a left shift in end-systolic volume, end-diastolic volume also shifts left (since the amount of diastolic filling remains unchanged). Finally, after a minute or two, end-systolic and end-diastolic volumes both return nearly to their original positions. Normal stroke volume is maintained in the face of increased afterload, without an appreciable increase in preload (*i.e.* without a prolonged Starling effect). The increased preload and Starling effect are gradually replaced by increased contractility. This phenomenon is called the Anrep effect or homeometric autoregulation.

The Anrep effect is probably caused by the gradual increase in Ca^{++} release from the sarcoplasmic reticulum following an increase in sarcomere length (see Chapter 4).

Topic 3: Left Ventricular Afterload Performance Curves

You were reminded in Part 2 of this chapter that one of the important characteristics of any pump is how its output responds to changes in the inflow pressure. Another important characteristic of any pump is how its output responds to changes in the outflow pressure.

Figure 15
This figure shows the effect of changing mean arterial pressure (MAP) on the output of the entire heart. In this experiment, inflow pressure (CVP, or MRAP) and heart rate are not allowed to change, and there is no change in extrinsic influences such as sympathetic and parasympathetic nerve activity. Therefore, this experiment shows how the pump can automatically cope with changes in afterload by changing its stroke volume.

The striking result is that the pump can automatically cope with changes in afterload exceedingly well. Only when MAP is elevated to over 200 mmHg, well beyond its normal range, is CO severely compromised. This is an important characteristic of the heart. It is able to increase its work output automatically to meet demands over the entire range of MAP normally encountered. This response is mediated at first by the Starling effect and then, more gradually, by the Anrep effect.

When the heart is made hypereffective (*e.g.* by sympathetic stimulation during exercise) it is able to cope with even higher afterloads. On the other hand, a heart that is hypoeffective because of reduced heart rate or contractility tends to fail at moderately elevated afterloads.

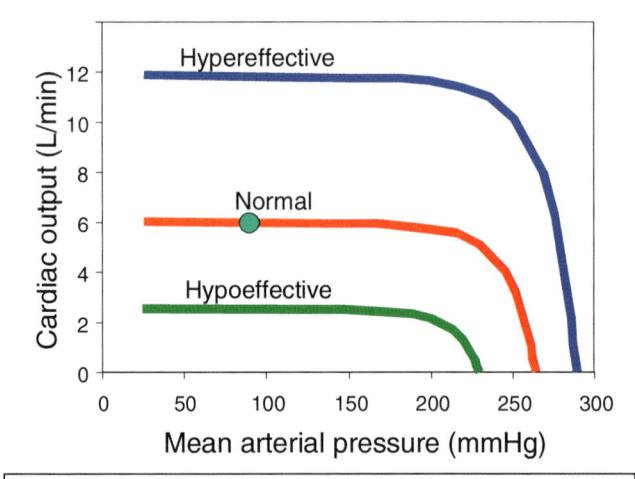

Figure 15. Afterload performance curves for the heart.

It should be pointed out that the marvelous ability of the heart to cope with a large increase in afterload, as illustrated in Figure 15, doesn't last forever. Chronically elevated afterload as in severe arterial hypertension or aortic stenosis, can eventually lead to cardiac deterioration and heart failure. Responses of the heart to chronic overload are discussed in Chapter 10.

Part 5: Effects of Exercise on Stroke Volume

Topic 1: Background

Figure 16
The increase in cardiac output during exercise is mediated partly by increased heart rate and partly by increased stroke volume. Heart rate increases directly with aerobic exercise intensity all the way to the highest intensities achievable. On the other hand, stroke volume is a linear function of aerobic exercise intensity only at low intensities. Beyond about 40-50% of maximum oxygen consumption, further increases in stroke volume make a relatively minor contribution to increased CO. In well-trained endurance athletes, exercising at 40% or more of maximum oxygen consumption, stroke volume can be increased by as much as 60% of its value at rest. Therefore, if an average size male distance runner

has a stroke volume at rest of 80 ml, his stroke volume during intense exercise might increase to about 130 ml. People who are only moderately active can increase their stroke volumes less. For example, in the group of subjects reported in Figure 16, intense exercise resulted in a 40% increase in stroke volume.

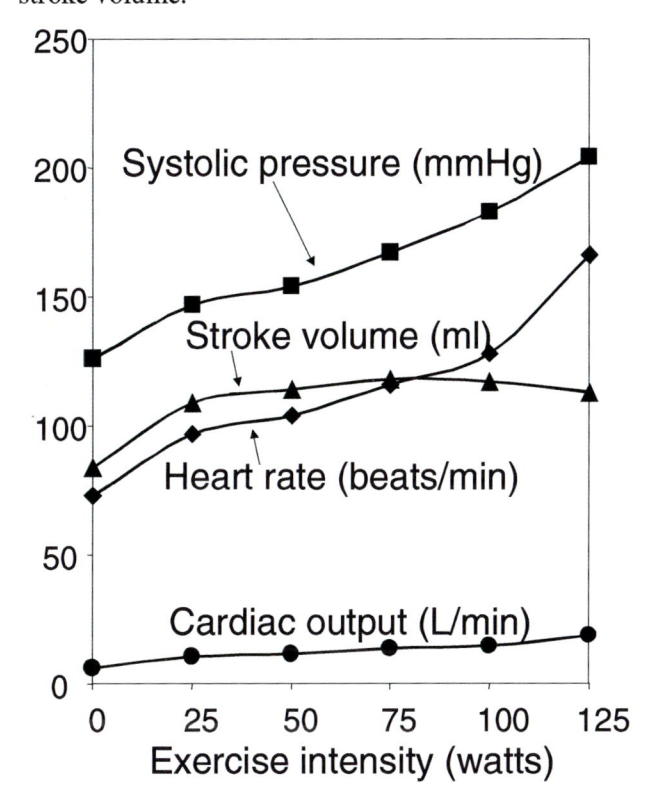

Figure 16. Effects of graded exercise on cardiovascular measurements. The subjects were moderately active males exercising on a stationary bicycle. The data are from G.D. Plotnik, et al., Am. J. Physiol. 251, H1101-H1105, 1986.

Topic 2: The Controversy

There was a prolonged debate about how stroke volume is increased during exercise: does it result from the Starling response to increased preload, or is it caused by increased contractility? In the first case, end-diastolic volume would be increased without a change in end-systolic volume. In the second case, end-systolic volume would be decreased without a change in end-diastolic volume. Some data seemed to support the Starling theory while other data supported the contractility theory. It turns out, of course, that both mechanisms are utilized. Which of the two mechanisms is most important depends upon the intensity of exercise and the posture during exercise (upright or horizontal).

Topic 3: Relative Roles of Preload and Contractility during Exercise

Figure 17

This figure shows values for end-systolic and end-diastolic volumes from the same study reported in the previous figure. The increased stroke volume at lowest exercise intensity resulted almost entirely from increased end-diastolic volume (Starling mechanism). As exercise intensity increased, end-systolic volume gradually decreased indicating a progressively important contribution of contractility to stroke volume. At highest intensity, end-systolic and end-diastolic volumes both decreased, implying that contractility increased so much that it was responsible for most of the increase in stroke volume, and a large Starling response was no longer needed.

↑contractility ↑ SV by ↓ ESV

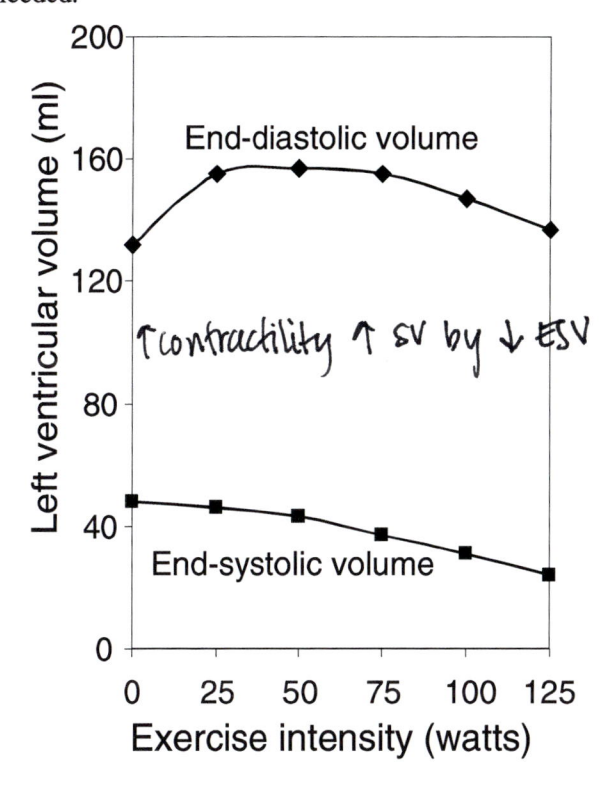

Figure 17. Effects of graded exercise on left ventricular end-diastolic and end-systolic volumes. Stroke volume is the difference between these two curves. Volumes were measured using a radionuclide angiography technique. The data are from G.D. Plotnik, et al., Am. J. Physiol. 251, H1101-H1105, 1986.

The end-diastolic and end-systolic volumes shown in Figure 17 under resting conditions are somewhat lower than shown in previous figures; this is because these studies were done on people in an approximately upright posture (stationary bicycle), and the values reflect the effect of gravity on distribution of blood. Exercise in the horizontal posture involves less Starling response than in the upright posture since the end-diastolic volume is already increased, even at rest.

See Figure 16 again.
Note the gradual rise in systolic arterial pressure, implying a gradual rise in afterload to the left ventricle. Increased afterload tends to reduce stroke volume. The positive effects of increased preload and increased contractility must overcome this negative effect of increased afterload.

Part 6: The Curious Effect of High Heart Rates on Stroke Volume and Cardiac Output

Consider a person who is not exercising. If heart rate increases moderately, blood is pumped a little faster out of the central veins and, consequently, CVP decreases a little. This causes a small decrease in stroke volume. However, the small decrease in stroke volume is not enough to prevent an increase in cardiac output. That's simple; a rise in heart rate leads to a rise in cardiac output.

A curious thing happens, however, if the heart rate of this resting person increases markedly – say to 120 or more. Now, stroke volume decreases so much that in spite of the increase in heart rate, cardiac output actually goes down. A good example of this effect is with the sudden onset of a supraventricular tachycardia in which heart rate jumps way up, often to 180 per minute or more. Cardiac output can go down enough to cause mild symptoms of heart failure. This paradoxical decrease in cardiac output is explained by the fact that at high heart rates there is so much less time available for diastolic filling of the ventricles that the filling curve is infringed upon all the way into its steep portion (see the filling curve for the left ventricle on the back cover). During exercise, this effect may not be obvious because of increased preload during mild exercise and increased contractility during intense exercise.

Chapter 8

Regulation of Cardiac Output

Here we examine the basic hydraulic relationships that control cardiac output. These relationships are complicated by the fact that we are dealing with a *circulatory* system. What goes around comes around. Cardiac output determines venous return and venous return determines cardiac output.

Part 1 describes the use of Guyton diagrams for summarizing how cardiac output is determined by the primary, independently adjustable parameters of the cardiovascular system.

Part 2 uses a Guyton diagram to summarize the factors that increase cardiac output during exercise.

Part 3 discusses the effects of changing from a horizontal to a vertical posture on the cardiovascular system. Guyton diagrams are used to summarize the responses.

Part 4 advertises a simulation for global control of the cardiovascular system.

Part 1: Introduction to Guyton Diagrams

Topic 1: The Primary Adjustable Parameters of the Cardiovascular System

The independently adjustable variables of the cardiovascular system operate together to regulate cardiac output, mean arterial pressure, and central venous pressure. They are:

- Heart rate
- Cardiac contractility
- Total peripheral resistance
- Venous capacity
- Total blood volume

In this chapter, we discuss the mechanisms by which alterations in the primary adjustable parameters control cardiac output. Control of mean arterial pressure and central venous pressure are discussed in later chapters.

In addition to the above adjustable parameters, changes in arterial compliance are important in aging, but probably not important with respect to shorter-term control.

Please restudy Chapter 1, Part 3 now (starting on p. 5) for an overview of cardiac output control. Understand how shifts of blood volume between systemic arteries and veins determine arterial and venous pressures and, therefore, afterload and preload.

Probably the best approach to understanding the control of cardiac output is with the use of Guyton diagrams, and this is the approach taken in this chapter. The Guyton diagram is a graphical method for analyzing and visualizing the effects of changing each of the primary adjustable parameters on cardiac output. The method was developed by Arthur C. Guyton *et al.*

Topic 2: Effect of Cardiac Effectiveness on the Operating Point of a Cardiac Function Curve

Cardiac Function Curves

Starling curves for the entire heart and lungs are called cardiac function curves. They show how changes in inflow pressure influence cardiac output. Everything else is held constant. Cardiac function curves were discussed in Chapter 7.

Figure 1

A set of cardiac function curves is shown in Figure 1. Each curve corresponds to a different cardiac effectiveness. Changes in cardiac effectiveness are accomplished by changes in heart rate and/or contractility. In this discussion, we will not distinguish between changes in cardiac effectiveness due to these two causes.

The Operating Point

The circles in Figure 1 represent the operating points; *i.e.*, the steady-state combination of cardiac output (CO) and central venous pressure (CVP) for any given cardiac effectiveness. These points can be determined experimentally in animals. Note that as cardiac effectiveness increases CO also increases and this causes a decrease in CVP. The operating point moves up and to the left. The fall in CVP results from a shift in blood volume from central veins to arteries. As cardiac effectiveness decreases, blood is pumped slower from central veins to arteries and CVP goes up as CO goes down.

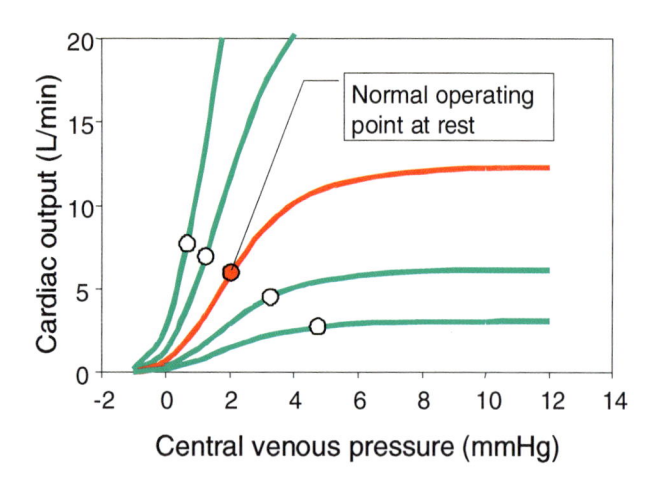

Figure 1. This is a set of cardiac function curves corresponding to different degrees of cardiac effectiveness. The operating point moves down and to the right as cardiac effectiveness decreases.

The Venous Return Curve
Figure 2

Now we connect the operating points with a line. This line is often called the venous return curve. It shows the effect of CO on CVP. Figure 2 is an example of a Guyton diagram.

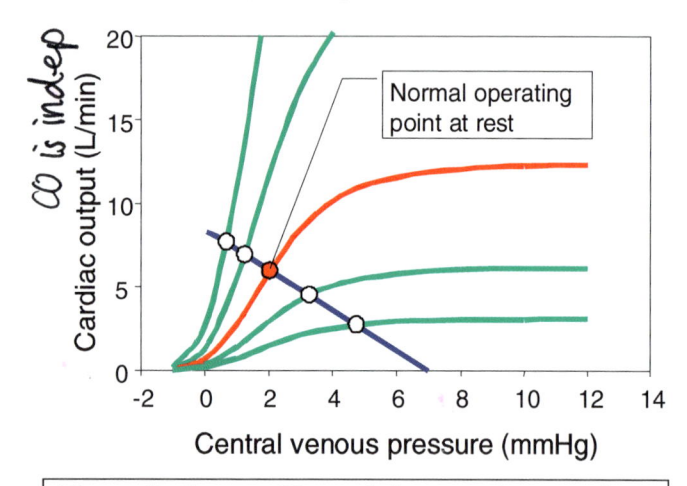

Figure 2. Same as Figure 1, but now the operating points are connected by a line called the venous return curve.

The Two Simultaneous Functions of a Guyton Diagram

Guyton diagrams depict two simultaneous functions: the effect of CVP on CO and the effect of CO on CVP. For the latter function, the independent variable, CO, is plotted on the ordinate. The system must always operate where these two functions intersect. This is a common method in engineering for predicting the operating point for two interacting variables. It's the graphical equivalent of solving two simultaneous equations.

General Static Pressure

If the heart is suddenly stopped, blood passively distributes throughout the entire system until the pressure is equal everywhere. This equilibrium pressure is given by the point where the venous return curve intercepts the CVP axis. This point has several names including mean circulatory filling pressure and general static pressure. The general static pressure is a measure of how tightly the whole system is filled with blood at zero flow. It can be measured in experiments on anesthetized animals. General static pressure is normally about 7 mmHg as seen in Figure 1.

Maximum cardiac output
Figure 3

Now we extrapolate the venous return curve to the left. Note the plateau. This plateau indicates that when cardiac effectiveness in increased enough to cause CVP to fall below about zero mmHg, further increases in cardiac effectiveness result in no further increase in CO. This phenomenon is caused by collapse of extrathoracic veins. As the transmural pressure in extrathoracic veins drops below zero, blood is sucked out and their oval cross-section becomes flatter. When extrathoracic veins partially collapse, their resistance to flow increases and limits the rate of venous return.

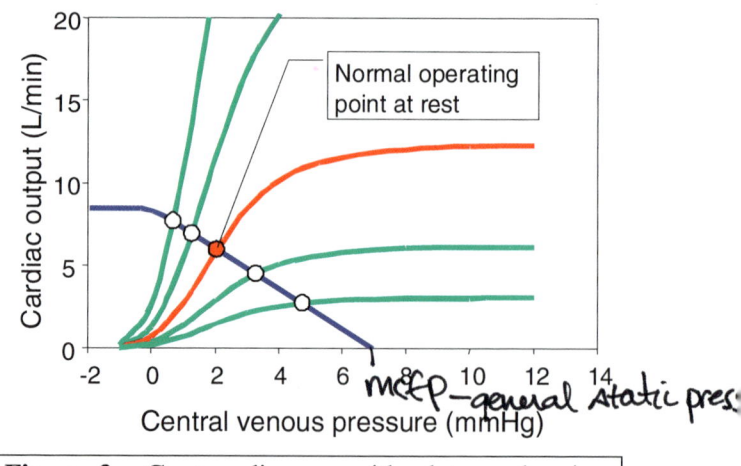

Figure 3. Guyton diagram with plateau showing the upper limit to which CO can be increased simply by increasing cardiac effectiveness.

Consequently, if the heart is already pumping hard enough that CVP is below zero mmHg, further increases in cardiac effectiveness cannot increase CO. The pressure within intrathoracic veins can drop a little below atmospheric before they begin to collapse, since negative intrathoracic pressure holds them open.

Topic 3: Effect of Total Peripheral Resistance on the Operating Point

Figure 4 (compare to Figure 3)

A decrease in total peripheral resistance (TPR) results in a shift of blood from arteries to veins. This volume shift causes venous pressures, including CVP, to rise. Thus, the operating point at any given cardiac effectiveness rises higher on the cardiac function curve as shown in the figure, and the venous return curve rotates clockwise. The plateau due to venous collapse also rises. An increase in TPR has the opposite effects.

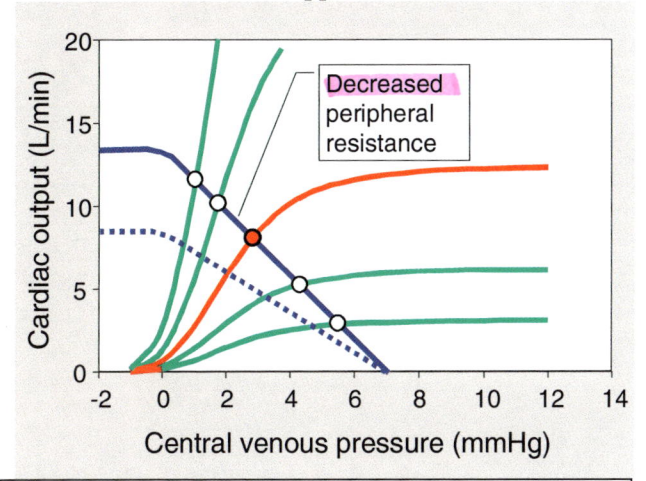

Figure 4. Effect of decreased TPR on the operating point. The venous return curve is rotated clockwise. In this example, TPR has been reduced to about 50% of its original value. Dotted line is control venous return curve.

Topic 4: Effect of Total Blood Volume on the Operating Point

Figure 5 (compare to Figure 3)

Increased total blood volume (TBV) increases pressures everywhere in the system, including CVP. Thus, the operating points move higher on all the cardiac function curves. The venous return curve moves higher. The venous return curve also shifts to the right, something it did not do when TPR was reduced. The shift to the right is caused by the fact that increased blood volume causes the general static pressure to rise (i.e. the whole system is more tightly filled with blood). Increased TBV also elevates the venous collapse plateau. A decrease in TBV, of course, has the opposite effects.

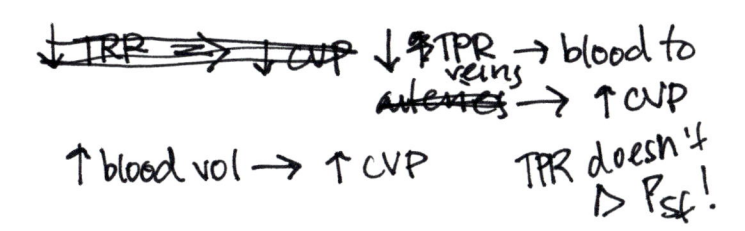

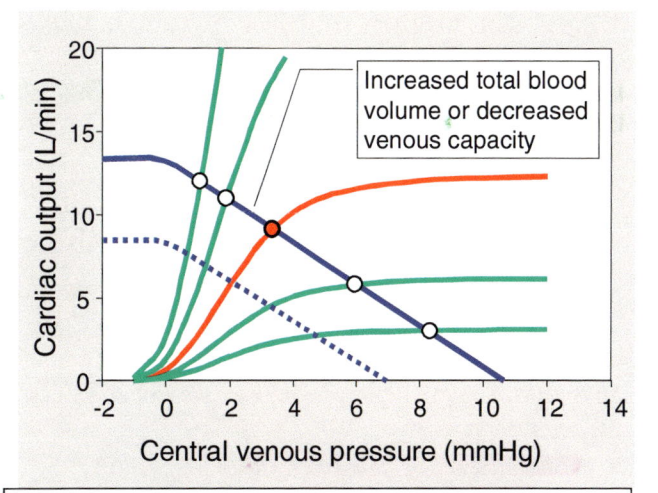

Figure 5. Effect of an increase in total blood volume or a decrease in venous capacity on the operating point. The venous return curve is shifted up and to the right.

Topic 5: Effect of Venous Capacity on the Operating Point

See Figure 5 again (compare to Figure 3)

Decreased venous capacity causes CVP to increase. Consequently, the operating points shift up along the cardiac function curves. The general static pressure also increases when venous capacity decreases (the system is filled more tightly with blood). The shift in the venous return curve is the same as that for an increase in TBV. The opposite shift occurs with increased venous compliance.

Topic 6: So What?

Guyton diagrams provide visual summaries of the changes in CO and preload induced by alterations of the primary adjustable parameters. You could probably figure out these changes without the Guyton diagrams, but they can be very helpful. [Note: Guyton diagrams are discussed (often extensively) in most major textbooks of physiology. Guyton diagrams are not usually mentioned in internal medicine or cardiology textbooks and you may never hear of them again, except perhaps in USMLE Part 1.]

Importance of systemic factors in the determination of cardiac output

Guyton diagrams are especially useful for illustrating the fact that the heart cannot increase cardiac output very much without the cooperation of the systemic adjustable features of the system. Notice in Figure 3 that increases in cardiac effectiveness can only increase CO to about 8 or 9

L/min. No matter how hard the heart tries, it cannot pump blood faster than the rate of venous return. Decreased TPR, decreased venous capacity, and increased TBV all result in operating points that lie higher up on the cardiac function curves. These alterations also raise the venous collapse plateau. Consequently, the systemic adjustments allow a hypereffective heart to go ahead and do its thing – pump blood.

The next two parts of this chapter utilize Guyton diagrams to summarize the factors that change CO during exercise and following a change in posture.

Part 2: Increased Cardiac Output during Exercise

Three primary cardiovascular changes occur during exercise. These are:
- Increased cardiac effectiveness, caused by:
  o increased sympathetic activity to the heart.
  o decreased parasympathetic activity.
  o increased circulating catecholamines.
- Decreased total peripheral resistance, caused by:
  o the local vasodilatory action of humoral agents released from active muscle fibers.
  o the local vasodilatory action of nitric oxide released from endothelial cells and perhaps from hemoglobin.
  o other local vasodilatory responses to exercise as discussed in Chapter 16.
- Decreased venous capacity, caused by:
  o venoconstriction (the result of increased sympathetic activity to veins). [It probably should be noted that the importance of this effect has been questioned: *J. Appl. Physiol.* 101: 1264-1265, 2006.]
  o venocompression (the result of skeletal muscle contractions).

Figure 6
All these changes contribute to the increase in cardiac output. The appropriate Guyton diagram is shown in Figure 6.
- Increased cardiac effectiveness is indicated by a shift in the cardiac function curve upward and to the left.
- Decreased TPR is indicated by a clockwise rotation of the venous return curve.
- Decreased venous capacity is indicated by a shift in the venous return curve upward and to the right.

The cardiac function curve and the venous return curve intersect at an operating point that is typical for strenuous exercise. CO is a little over four times greater than it is at rest. In endurance athletes, CO can go as much as six times above its value at rest. CVP is only slightly elevated; therefore, you can conclude that the intensity of exercise is such that the Starling effect does not account for much of the increase in stroke volume.

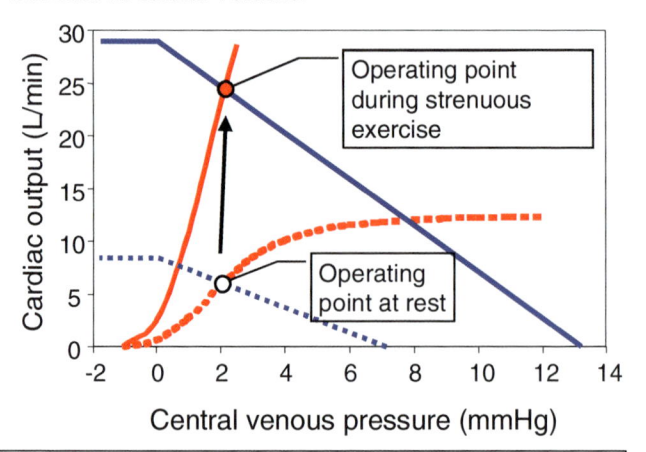

Figure 6. Effect of exercise on the operating point.

Figure 6 should make it quite clear that the real effectiveness of a sympathetically stimulated heart can be brought into play if, and only if, the changes in peripheral resistance and venous capacity occur.

Regulation of Cardiac Output

Part 3: Effect of Postural Changes on Cardiac Output

Topic 1: Blood Redistributes upon Changing from a Horizontal to a Vertical Posture

When a person is reclining in a horizontal position, we can usually ignore effects of gravity, but when a person stands upright, the influence of gravity becomes important.

If a completely relaxed person is suddenly tilted from a horizontal to an upright posture, blood shifts toward the feet. Arterial and venous pressures in the upper body decrease, while they increase in the lower body. This effect develops over a period of seconds as blood flows into veins of the lower body from the microcirculation faster than it flows up toward the heart. Blood does not actually shift directly from upper veins to lower veins because of the venous valves. A new steady state is reached in roughly 30 seconds.

The translocation of blood from the upper parts of the body to the legs is often called "venous pooling." This blood is still circulating, but with respect to CO, it is as though this blood were temporarily out of circulation. In the absence of compensatory adjustments, roughly 500 ml of blood are pooled in the legs upon standing. Far more than this would be pooled if veins were as distensible at high pressures as they are at low pressures. Fortunately, venous pooling is limited by the veins becoming almost completely nondistensible in the high-pressure range.

Topic 2: The Hydrostatic Indifference Point

There is a point located a few centimeters below the diaphragm at which the venous pressure is the same in the vertical posture as it is in the horizontal posture. This point is sometimes called the hydrostatic indifference point.

In the upright posture, the venous and arterial systems have the hydrostatic properties of long vertical columns of blood. Pressure increases with depth below and decreases with height above the hydrostatic indifference point. These changes in hydrostatic pressure are proportional to distance from the hydrostatic indifference point. Thus, pressure in the foot vessels of a 5'9" person is raised by about 120 cm of blood, which is about 90 mmHg. This hydrostatic effect is added to the usual hydraulic pressures in the arteries and veins of the feet, so the total pressures become about 180 mmHg and 105 mmHg respectively. This, in itself, does nothing to impede blood flow through the feet or legs since the arterial and venous pressures are both increased equally.

Topic 3: Upon Standing, Preload and Cardiac Output Decrease

Figure 7
Nevertheless, taking an upright posture has a serious effect on the cardiovascular system. Since the hydrostatic indifference point is below the heart, when a person stands the right atrial pressure decreases and, consequently, cardiac output decreases.

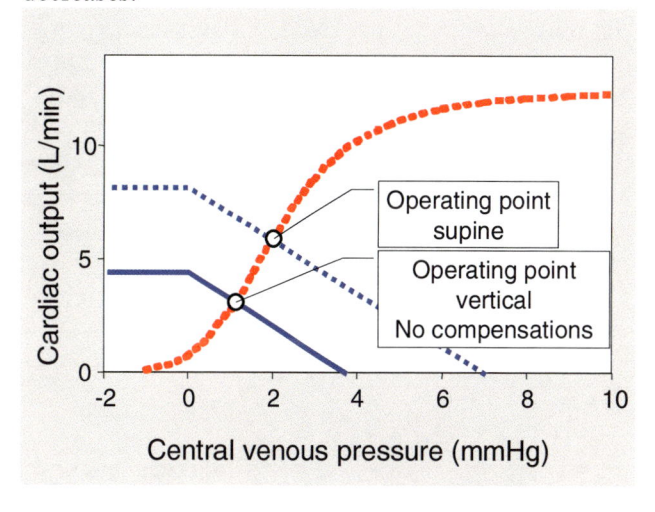

Figure 7. Effect of changing from a reclining to an upright posture – no compensatory mechanisms.

Unless compensatory mechanisms promptly come into play, CO decreases by roughly 2 L/min, and the subject faints. The Guyton diagram in Figure 5 will be helpful for visualizing this effect; it shows a normal operating point for a supine subject. Upon standing, the venous return curve shifts to the left, thus lowering CO and right atrial pressure. The change in the venous return curve is qualitatively similar to the change that would result from a reduction of blood volume.

Topic 4: Elevated Capillary and Venular Pressures in the Feet and Legs during Standing Tend to Promote Edema

In addition to problems resulting from reduced CO upon standing, elevated pressures in the microcirculation of the feet and lower legs cause increased filtration of fluid across the endothelium of capillaries and venules into the interstitial spaces. If this situation prevails for any length of time, edema of the feet and lower legs can occur.

Topic 5: Compensatory Mechanisms – Skeletal Muscle Contraction

Figure 8 (compare to Figure 7)
Of course, we do not faint every time we stand. There are compensatory mechanisms. One of these is tensing of leg and abdominal muscles; this ordinarily occurs along with standing and causes venous compression in the legs and abdomen. Consequently, venous capacity and venous pooling in these regions are reduced, and the venous return curve moves to the right. Right atrial pressure is elevated.

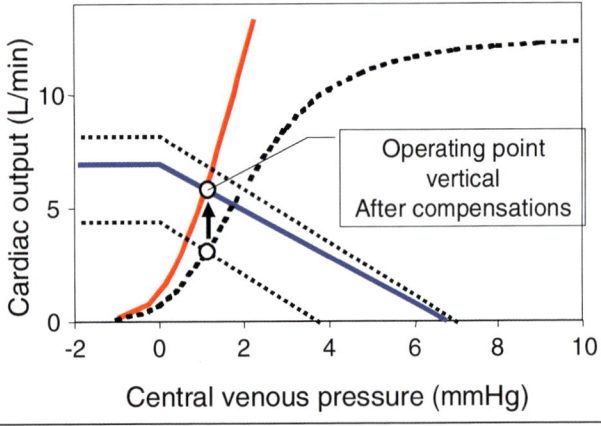

Figure 8. Compensatory mechanisms in response to standing lead to elevation of the operating point. The venous return curve shifts to the right because of venous constriction and venous compression. The venous return curve also rotates slightly counterclockwise because of increased TPR. The cardiac function curve is elevated because of increased cardiac effectiveness (increased heart rate and contractility).

In addition to tensing of skeletal muscles, phasic contraction-relaxation cycles, as in walking, pump blood toward the heart. This process reduces average intramuscular venous and capillary pressures and helps to prevent edema.

Topic 6: Compensatory Mechanisms – Arterial Baroreceptor Reflexes

See Figure 8 again (compare to Figure 7)
Certain autonomic reflexes also assist in adjusting the cardiovascular system to changes in posture — in particular, the arterial baroreceptor reflexes. These reflexes will be described in Chapter 15. All we need to point out here is that if CVP, MAP, and arterial pulse pressure are reduced during standing, a generalized increase in sympathetic nervous activity occurs. This increase in sympathetic activity is caused by baroreceptor reflexes and results in:

- Increased cardiac effectiveness
- Decreased venous capacity
- Increased TPR

The first two of these effects increase CO. The third effect reduces CO slightly, but increases MAP. The effect on MAP is important since it helps to keep the brain and heart perfused adequately with blood.

Some of the receptors involved in the baroreceptor reflexes are located in the carotid sinuses. The carotid sinuses are roughly 40 cm above the hydrostatic indifference point; so upon standing, MAP in the carotid sinuses drops from about 95 mmHg to about 65 mmHg. This decrease would reflexly induce increased sympathetic activity even if CO did not go down. The carotid sinus reflex helps maintain CO and MAP during periods of quiet standing and sitting at values not much below those that exist while reclining.

Topic 7: Effects on Cerebral Circulation

When an upright posture is taken, pressures in the cerebral blood vessels fall by roughly 40 mmHg. This drop has no effect on blood flow through the brain since arterial and venous pressures are affected equally. Flow continues to be driven by the difference between inflow and outflow pressures, as it would be through any other siphon.

Note that a 40 mmHg drop in pressure results in cerebral venous pressures that are considerably subatmospheric. The cerebral veins do not collapse since they are held open by surrounding tissues and ultimately by the rigid cranium. The superficial veins in the neck collapse during standing since there is nothing to hold them open, and venous return from the head occurs mainly through deeper cervical veins.

If MAP decreases very much cerebral perfusion may become inadequate and the individual may feel faint. Fainting can often be avoided by taking lying down. This maneuver is effective not because it makes it easier for blood to flow through the brain, but by raising right atrial pressure and, consequently, CO. The most effective position should be the one at which right atrial pressure is maximal, and this occurs at a slightly head down position.

Part 4: A Simulation of Cardiovascular Control

Simulation: Global Control [electronic edition]
You are the wisdom of the body. Figure out what the body would do to cope with various situations. You can use this simulation to construct Guyton diagrams before and after making your wise adjustments. For example:
- Decrease blood volume to simulate hypovolemia.
- Decrease cardiac effectiveness as in heart failure.
- Decrease total peripheral resistance as in exercise.
- Increase arterial capacity as in aging (Chapter 18).

In each case, what compensations will you perform?

You can also simulate a generalized increase in sympathetic activity (fight or flight response). You can simulate the effects of vasodilator drugs, *etc.*

Chapter 9

Myocardial Energetics

This chapter treats myocardial energy transfer and oxygen consumption.
Part 1 describes ATP supply
Part 2 discusses ATP use
Part 3 discusses myocardial hypoxia

Part 1: ATP Supply

Topic 1: Introduction

Figure 1
ATP mediates transfer of energy from chemistry to mechanics. Nearly all of it is generated in mitochondria by oxidative phosphorylation. Cardiac myocytes are loaded with mitochondria, which are lined up longitudinally directly alongside the myofibrils as shown in Figure 1.

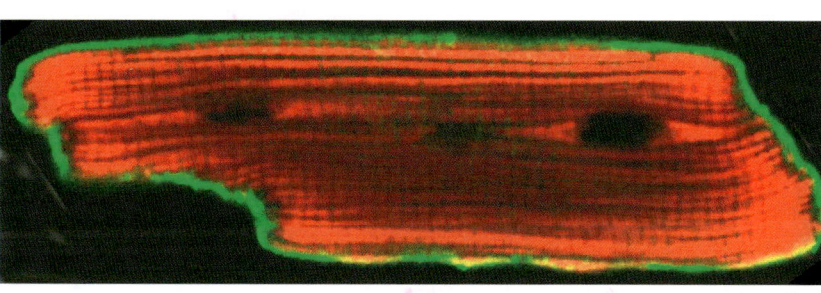

Figure 1. Rat ventricular myocyte from an enzymatically dispersed cell preparation. This is a confocal fluorescence image obtained after staining the mitochondria with MitoTracker Red (Molecular Probes) and the glycocalyx with Alexa488-Wheat Germ Agglutinin (Molecular Probes). Rows of mitochondria (red) are longitudinally arranged in line with myofibrils. Each mitochondrion is the same length as a sarcomere. Three nuclei are evident. The cardiomyocyte is the same one shown in Figure 1 of Chapter 2. Courtesy of Dr. Phillip Palade (myocyte preparation) and Dr. Leoncio Vergara (imaging), Dept. of Physiology and Biophysics, UTMB, Galveston, TX.

Figure 2
The mitochondria generate ATP at just the rate necessary to support crossbridge cycling, Na$^+$-K$^+$ pumping, Ca^{++} pumping, plus synthesis of new protein. In the short term (msec), the concentration of ATP is buffered by a comparatively large store of creatine phosphate that can supply ATP in times of need, and be replenished from ATP in times of plenty.

Topic 2: Substrates

Figure 3
The principle substrates used by the heart for energy metabolism are fatty acids, glucose, and lactate. Relative use of these substrates depends mainly on their availability in blood. At rest, most substrate supply comes from fatty acids and almost none from lactate (since there is very little lactate in blood at rest). During some types of exercise, lactate increases in blood and is prominently used by the heart. Glucose use is also increased during exercise because of increased release of glucose from the liver, and because of a circulating factor that increases glucose transport into myocardial cells. During the final stages of endurance exercise (the wall), use of fatty acids increases greatly due to depletion of the glucose supply.

Topic 3: Overview of the ATP Factory

Figure 4
Here we open the black box of Figure 2 and find several more black boxes. These black boxes hide much detail that is ordinarily covered in biochemistry courses, but will not be described here. Figure 4 is very complex, even without opening its black boxes.

The outer mitochondrial membrane is studded with large channels that make it quite permeable to small molecules at least up to the size of ATP. The inner mitochondrial membrane, however, does not have such channels. Anything that crosses the inner mitochondrial membrane requires specific membrane transport proteins or vectorial shuttles.

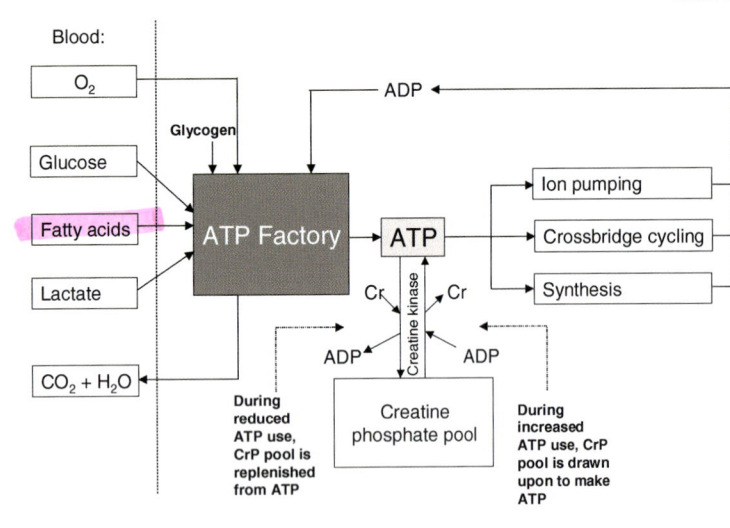

Figure 2. Zoomed out view of ATP generation and use.

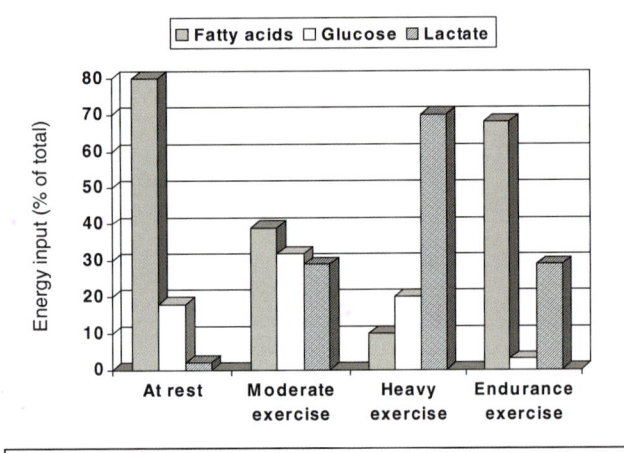

Figure 3. Relative substrate use in different conditions.

Trace the following sequences using Figure 4:

Fatty Acids in Extracellular Space → Acetyl-CoA in Mitochondrial matrix

Fatty acids (upper left of figure) diffuse across the plasma membrane and are converted to acyl-CoA by acyl-CoA synthetase in the cytoplasm and on the surface of the outer mitochondrial membrane. This step utilizes one ATP. Acyl-CoA readily diffuses across the outer mitochondrial membrane. It is then transported across the inner mitochondrial membrane by the carnotine shuttle.

Within the mitochondrial matrix, acyl-CoA enters the pathway for β-oxidation of fatty acids. The output from this black box (for each 16 carbon palmitate) is 8 acetyl-CoA, 7 NADH, and 7 FADH$_2$. The cost has been two high-energy phosphate bonds at the acyl-CoA synthetase step. The acetyl-CoA, NADH, and FADH$_2$ molecules will generate many ATP molecules during subsequent steps (Krebs cycle and oxidative phosphorylation).

Lactate in Extracellular Space → Acetyl-CoA in Mitochondrial Matrix

Circulating lactate from exercising skeletal muscle enters cardiac myocytes by means of a lactate-H$^+$ cotransporter (symporter) in the plasma membrane. In the cytoplasm, lactate is converted to pyruvate by the action of lactate dehydrogenase, with generation of one NADH. Pyruvate passively diffuses across the outer mitochondrial membrane. It is then transported across the inner mitochondrial membrane by a pyruvate-H$^+$ cotransporter.

Within the mitochondrial matrix, pyruvate enters the pyruvate dehydrogenase complex, which is associated with the inner mitochondrial membrane. The output from this black box (for each pyruvate molecule) is 1 acetyl-CoA, 1 NADH, and 1 CO$_2$.

Glucose in Extracellular Space → Acetyl-CoA in Mitochondrial Matrix

Circulating glucose enters cardiac myocytes by Glut 4 transporters in the plasma membrane. In the cytoplasm, glucose is phosphorylated to glucose-6-phosphate by the action of hexokinase. Glucose-6-phosphate enters the glycolytic pathway. Net output from glycolysis (including the hexokinase step) is 2 pyruvate, 2 NADH, and 2 ATP.

Both pyruvate molecules enter the mitochondrial matrix and then the pyruvate dehydrogenase complex. Output from the entire pathway (hexokinase, glycolysis, pyruvate dehydrogenase complex) is 2 acetyl-CoA, 4 NADH, and 2 ATP.

Glycogen in Cytoplasmic Granules → Acetyl-CoA in Mitochondrial Matrix

Glycogenolysis produces glucose-6-phosphate, which follows the same path as just described. There is relatively little glycogen in cardiac muscle compared to skeletal muscle. It is not a major source of energy in cardiac muscle.

v. little E from glycogen

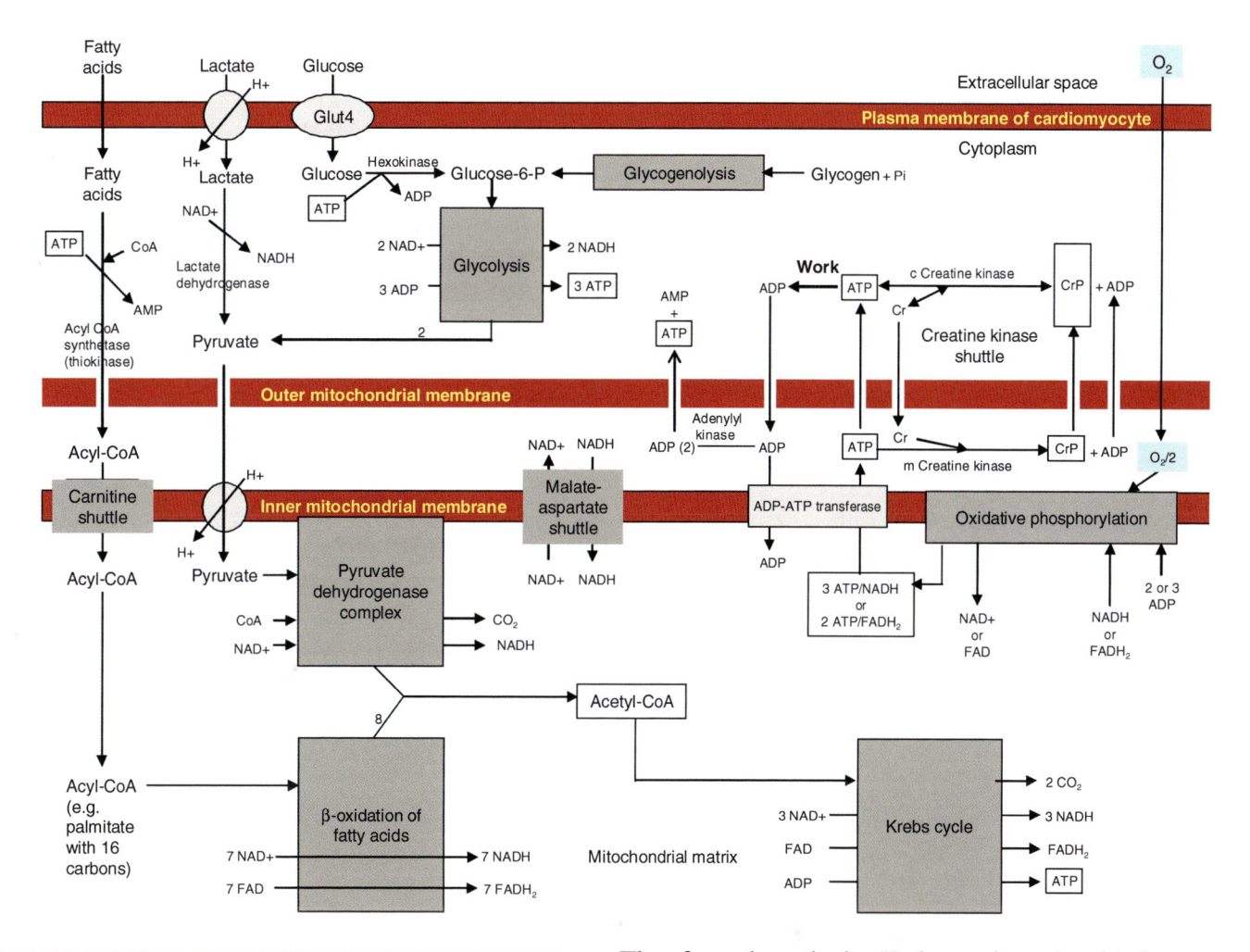

Figure 4. Overview of ATP production in cardiac myocytes.

The Krebs Cycle
Now we have generated a lot of acetyl-CoA in the mitochondrial matrix. Acetyl-CoA enters the Krebs cycle. For energy transfer, this is the only fate of acetyl-CoA that we need to consider. Output from the Krebs cycle (for each molecule of acetyl-CoA) is 3 NADH, 1 $FADH_2$, 1 ATP, and 2 CO_2.

Oxidative Phosphorylation
Now we have generated a whole lot of NADH and some $FADH_2$. These so-called reducing equivalents enter the system for oxidative phosphorylation, which is associated with the inner mitochondrial membrane. For each molecule of NADH that enters oxidative phosphorylation, three ATPs are generated from three ADPs, and half an O_2 molecule is consumed. For each $FADH_2$ molecule that enters, two ATPs are generated from two ADPs, and half an O_2 molecule is consumed.

Therefore, through the Krebs cycle and oxidative phosphorylation, twelve ATPs are generated for each molecule of acetyl-CoA.

It is important to note that all the ADP that is phosphorylated is supplied from the mitochondrial matrix, not from the space between the mitochondrial membranes. All of the ATP is generated at the inner surface of the inner mitochondrial membrane.

What normally determines the rate of oxidative phosphorylation?
Let's assume that everything is normal. The respiratory system and the coronary arteries are functioning normally, so we have an adequate supply of oxygen. We have been eating our vitamins, so we have enough NADH and $FADH_2$. Under these conditions, the supply of ADP to oxidative phosphorylation determines the rate of ATP production.

Topic 4: ATP: Summary of Sources

You could do the calculations yourselves from the above data, but why bother? Here are the results. [The numbers are for reference. I don't recommend memorizing them.]

Fatty Acids (*e.g.* palmitic acid with 16 carbons)
Complete oxidation results in 129 ATPs/palmitate = 8 ATPs/carbon. [Without oxygen, the yield would be only 7 ATPs/palmitate, 8 generated by the Krebs cycle minus 1 used at the acyl CoA synthetase step.]

Lactate
Complete oxidation results in 18 ATPs/lactate = 6 ATPs/carbon. [Without oxygen, the yield would be only 1 ATP/lactate from the Krebs cycle.]

Glucose
Complete oxidation results in 38 ATPs/glucose = 6.3 ATPs/carbon. [Without oxygen, the yield would be only 4 ATPs/glucose, 2 by glycolysis and 2 by the Krebs cycle.]

Topic 5: Need for Continuous Supply of Oxygen

In order to make use of the energy stored in the reducing equivalents (NADH and FADH$_2$), they must be processed by the oxidative phosphorylation system. This system cannot do anything without oxygen.

It is obvious from the above data that relatively little ATP can be generated without oxygen. The heart consumes ATP so fast that the meager supply from anaerobic sources is insufficient. Anaerobic metabolism cannot generate ATP fast enough to support essential crossbridge cycling and ion pumping for more that a few seconds. A myocardium without oxygen quickly succumbs. This is in contrast to fast twitch skeletal muscle, which can perform with strength and speed over short periods (sprints, weight lifting, etc.) using ATP at a rate far faster than it can be produced by oxidative phosphorylation. The deleterious results of cardiac hypoxia will be discussed below.

Topic 6: ATP-ADP Transferase

In order to reach the cytoplasm, ATP must first be transported across the inner mitochondrial membrane. The transporter that performs this function catalyzes the outward movement of ATP simultaneously with the inward movement of ADP. The coupling between the fluxes of ATP and ADP is obligatory: ATP can't get out unless, molecule for molecule, ADP gets in. This transporter is called ADP-ATP transferase. It is an example of a class of transporters called obligatory countertransporters.

Where does this ADP come from? It comes from ATP that has been used in the cytoplasm for processes like crossbridge cycling and ion pumping.

Topic 7: Regulation of the Rate of ATP Generation

It was mentioned above that the rate of oxidative phosphorylation is normally determined by the supply of ADP from the mitochondrial matrix. But the supply of ADP to the mitochondrial matrix is determined by the rate at which ATP is used in the cytoplasm. Therefore, ATP is generated by oxidative phosphorylation at just the rate that it is used in the cytoplasm. Tight coupling between ATP use and ATP generation is assured by the ADP-ATP transferase reaction across the inner mitochondrial membrane – impressive arrangement.

Topic 8: The Creatine Kinase Shuttle and the Cytoplasmic Creatine-Phosphate Pool

After ATP is transported into the mitochondrial intermembrane space, some of it simply diffuses through the large pores in the outer membrane into the cytoplasm. A sizeable fraction, however, is immediately used to make creatine phosphate (CrP) from creatine (Cr). The enzyme catalyzing this reaction is mitochondrial creatine kinase. The CrP formed in the intermembrane space diffuses into the cytoplasm across the outer mitochondrial membrane. In the cytoplasm, CrP phosphorylates ADP to reform ATP under the action of cytoplasmic creatine kinase. It can be shown (though not easily) that this so-called creatine kinase shuttle results in faster delivery of ATP to the cytoplasm than would be the case with direct diffusion of all the ATP.

There is roughly five times more CrP in the cytoplasm than ATP. Creatine kinase maintains equilibrium between cytoplasmic CrP and ATP. The result of this arrangement is that the concentration of ATP in the cytoplasm remains nearly constant in the face of sudden changes in the rate of ATP use. The large CrP pool buffers the size of the smaller ATP pool.

CrP keeps cytoplasmic [ATP] constant

Topic 9: Regeneration of ATP by the Adenylyl Kinase Reaction

Another way the myocyte protects against a decline in the concentration of cytoplasmic ATP is by converting two ADPs to one ATP plus one AMP. This reaction is catalyzed by adenylyl kinase located in the intermembrane space.

Topic 10: The Malate-Aspartate Shuttle

For every NADH produced in the cytoplasm during glycolysis and during conversion of lactate to pyruvate, an NADH appears in the mitochondrial matrix and a new NAD^+ appears in the cytoplasm. This exchange is a function of the malate-aspartate shuttle associated with the inner mitochondrial membrane.

If you want to peek into any of the black boxes shown in Figure 4, you will have to consult a biochemistry text.

Topic 11: Myoglobin

The cytoplasm of cardiac myocytes is rich in myoglobin. Myoglobin stores some oxygen that mitochondria can draw upon during brief periods of increased oxygen use or decreased oxygen delivery. However, the main function of myoglobin is probably to facilitate the diffusion of oxygen through the cytoplasm.

Part 2: ATP Use

Topic 1: Distribution of ATP Use

Figure 5
About 60% of total ATP utilization by cardiac muscle is for crossbridge cycling, about 15% for Ca^{++} pumping, about 5% for Na^+-K^+ pumping, and about 20% for other cell functions including protein synthesis and protein phosphorylations.

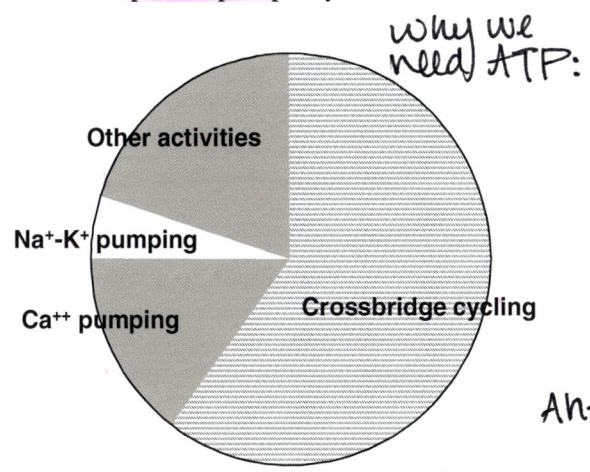

Figure 5. Distribution of ATP use.

Topic 2: Factors that Determine the Rates of ATP and Oxygen Consumption

The most important primary factor determining the rate of ATP utilization by a cardiac chamber is the amount of active tension generated in its wall during systole. Another primary factor is the amount of shortening of its muscle fibers.

Active Wall Tension
Contraction of any cardiac chamber produces active tension in its wall. The magnitude and the duration of active wall tension are both important in determining ATP consumption. Most of the ATP is consumed by crossbridge cycling, which increases as active tension increases. Restorative Ca^{++} pumping and Na^+-K^+ pumping consume the rest.

The magnitude of active wall tension depends on afterload. Active tension abruptly increases during the isovolumetric contraction period until chamber pressure just exceeds the afterload. It remains about constant during the rapid ejection period, subsides during the reduced ejection period, and finally vanishes during the isovolumetric relaxation period.

When heart rate increases, the duration of diastole is reduced more than is the duration of systole. Therefore, when heart rate increases, active wall tension is exerted for a larger fraction of the time. Consequently, ATP utilization increases with increased heart rate.

The Laplace Equation

It is important to understand the relationship between wall tension and chamber pressure. Imagine a soap bubble. The pressure inside a soap bubble is slightly higher than the pressure outside. What keeps the bubble from expanding? The answer is wall tension. Imagine a line anywhere along the wall of this bubble. A force exists from one side to the other of such a line. This force holds the wall together. Wall tension is defined as the force per unit distance along such an imaginary line anywhere on the surface.

For a soap bubble to be stable, transmural pressure (inside pressure minus outside pressure) must be perfectly balanced by wall tension. The famous 19th century mathematician, Laplace, derived the relationship between transmural pressure and wall tension that is required for stability of any curved surface, including that of a soap bubble. The Laplace equation is:

$$P = T/R_1 + T/R_2 \qquad (1)$$

P = transmural pressure
T = wall tension (assumed to be the same in all directions)
R_1 and R_2 = the major and minor radii of curvature of the curved surface

For a sphere, R_1 and R_2 are identical and the Laplace equation becomes

$$P = 2T/R \qquad (2)$$

For a cylinder, one of the radii is infinite and the Laplace equation is

$$P = T/R \qquad (3)$$

The Laplace equation was originally derived under the assumption that the wall is exceedingly thin compared to the radii of curvature (true for soap bubbles, but not for hearts and blood vessels). Fortunately, it has been demonstrated (by Dr. Alan Burton) that the Laplace relationship still holds for structures with finite wall thickness as long as R is regarded as the average radius over the entire thickness of the wall, and T is regarded as the average wall tension.

For blood vessels, equation 3 is appropriate. For the chambers of the heart, equation 2 is usually used, incorrectly assuming spherical geometry for cardiac chambers, but qualitatively OK. Thus, for a cardiac chamber, the Laplace equation is approximately

$$T = P \cdot R/2 \qquad (4)$$

If $T > P \cdot R/2$ due to generation of active tension, blood is ejected. If $T < P \cdot R/2$ due to relaxation during diastole, the chamber fills with more blood.

Equation 4 makes an extremely important point. Wall tension not only increases as chamber pressure increases, it also increases as chamber radius increases.

It should be clear, therefore, that the rates of ATP and O_2 consumption increase if
- Chamber pressure increases during systole due to increased afterload, or if
- Chamber radius increases during diastole due to increased preload.

A Modification of the Laplace Equation – Wall Stress

If we divide both sides of equation 4 by wall thickness, we get

$$T/d = P \cdot R/2d \qquad (5)$$

d = wall thickness

T/d is called wall stress, σ. Therefore,

$$\sigma = P \cdot R/2d$$

Wall stress decreases as wall thickness increases. [Note that wall stress is force divided by area, while wall tension is force divided by distance.]

The total rate of oxygen consumption is proportional to active wall tension as noted above. The rate of oxygen consumption per unit of myocardial mass is proportional to wall stress.

Shortening

When a muscle fiber shortens, it consumes more ATP than it does if it merely contracts isometrically. The amount of additional ATP consumed is proportional to the amount of shortening.

Since an increase in contractility results in more shortening (see Chapter 7), increased contractility causes increased ATP and oxygen consumption. This effect is sometimes called the oxygen cost of contractility.

Increased preload also results in more shortening with each beat. This is the Starling effect. Therefore, increased preload causes more ATP utilization not only because it increases chamber radius, but also because it increases the amount of shortening.

Summary of Factors that Determine ATP and Oxygen Consumption
Figure 6

The fundamental variables that determine the need for ATP and O₂ are active wall tension and fiber shortening.

- Active wall tension depends on chamber pressure and chamber radius and, therefore, on preload, afterload, and any pathological dilation that might be present (see Chapter 10). Active wall tension summed over time also depends on heart rate.
- The amount of fiber shortening depends on preload, afterload, and contractility (see Chapter 7).

Therefore, myocardial ATP and O₂ consumption are increased by increases in:
- Preload
- Afterload
- Contractility
- Heart rate
- Pathological dilation

Medical attempts to reduce the need for oxygen in cases of myocardial ischemia can be aimed at any of the above factors.

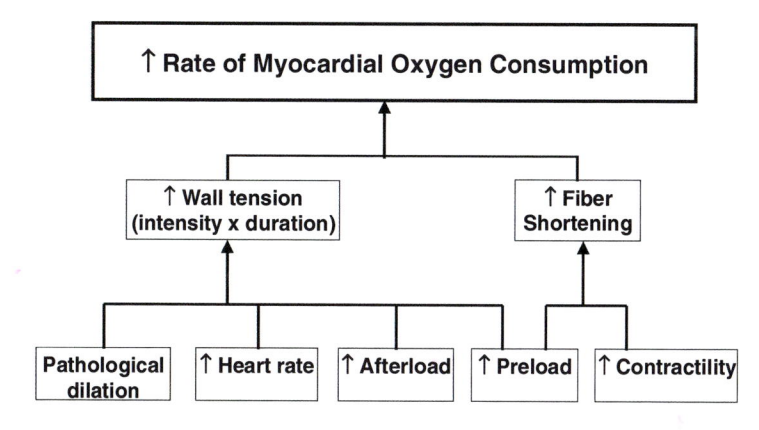

Figure 6. Summary of the factors that determine the rate of myocardial oxygen consumption.

Topic 3: Energetic Efficiency

Mechanical efficiency is defined as the amount of work accomplished divided by the amount of energy consumed. The area within a pressure-volume loop equals stroke work, but is not routinely measured. A rough estimate of stroke work can be obtained simply by multiplying stroke volume by mean aortic pressure. Energy consumed per beat can be calculated from measurements of cardiac oxygen consumption. Normal mechanical efficiency of the heart is roughly 15%, about the same as an internal combustion engine.

Topic 4: The Extremely Important Difference between Increased Pressure Load and Increased Volume Load

The rate at which a cardiac chamber performs work increases when afterload increases and when preload increases. Increased afterload increases cardiac work by increasing active wall tension. The rate of oxygen consumption increases in proportion to the increase in active wall tension and, therefore, to the increase in afterload. Efficiency is not changed much.

Increased preload increases cardiac work by increasing stroke volume; active wall tension is not increased much. The rate of oxygen consumption increases in proportion to the increase in amount of fiber shortening. The increase in fiber shortening is very little compared to the increase in stroke volume since the change in volume of a sphere is proportional to the change in its radius to the third power. Therefore, there is relatively little increase in oxygen consumption with increased volume work compared to increased pressure work. Mechanical efficiency increases with increased volume work.

There is much practical consequence of the above facts. A person with some degree of myocardial ischemia due to coronary artery disease may suffer occasional bouts of angina pectoris and be at risk for acute myocardial infarction. Increased pressure work resulting from increased arterial pressure related to sudden emotional stress or excitement causes a larger increase in oxygen demand than an equivalent increase in volume work resulting from exercise, and can be more dangerous.

Topic 5: Effect of Hypertrophy on Myocardial Oxygen Consumption

Responses of the heart to chronic overload are discussed in the next chapter. A common response to increased left ventricular afterload (due, for example, to arterial hypertension or aortic stenosis) is concentric hypertrophy in which the walls of the left ventricle thicken. What is the effect of wall thickening in response to increased afterload on myocardial oxygen consumption and efficiency?

The elevated afterload, of course, necessitates generation of greater active wall tension during systole and, therefore, the rate of oxygen consumption increases. This is true whether the left ventricle hypertrophies or not. If the left ventricle does not hypertrophy, oxygen consumption increases in proportion to the increase in work output and efficiency is practically unchanged. If the left ventricle hypertrophies, its walls can generate greater active tension and this helps it cope with the increased afterload. Since active tension and wall thickness both increase, wall stress (σ) and, therefore, oxygen consumption per unit of myocardial mass, do not change much. The change in mechanical efficiency depends on which increases more, work output or total oxygen consumption. Evidence from patients with left ventricular hypertrophy caused by arterial hypertension shows that total oxygen consumption increases more than work output [L.H. Katoh, *et al.*, *Circulation* 100:2425-2430, 1999].

Thus, the pathologically hypertrophied ventricle is a less efficient machine than the non-hypertrophied ventricle. It is not known if the physiological ventricular hypertrophy of endurance athletes (see next chapter) changes cardiac efficiency.

Topic 6: Clinically Useful Predictors of Myocardial Oxygen Consumption

It is often useful to be able to predict a person's rate of myocardial oxygen consumption from easily measured variables. One commonly used index is obtained simply by multiplying heart rate by peak systolic pressure measured at a brachial artery. This index, called the rate-pressure product or double product, is non-invasive and quite satisfactory for predicting changes in myocardial oxygen consumption in normal people who are exercising at various intensities.

Multiplying the rate-pressure product by systolic ejection time provides an index called the triple product, which is also non-invasive but not usually worth the extra trouble. Heart rate alone is reasonably well correlated with myocardial oxygen consumption, but is not as accurate an index as the rate-pressure product. Other classically important measures, such as the time-tension index have little modern use.

Part 3: Myocardial Hypoxia

Topic 1: Oxygen Supply

Principles of Oxygen Delivery
Coronary blood flow and oxygen delivery to the myocardium are treated in Chapter 16. There are two principles of normal coronary blood flow that are important now; details can wait until later. The first principle is that coronary blood flow is automatically adjusted to meet metabolic demand over a wide range of myocardial work outputs. Changes in resistance to flow through the cardiac arterioles accomplish these adjustments. The second principle is that oxygen extraction from coronary blood is normally so high (about 70%) that little further oxygen can be supplied in times of need by increased extraction. The result of this second principle is that changes in oxygen need by the myocardium must be met almost entirely by changes in coronary blood flow.

Causes of Myocardial Hypoxia
The term myocardial hypoxia means a deficiency of oxygen supply to the working myocardial cells. The principal cause of myocardial hypoxia is occlusion of a main coronary artery or one of its branches by an atherosclerotic plaque or a blood clot. Another cause is spasm of a coronary artery. In either case, we refer to the condition as myocardial ischemia (deficient blood flow). Other causes of myocardial hypoxia include anemias, circulatory shock, and certain pulmonary diseases that lead to decreased partial pressure of oxygen in arterial blood.

Even with normal oxygen delivery to the myocardium, relative myocardial hypoxia can occur with various cardiovascular diseases that require the heart to work much harder than normal, thereby increasing the need for oxygen beyond normal limits. Such conditions include valvular diseases, hypertension, hypertrophic obstructive cardiomyopathy, and hyperthyroidism.

Topic 2: Consequences of Myocardial Hypoxia

Systolic Dysfunction
Contractility is reduced in myocardial hypoxia due to decreased availability of ATP to myosin S_1 heads.

Diastolic Dysfunction
Diastolic relaxation and filling of the ventricles can be impaired due to failure of Ca^{++} pumps in the sarcoplasmic reticulum to remove enough Ca^{++} from the cytoplasm after excitation is finished.

Heart Failure
The most common cause of heart failure is systolic and/or diastolic dysfunction due to myocardial hypoxia.

Angina Pectoris
Myocardial hypoxia often leads to chest pain. The pain is usually substernal but may be much more diffuse. It is usually characterized as an ominous pressure-like or crushing-like discomfort rather than sharp or stabbing. It often radiates to the left arm and sometimes to the lower jaw.

Myocardial Hibernation
When a region of myocardium becomes moderately ischemic for an extended period, its contractility diminishes and remains at a reduced level as long as the problem remains. It generates subnormal active wall tension during each systole and, therefore, its rate of oxygen consumption decreases. This condition is appropriately called myocardial hibernation. Heart failure can result if the region is large, but oxygen is conserved. The myocardium is not irreversibly damaged during hibernation since its need for oxygen is reduced to match the available supply. When normal blood flow is restored (*e.g.* by coronary bypass surgery or percutaneous balloon angioplasty), contractility quickly returns to normal.

Myocardial Stunning
Severe ischemia leads to infarction. However, if the duration of severe ischemia is brief (perhaps relieved by prompt medical and/or surgical intervention), infarction can be aborted. Myocardial contractility is temporarily depressed but eventually fully recovers. Recovery may take several weeks. In the meantime, regional contractility is depressed – the myocardium is said to be stunned.

Myocardial Infarction
An infarct is a region of myocardium that has become permanently necrotic due to severe and prolonged ischemia. See your pathology and pathophysiology textbooks for details.

Mechanisms of Hypoxic Effects
The biochemical and physiological mechanisms of the above effects are extremely complex, incompletely understood, controversial, and beyond the scope of this chapter. Interested readers are referred to J.I. Goldhaber, <u>Metabolism in Normal and Ischemic Myocardium</u>, in G.A. Langer, *The Myocardium, 2nd Ed.*, Academic Press, 1997.

Topic 3: Reperfusion Injury

It sometimes happens that after a period of severe ischemia the affected region gets suddenly worse when blood flow is restored (*e.g.* by balloon angioplasty). This phenomenon is called reperfusion injury. Before reperfusion, the ischemic region might appear anatomically normal and would seem to be ready to survive. But reperfusion precipitates sudden contracture (shortening and stiffening that does not relax) and deterioration that at a minimum contributes to stunning and at most ends in irreversible necrosis.

Reperfusion injury is associated with a large influx of Ca^{++} into the myocytes. It is thought that the consequent rise in intracellular Ca^{++} concentration (calcium overloading) causes the contracture and cellular deterioration.

Apparently during ischemia, something happens that opens Ca^{++} channels in the cell membrane. Just what happens is not known. As long as the region is ischemic, not much Ca^{++} can enter the cells since not much is available in the small extracellular spaces. As soon as the region is reperfused with blood, the supply of extracellular Ca^{++} becomes essentially infinite and Ca^{++} overload results. If reperfusion is done with a Ringer's solution having no Ca^{++}, reperfusion injury is greatly diminished.

The increase in Ca^{++} permeability has been attributed to various substances that build up in the myocardium during ischemic periods. The main culprits are thought to be oxygen free radicals, inflammatory cytokines, and amphiphiles such as lysolecithin. There are probably other deleterious effects of these substances besides their effects on Ca^{++} permeability. Again, for more information the interested reader is encouraged to consult the Goldhaber reference (see p. 89).

Topic 4: Protection by Subclinical Hypoxic Episodes

Brief periods of ischemia condition the myocardium so that it becomes less sensitive to hypoxia. This phenomenon is called ischemic preconditioning. Necrosis and arrhythmias become less likely during subsequent more severe and prolonged ischemic attacks and during reperfusion. The mechanism of ischemic preconditioning is not understood. It appears to require activation of adenosine receptors on cardiomyocyte membranes.

Chapter 10

Responses of the Heart to Chronic Overload

This chapter describes:
- Types of Overload
- Responses to Overload
- Concentric and Eccentric Hypertrophy
- Cardiac Hypertrophy Resulting from Exercise
- Mechanisms of Hypertrophy

Part 1: Responses of the Heart to Chronic Overload

Topic 1: Types of Overload

Excessive Afterload (Pressure Overload)

Chronic, excessive afterload can result from arterial hypertension (systemic or pulmonary) or from stenosis of an outflow valve. This kind of overload is called pressure overload since systolic ventricular pressure must be greater than normal in order to eject blood.

Excessive Preload (Volume Overload)

Chronic, excessive preload can result from a variety of disorders, including leaky outflow valves (aortic or pulmonic regurgitation), leaky inflow valves (mitral or tricuspid regurgitation), myocardial infarction, and various other causes of heart failure. This kind of overload is called volume overload since end-diastolic ventricular volume is greater than normal.

Topic 2: Responses to Overload

Chronic overload results in myocyte hypertrophy. Hypertrophy is an increase in cellular volume due to a greater number of thick and thin myofilaments. Increase in cell volume resulting from swelling (cellular edema) is not regarded as hypertrophy. Increase in tissue volume resulting from more cells is called hyperplasia rather than hypertrophy. Non-myocyte cardiac cells (vascular, interstitial) undergo both hypertrophy and hyperplasia in response to overload. There is evidence that hyperplasia of myocytes can also occur in extreme circumstances, probably due to longitudinal splitting of cells.

Topic 3: Concentric and Eccentric Hypertrophy

Concentric Hypertrophy

Hypertrophy can result from addition of myofilaments alongside preexisting myofilaments. The sarcomeres and, therefore, the myofibrils, become thicker. Eventually thickened myofibrils split and form additional myofibrils. This is the dominant response to pressure overload. The consequence is a thicker and stronger myocardium. This phenomenon is called concentric hypertrophy. The term, concentric remodeling is also used.

Concentric hypertrophy results in a thickened myocardium, reduced internal diameter, and some degree of interstitial fibrosis. All of these responses lead to reduced compliance of the chamber. There may also be slower relaxation and reduced diastolic suction.

For example, systemic arterial hypertension induces the left ventricle to undergo concentric hypertrophy. The thicker left ventricular myocardium can generate greater active tension during systole and, therefore, higher chamber pressure. This effect is good since it allows a normal stroke volume in spite of the elevated afterload. The bad news is that a left ventricle with decreased compliance requires a chronically elevated preload in order to obtain a normal amount of diastolic filling. There is more bad news. Increased coronary vascularization does not keep pace with myocyte hypertrophy. The myocytes, whose work load and oxygen requirements have increased, may become ischemic. Myocardial ischemia can lead to a further decrease in compliance due partly to slower reuptake of Ca^{++} by the SR with consequent slowing of relaxation. It can also cause angina pectoris. There is even more bad news. Eventually, after years of overload and ischemia, myocytes begin to self-destruct by apoptosis or necrosis and the myocardium becomes even more fibrotic. Thus, responses to increased afterload that are initially helpful eventually contribute to the problem.

pathogenic – MAP IT!

Eccentric Hypertrophy

Hypertrophy can also result from addition of sarcomeres in series with preexisting sarcomeres, resulting in longer myofibrils and longer myocytes. Presumably, series addition of sarcomeres occurs at the ends of myofibrils. This is the dominant response to volume overload. The consequence is a dilated cardiac chamber and the condition is called eccentric hypertrophy. Slippage of myocytes with respect to other myocytes might also occur, possibly providing a minor contribution to chamber dilation during chronic volume overload. Dilation of a cardiac chamber due to longitudinal hypertrophy and cell slippage can be called eccentric remodeling. Eccentric hypertrophy can be accompanied by wall thickening or thinning, depending on the situation.

For example, in mitral valve regurgitation (incompetence) total left ventricular stroke volume includes blood pumped into the aorta plus blood pumped back into the left atrium through the leaky valve. Diastolic filling equals the normal volume of venous return plus the additional volume that was ejected into the left atrium during the previous systole. Consequently, end-diastolic volume is greater than normal. This volume overload induces eccentric hypertrophy of the left ventricle. Ventricular diameter increases because of myofibril lengthening (due to series addition of sarcomeres) and perhaps cell-to-cell slippage. Ventricular wall thickness may also increase because of parallel formation of myofibrils. Increased chamber volume results in greater compliance and end-diastolic pressure remains normal. The increase in diameter allows a normal amount of sarcomere shortening to eject a larger than normal stroke volume. This result follows from the fact that the change in volume of a cylinder is proportional to the change in circumference squared. Alternatively, if the ventricle is modeled as a sphere instead of a cylinder, the change in volume is proportional to the change in circumference cubed. The bad news is that with increased chamber diameter the amount of active tension generated in the wall must be greater for a given amount of chamber pressure (Law of Laplace). The good news is that the left ventricular wall may be thickened enough to generate the required active tension (albeit with increased oxygen consumption) and the patient may remain asymptomatic for years. This situation is called compensated mitral regurgitation. Eventually, the situation deteriorates into uncompensated mitral regurgitation in which there is a further increase in ventricular diameter, a decrease in compliance, and a decrease in contractility.

It is important to realize that pathological dilation of the ventricle, as in mitral regurgitation, does not improve stroke volume by the Starling effect. After dilation, the operating range of sarcomere lengths remains about what it was in the normal myocardium. The Starling effect still operates within this range, as it must in order to have a stable circulatory system. Lengthening of myofibrils during eccentric hypertrophy is due to addition of more sarcomeres in series, not to stretching each sarcomere to a more optimal length.

Topic 4: Cardiac Hypertrophy Resulting from Exercise

Endurance training induces a type of cardiac hypertrophy that is sometimes called physiological hypertrophy. The stimulus is more of a volume overload than a pressure overload. Thus, the hypertrophy is more eccentric than concentric with substantial dilation and some wall thickening. The increase in left ventricular mass can be as much as 50%. End-diastolic left ventricular volume can increase by as much as 80%. Systolic function is augmented with end-systolic volume remaining normal or even less than normal, and a large increase in stroke volume occurs both during exercise and at rest. Cardiac output remains normal at rest due to increased parasympathetic tone to the SA node, which reduces heart rate. The physiologically hypertrophied heart exhibits especially forceful early diastolic suction. Thus, diastolic function is improved. There is an increase in the number and length of capillaries resulting in an increased ratio of capillaries to myocytes and a reduced diffusion distance between capillaries and myocyte mitochondria. Also, some collateralization probably develops. The ischemia, fibrosis, diastolic dysfunction, and eventual myocyte deterioration commonly seen in pressure overload hypertrophy are avoided. Physiological hypertrophy is reversible, largely disappearing after several weeks of inactivity.

Topic 5: Mechanisms of Hypertrophy

Increased active tension during systole is probably the stimulus for inducing concentric hypertrophy. The stimulus for eccentric hypertrophy is probably increased passive tension and/or stretch during diastole. In both cases, the response is increased synthesis of myofilament proteins. The process is promoted by various agents including angiotensin II, endothelin-1, several growth factors, several cytokines, and by norepinephrine. Hypertrophy is suppressed by a member of the transforming growth factor-β superfamily called myostatin. These agents are mostly of local origin and, therefore, act as paracrines or autocrines. Their receptors are G-protein-linked 7-transmembrane proteins.

The myosin that is synthesized during hypertrophy tends to be the V_3 isoform (β myosin heavy chain). The crossbridge cycle is slower with the V_3 isoform than with the faster V_1 isoform (α myosin heavy chain). Some experimental animals such as adult rats normally have predominantly the V_1 isoform. When their ventricles hypertrophy there is a shift toward V_3 and ventricular contraction tends to become slower and weaker. In adult humans, the predominant ventricular isoform is normally V_3, so during ventricular hypertrophy there is no shift to the slower isoform. The predominant isoform in human atria is normally V_1, so a shift toward V_3 could conceivably contribute to compromised atrial function during atrial hypertrophy.

Further discussion of the mechanisms involved in hypertrophy is beyond the scope of this chapter. .

Selected References for Chapter 10

- J.N. Cohn, R. Ferrari, and N. Sharpe, Cardiac Remodeling – Concepts and Clinical Implications: A Consensus Paper from an International Forum on Cardiac Remodeling, *J. Am. College of Cardiology* 35: 569-582, 2000.
- B. Swynghedauw, Molecular Mechanisms of Myocardial Remodeling, *Physiol. Rev.* 79: 215-262, 1999.
- T. Tamura, T. Onodera, S.Said, and A.M. Gerdes, Correlation of Myocyte Lengthening and Chamber Dilation in the Spontaneously Hypertensive Heart Failure Rat, *J. Molec. Cell. Cardiology* 30: 2175-2181, 1998.
- H. Zhu, Myocardial Cellular Development and Morphogenesis, in G.A. Langer, *The Myocardium, 2nd Ed.*, 1998, p57-71.
- L.H. Opie, *The Heart: Physiology from Cell to Circulation, 3rd Ed.*, 1998, Chapter 13.
- N. Frey and E.N. Olson, Cardiac Hypertrophy: The Good, the Bad, and the Ugly, *Annu. Rev. Physiol.* 65:45-79, 2003.
- P.M. Buttrick and J.Scheuer, Exercise and the Heart: Acute Hemodynamics, Conditioning Training, the Athlete's Heart, and Sudden Death, in *Hurst's, The Heart: Arteries and Veins, 8th Edition*, Edited by R.C. Schlant and R.W. Alexander, McGraw-Hill, 1994, Chapter 114.
- M.K. Miller, *et al.*, The sensitive giant: the role of titin-based stretch sensing complexes in the heart, *Trends in Cell Biology* 14: 118-126, 2004.

Chapter 11

Principles of Blood Flow

In this chapter, we examine those elementary principles of fluid dynamics and the properties of blood and of blood vessels that are required for understanding the mechanics of blood flow in the vascular system.

Part 1 of this chapter treats some principles of fluid flow through tubes. These principles are generally applicable to flow of any liquid through any kind of tubing, but are selected here for their relevance to blood flow in the vascular system.

Part 2 deals with certain special properties of blood that influence its flow through tubes; these properties result from the fact that blood is a suspension of cells in plasma rather than a homogeneous liquid.

Part 3 treats some unique properties of blood flowing through very small tubes such as those in the microcirculation.

Part 4 addresses special features of vascular beds that influence blood flow in ways not expected in a system of rigid tubes.

Part 1: General Principles of Fluid Flow through Tubes

Topic 1: The Driving Force for Fluid Flow is Pressure Difference [Figure 1]

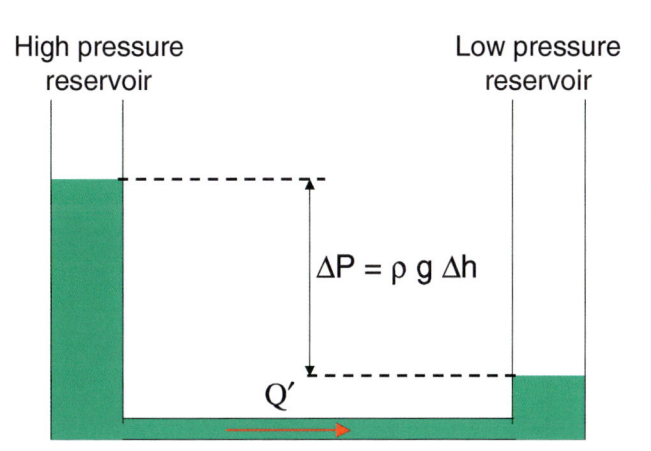

Figure 1. The difference in pressure between the ends of the horizontal tube provides the force to drive flow from left to right. In this case, the pressures are hydrostatic pressures created by columns of fluid in the two reservoirs; therefore, the pressure difference is given by the difference in height of the columns (Δh) multiplied by the acceleration of gravity (g) and the density of the fluid (ρ). In the cardiovascular system, pressure differences are generally created by the pumping action of the heart.

Flow of fluid through tubes is driven by pressure differences. For example, in Figure 1 flow occurs from the high-pressure reservoir to the low-pressure reservoir *via* the tube between them. Blood flow from arteries to veins is driven by the pressure difference between them. Blood flow through a capillary is driven by the pressure difference between the arterial and venous ends of the capillary. Cardiovascular pressures are usually given in millimeters of mercury (mmHg). If you need to convert among various units of pressure, see [Pressure conversions].

Topic 2: Resistance to Flow [Figure 2]

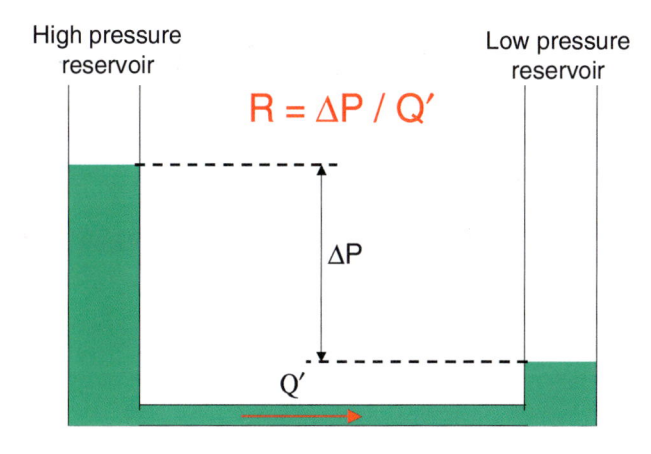

Figure 2. The definition of resistance to flow, R.

Resistance to flow is defined as the ratio between the driving pressure difference and the flow rate:

$$R = \Delta P / Q' \qquad (1a)$$

$R =$ resistance to flow
$\Delta P =$ pressure difference
$Q' =$ flow rate

$$flow = \frac{\Delta P}{R}$$

This definition is analogous to that for electrical resistance.

In physiology and medicine, the unit often used for resistance is mmHg/(ml/sec), which is called the peripheral resistance unit, PRU. However, other units are also used [Units of resistance for blood flow].

Topic 3: Flow Rate is Determined by Pressure Difference and Resistance [Figure 3]

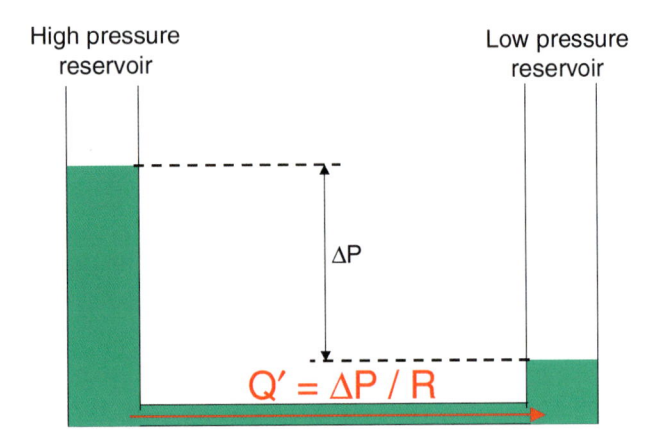

Figure 3. The fundamental equation of flow:
$Q' = \Delta P/R$

Rearranging equation 1a;

what factors affect R?

$Q' = \Delta P / R$ (1b)

This is the fundamental equation of flow. It tells us that flow rate increases as ΔP increases or as R decreases. If resistance increases, a greater pressure difference is required to achieve any given flow rate.

In the cardiovascular system, changes in R are extremely important in regulating blood flow through specific tissues and for regulating total blood flow (*i.e.* cardiac output). R is changed mainly by changes in caliber of precapillary resistance vessels, and occasionally by changes in blood viscosity.

what are precap vessels?

Topic 4: Viscosity

The shape of a fluid changes in response to even the slightest shearing force. However, the rate of change in response to any given shearing force varies from one fluid to another. The property of fluids underlying this variation is called viscosity. Newton aptly called viscosity "a defect of slipperiness between adjacent layers of fluid."

Figure 4

Picture thin layers of liquid on top of each other, and imagine that we can push horizontally on the top layer without deforming it so that it slides over the next layer. The amount of force we apply divided by the area of contact between the two layers is called the shear stress. Because of viscosity, as the first layer slides, it pulls the second layer along with it; but the second layer does not move as fast as the first layer – it lags behind. The forward motion of the second layer pulls on the third layer, but the third layer lags behind even more. A gradient of velocities is instantly established, with the top layer moving the fastest and the bottom layer moving the slowest. The velocity gradient is called the shear rate. We can use a viscometer to measure shear stress and shear rate, and then calculate viscosity (η) as

η = shear stress / shear rate   (2)

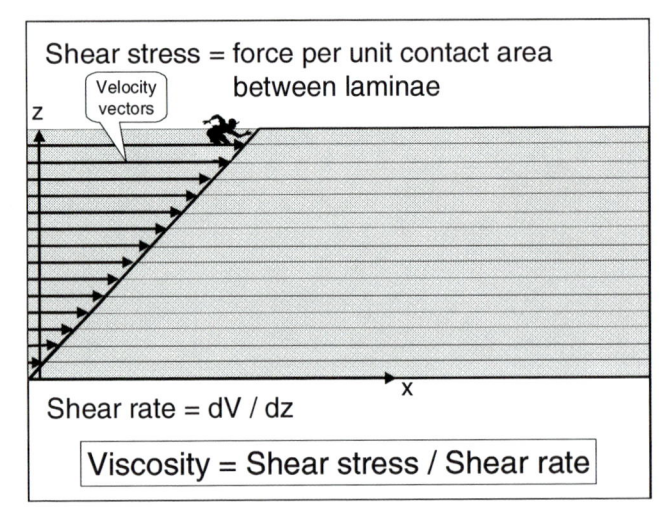

Figure 4. This diagram illustrates the concepts of shear stress and shear rate, and gives the formal definition of viscosity.

Equation 2 is the formal definition of viscosity. Shear stress is force per unit area, which (in cgs units) is dynes/cm^2. Shear rate is velocity per unit distance, which is sec^{-1}. Therefore, viscosity has units of dyne-sec/cm^2, which is called the poise. A centipoise is 0.01 poise and is the unit that is usually used for viscosity. For people who insist on SI units, viscosity is in Newton-sec/m^2 (1 centipoise = 0.001 N-sec/m^2).

Principles of Blood Flow

Water has a viscosity of 1.00 centipoise at 20° C and 0.69 centipoise at 37° C. Blood plasma has a viscosity about 1.8 times that of water. Whole blood normally has a viscosity about 4 times that of water when it is flowing in relatively large vessels, but a viscosity only about twice that of water when it is flowing through the microcirculation. This amazing fact will be discussed in Part 3 of this chapter.

Viscosity is analogous to friction between solid objects. Because of viscosity, heat is produced during flow. Heat is produced at the expense of other forms of fluid energy, most notably pressure.

Topic 5: As a Fluid Flows through a Resistance the Pressure Drops [Figure 5]

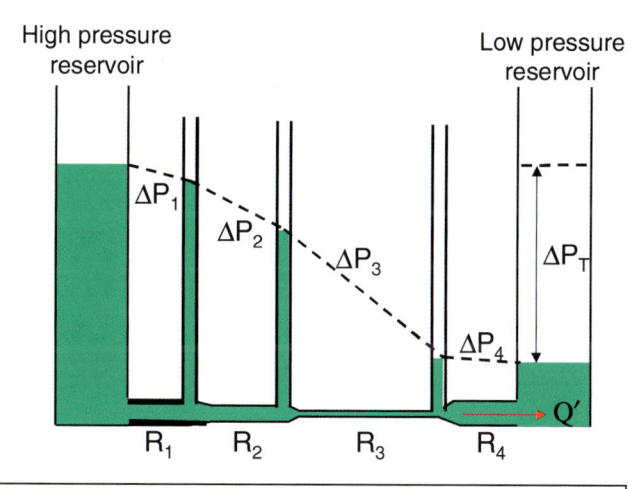

Figure 5. Through any section of tubing, the drop in pressure (ΔP) is given by the flow rate (Q') multiplied by the resistance (R).

Picture a tube through which a liquid is flowing under the influence of a pressure difference. The tube consists of four sections in series, each contributing its own resistance to flow. It should be obvious that regardless of the diameter of each section, the flow rate must be the same in all sections. Again rearranging equation 1:

$$\Delta P_T = R_T \cdot Q' \qquad (1c)$$

ΔP_T = total pressure drop from inflow end to outflow end of the tube
R_T = total resistance to flow
Q' = flow rate

The pressure drops because of the viscous (frictional) loss in fluid energy as heat.

For each section of tubing, we can write a similar equation. For section 3 for example:

$$\Delta P_3 = R_3 \cdot Q' \qquad (1d)$$

$\Delta P \propto Q$
$\Delta P \propto R$

There are two important points:
- For any given flow rate, the pressure drop from the inflow end to the outflow end of each section of tubing increases as its resistance increases.
- If the flow rate is increased (by increasing ΔP_T), the pressure drop through each section of tubing increases.

The sum of the individual ΔP values must, of course, equal ΔP_T, and the sum of the individual R values must equal R_T.

Topic 6: Cross-Sectional Area Influences Velocity [Figure 6]

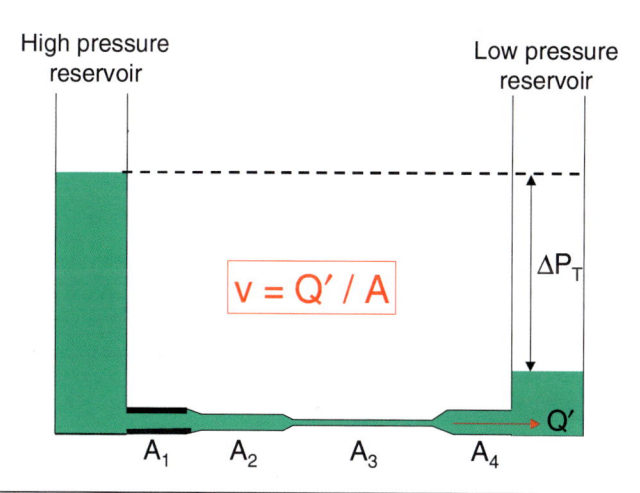

$$v = Q' / A$$

Figure 6. The continuity equation. Through any section of tubing, the average velocity of flow is inversely proportional to the cross-sectional area of the tube. Thus, in a series of tubes, the velocity is least in the thickest tube.

The flow rate through a tube is the product of average velocity of flow (v) and cross-sectional area (A).

$$Q' = v \cdot A$$

↑ area = ↓ velocity
flow = velocity × area

Again picture a tube with several sections (Figure 6). The sections have different cross-sectional areas. The flow rate must be the same in all sections (since liquids are incompressible). Consequently, the velocities cannot be the same in all sections. The greater the cross-sectional area, the slower is the average velocity.

Q is the same across a tube
· velocity ≠ across tube

The reciprocal relationship between cross-sectional area and average velocity also applies when the change in total cross-sectional area results from branching rather than from simple expansion. You will recall that the velocity of blood flow in each section of the systemic system is inversely related to the total cross-sectional area of that section (Chapter 1, Figure 4).

Topic 7: Changes in Velocity Influence Pressure: Bernoulli's Principle

The types of energy involved in fluid flow are:

- potential energy of position in the gravitational field, E_g
- potential energy of pressure, E_p
- kinetic energy, E_k
- heat, E_h

The Law of Conservation of Energy (1st Law of Thermodynamics) allows us to state:

$$\Delta E_g + \Delta E_p + \Delta E_k + \Delta E_h = 0 \qquad (4a)$$

Δ = a change incurred while flowing from one location to another

ΔE_h = the amount of heat lost from the system due to viscosity.

This equation implies that there can be exchanges of energy from one form to another, but there can be no change in total energy. Heat production, because of viscosity (friction), must be at the expense of other forms of fluid energy, generally pressure.

Let's assume that we are dealing with a horizontal tube so that ΔE_g is zero. Now if we ignore viscosity for a moment so that we can assume there is no heat production during flow, equation 4 can be written

$$\Delta E_p + \Delta E_k = 0 \qquad (4b)$$

The pressure energy per unit volume of fluid is simply the pressure, P. Kinetic energy per unit volume of fluid is ½ ρ v², where ρ is density of the fluid and v is average velocity. Thus

$$\Delta P + \Delta(\tfrac{1}{2} \rho v^2) = 0 \qquad (4c)$$

Equation 4c is the Bernoulli equation, one of the most important equations in all of physical science. It tells us that as velocity decreases, pressure increases.

Figure 7
This figure illustrates the Bernoulli Effect. Pressure in the widest section of the tube is higher than in the preceding section.

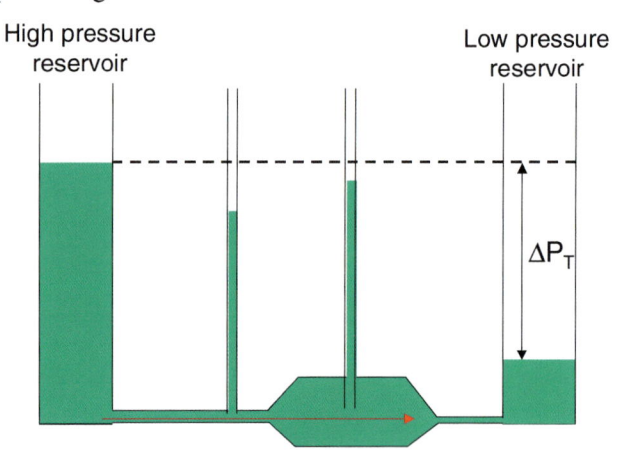

Figure 7. This diagram illustrates the Bernoulli Effect. The lateral pressure is highest in the thickest tube, since that is where the velocity (and, therefore, the kinetic energy) is lowest.

Topic 8: The Difference between End Pressure and Lateral Pressure
[Figure 8]

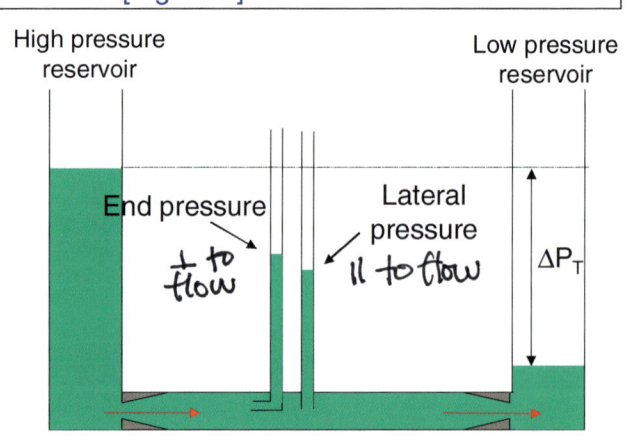

Figure 8. Measurement of end pressure and lateral pressure. Whenever flow is not zero (i.e. whenever some of the fluid energy is in the form of kinetic energy), end pressure is greater than lateral pressure.

Two manometers are inserted into a tube such that the opening of one is perpendicular to the flow (i.e., faces the oncoming flow of fluid), and the opening of the other is parallel to the flow. The pressures registered by these manometers are called end pressure and lateral pressure respectively. We will assume that the two manometers are close enough together that there is no appreciable viscous energy loss between them. It is found that during flow the end pressure is greater than the lateral pressure. This discrepancy results from the fact that just at the tip of the perpendicular manometer there is no flow (it presents a so-called stagnation point). Here, all of the kinetic energy is converted to pressure energy. Flow proceeds past the parallel manometer with undiminished velocity, and, therefore, undiminished kinetic energy. Consequently, only a portion of the total fluid energy is registered as lateral pressure. This principal has often been used in engineering and physiology to measure flow velocities (solving Bernoulli's equation for v).

In most parts of the cardiovascular system, flow velocities are not normally great enough to make end pressure importantly higher than lateral pressure. The difference may be considerable, however, in the *venae cavae*, pulmonary artery, and aorta, especially during exercise.

Topic 9: Laminar Flow

The subject of fluid dynamics deals with various kinds of flow, the most common being laminar, turbulent, and inviscid. The most important type of flow in most engineering problems is turbulent flow. In physiology, however, we deal mainly with laminar (or streamline) flow. Turbulent flow is involved in creating murmurs near abnormal heart valves and bruits at sites of abnormal narrowing of arteries, but otherwise is rare in the cardiovascular system.

Figure 9
Blood flow in the vascular system is almost exclusively laminar. In laminar flow through a cylindrical tube, the fluid behaves as though it is composed of a large number of very thin concentric layers. During flow, these concentric layers do not mix with each other; instead, they slide quietly past each other. The outermost layer is usually assumed to adhere to the vessel wall and not move at all; this is called the no-slip assumption. The no-slip layer is probably only a few molecules thick. The next layer moves over the no-slip layer, but only very slowly. The next layer moves a little faster, etc., until finally the layer at the center of the vessel (the axial stream) moves the fastest. Thus, a transverse velocity gradient exists during flow. If dye is discretely injected into the axial stream it can be seen to flow much faster than if it is injected more laterally. Regardless of where such an injection is made, the dye will remain at the same lateral position; it will not mix with adjacent layers, nor will it follow a corkscrew path. For a simulation of this dye experiment see [StripChart: Laminar flow].

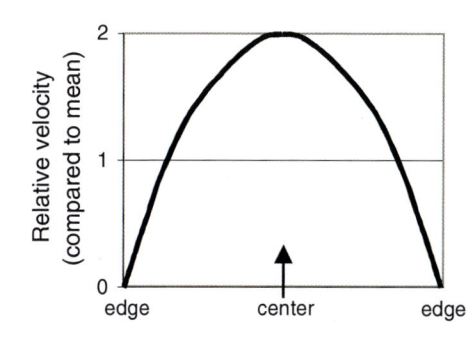

Figure 9. The parabolic relationship between velocity and transverse position in laminar flow. Velocity is assumed zero at the surface (although it probably is not truly zero in blood vessels). Velocity then increases parabolically to a maximum at the center of the tube. The maximum velocity is twice the average velocity.

In a cylindrical tube, anywhere beyond the entrance region, the velocity gradient has a parabolic shape as illustrated in Figure 9. Therefore, shear rate (the slope of the velocity gradient) is greatest at the inner wall of the vessel (just beyond the no-slip layer), and zero at the center of the vessel. The maximal velocity (*i.e.* in the axial stream) is twice the average velocity. The entrance region is defined as the part of the tube through which the parabolic velocity profile gradually develops. In the cardiovascular system, a nearly parabolic velocity profile is present in all large vessels beyond the arch of the aorta.

Topic 10: The Components of Resistance (Poiseuille's equation)

The flow rate (Q′) of a Newtonian fluid in steady, laminar flow through a long, straight, unbranched, rigid, cylindrical tube is given by the following equation:

$$Q' = (\pi r^4 \Delta P) / (8 \eta \ell) \qquad (5)$$

η = viscosity
ℓ = length of the tube
r = radius of the tube

This is the famous Poiseuille equation. It can be obtained by experiment or by theory and is absolutely correct – but only when all of the above qualifications are true. Blood vessels are not long, straight, unbranched, rigid, cylindrical tubes. Blood flow is often not steady. Nevertheless, the Poiseuille equation provides us with important qualitative insight into the physical factors that regulate blood flow through each individual blood vessel.

Note that flow increases as viscosity or length decrease or as radius increases. These effects might have been anticipated. The surprise is that flow is related to the fourth power of the radius. Thus, small changes in tube radius lead to surprisingly large changes in flow. For example, doubling the tube radius increases flow 16-fold. If tube radius decreases by 50%, flow decreases by 94%. A mere 20% reduction in radius is expected to decrease flow by nearly 60%.

Recall that by definition $R = \Delta P/Q'$. Therefore, for steady, laminar flow of a Newtonian fluid through a long, straight, unbranched, rigid, cylindrical tube:

$$R = (8 \eta \ell) / \pi r^4 \quad (6)$$

Again note the importance of tube radius. Blood vessels do not ordinarily change length much. Blood viscosity normally remains practically constant. But the caliber of blood vessels is variable, especially that of the precapillary resistance vessels and the veins. Total peripheral resistance is primarily regulated by changes in the caliber of precapillary resistance vessels, especially arterioles, since these are the vessels that provide most of the total resistance and since their caliber is adjustable over a wide range. *target arterioles to adjust TPR*

Changes in caliber of veins have important effects on venous capacity, and therefore on cardiac output and mean arterial pressure. However, changes in the caliber of veins have very little impact on total peripheral resistance since the veins provide such a small fraction of total peripheral resistance. *diff b/t arterioles & venous targets*

Topic 11: Effect of Branching on Resistance to Flow

When an artery branches the resulting vessels are usually each of smaller caliber than the stem; therefore, the resistance per unit length of each individual branch is greater than that of the stem. The total resistance of all parallel branches combined (R_T) is given by:

$$1/R_T = 1/R_1 + 1/R_2 + 1/R_3 + \ldots \quad (7)$$

Equation 7 is identical to the familiar equation for electrical resistances in parallel. This equation tells us that the total resistance of vessels arranged in parallel with each other is less than the resistance of any one of them. The total resistance per unit length of all branches in parallel can be greater or less than that of the stem depending on their relative numbers and calibers.

In general, as arteries progressively branch to the level of arterioles, total resistance markedly increases in spite of having millions of arterioles in parallel with each other. Total resistance at the level of capillaries is less than that at arterioles even though each capillary is smaller than each arteriole, since there are so many more capillaries in parallel than there are arterioles in parallel.

Topic 12: Turbulent Flow

Laminar flow is precarious. There is always a tendency toward loss of orderliness. This tendency is strengthened by increased velocity and by increased radius of the tube. Viscosity counteracts this tendency and helps maintain laminar flow. However, if velocity and/or radius increase too much, flow can become turbulent. In turbulent flow, lamellae often sweep off into eddies (swirls), which flow for considerable distances like little dust devils, shearing against the more linear laminae around them. In fully developed turbulent flow, these eddies can occupy most of the tube, but are random in frequency and in amplitude. The following nondimensional number, called the Reynolds number (Re), expresses the ratio of dispersive influences to restorative influences:

$$Re = (v \rho r) / \eta \quad (8)$$

v = average velocity of flow
r = radius of the tube
ρ = density of the fluid
η = viscosity

For steady flow through cylindrical tubes, fully developed turbulence never occurs unless the Reynolds number exceeds a value of roughly 1000. Local eddies may appear near rough sites on the tube surface, small obstructions, branches, bends, etc., but these soon disappear as viscosity smoothes things out again. When the Reynolds number exceeds the critical value of about 1000, these eddies can persist and dominate the flow well beyond the site where they began; in other words,

Principles of Blood Flow

true turbulence can occur.

At the moment the left and right ventricles begin ejecting blood during systole, flow rates in the ascending aorta and main pulmonary artery reach their maximal values. At this instant the Reynolds number can exceed 2000. Consequently, a transient type of turbulence (sometimes called disturbed flow) can occur in these locations, especially during exercise. These are the only locations in the entire cardiovascular system where Reynolds number can normally exceed its critical value. In the femoral artery, for example, Reynolds number is only about 500 at peak flow rate. It is much less than this in most other locations. Thus, laminar flow is the rule in arteries and veins.

Just beyond constrictions or irregularities there may be local eddies which normally do not develop into real turbulence. This condition normally exists around heart valves when they are open and blood is flowing through them. When a valve is diseased or damaged so that it either does not fully open when it is supposed to open (stenosis), or it leaks when it is supposed to be closed (incompetence), these eddies may become exaggerated and even develop into turbulent flow for some distance beyond the valve.

Flow through a stenotic or incompetent valve is an example of so-called orifice flow. Turbulence is much more likely just distal to an orifice than in a straight tube with no constriction. There are two reasons for increased likeliness of turbulence in orifice flow:

- Since the orifice has a reduced cross-sectional area, the velocity of flow is elevated.
- In orifice flow, the critical Reynolds number is much less than it is for flow through a straight tube.

Topic 13: Murmurs and Bruits

Laminar flow is silent since no vibrations are induced. In contrast, turbulent flow is noisy since it is characterized by oscillations of random frequency and amplitude that set the walls of blood vessels and surrounding tissues into vibrations at audible frequencies. Thus, the turbulence downstream from stenotic or incompetent valves can be heard with a stethoscope on the chest wall as murmurs. Sounds heard from turbulent flow distal to narrowing of the lumen of blood vessels (*e.g.* by atherosclerotic plaques) are called bruits.

The normal heart sounds are probably caused mainly by vibrations of the valves upon closing, rather than by turbulence, although there may still be some controversy about this.

Part 2: Special Features of Blood Flow through Tubes

Topic 1: Axial Accumulation of Red Cells

As blood flows through blood vessels, red cells tend to accumulate in the central portion of the stream. As a result, the hematocrit increases in the central laminae and decreases in the outer laminae. This behavior is thought to result from spin imparted to cells in the outer laminae by the velocity gradient of the plasma. As the cells spin their paths curve by a Bernoulli effect analogous to that of a curveball. As the cells accumulate in the more central laminae where the shear rate is less, they tend to quit spinning and line up with their long axes parallel to the direction of flow. Their shape also changes; they get longer and skinnier. Axial accumulation of red cells is a prominent feature only in vessels of less than about 1 mm in diameter.

Topic 2: Blood is Not Quite a Perfect Newtonian Fluid

Figure 10

We can measure flow rate through a straight glass tube as a function of the pressure difference applied. Figure 10 shows a plot of the results. When water is the liquid, the relationship is perfectly linear. The reciprocal of the slope of this line equals the resistance to flow. We note that for water the resistance is constant. This result implies that the viscosity is constant – it does not depend on flow rate. A fluid having constant viscosity over a wide range of flows is called a Newtonian fluid. When this same experiment is done with blood plasma the relationship is still linear, demonstrating that blood plasma is also a Newtonian fluid. The slope is less with plasma than with water since plasma has a viscosity about 1.8 times that of water (due to the presence of plasma proteins).

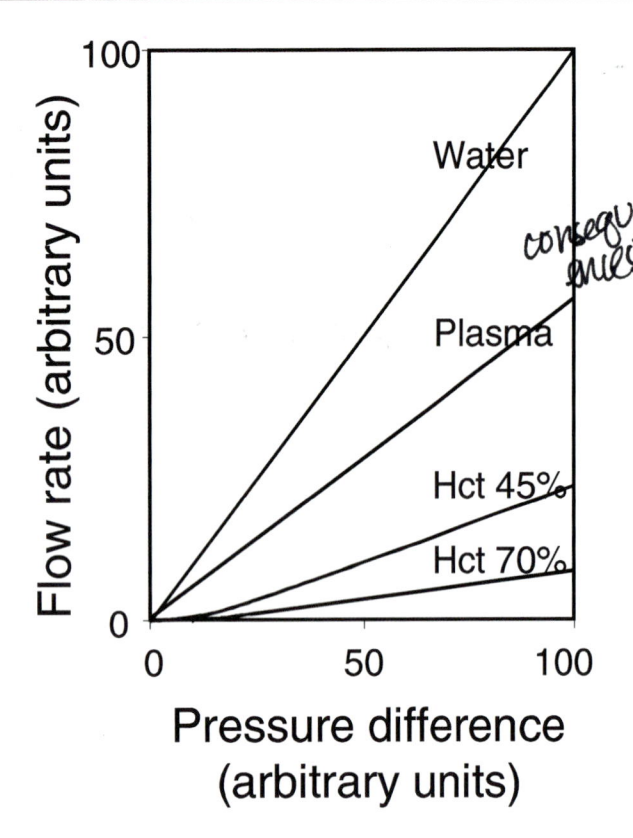

Figure 10. Pressure-flow curves for flow of water, blood plasma, and whole blood through a rigid tube with diameter far greater than that of blood cells. Data are shown for whole blood at two different hematocrits (Hct), 45% and 70%.

When whole blood with a normal hematocrit is used, the relationship between ΔP and Q′ shows a slight departure from perfect Newtonian behavior. At very small flows the curve is not linear; viscosity decreases as flow rate increases; viscosity then becomes constant at higher flow rates, and has a value about 4 times that of water.

It is generally thought that this departure from ideal Newtonian behavior is of no importance in the cardiovascular system because the shear rates are everywhere too high. Nevertheless, the explanations for this so-called anomalous viscosity might be of interest [Anomalous viscosity]. The influence of turbulence on the pressure-flow relationship might also be of interest [Pressure-flow curve during turbulence].

Topic 3: Effect of Hematocrit on Viscosity of Blood

Figure 11
The viscosity of blood is markedly influenced by the fraction of its volume occupied by red cells (*i.e.* its hematocrit). Normal hematocrit is roughly 45%. Patients with low hematocrits (anemia) have low blood viscosity; patients with high hematocrits (polycythemia) have high blood viscosity. In severe anemia the hematocrit can get as low as 10%; in some forms of polycythemia it can get as high as 80%. The curve in Figure 11 gets very steep in the hematocrit range above normal, so even mild polycythemia can have a marked effect on viscosity.

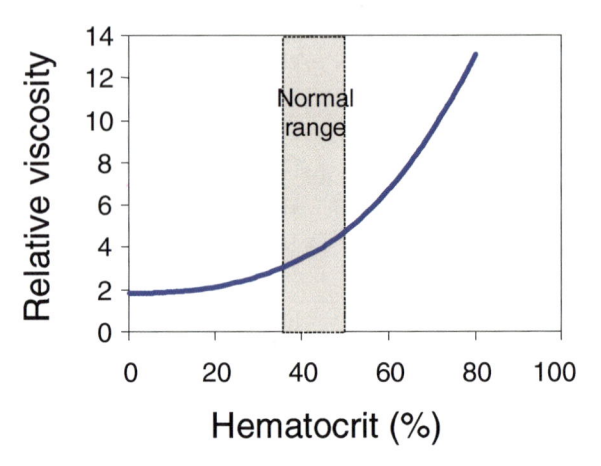

Figure 11. Effect of hematocrit on viscosity of blood flowing through relatively large tubes. The term relative viscosity means the viscosity of the fluid compared to that of water.

Anemia usually results in increased cardiac output. Part of the mechanism for this effect is related to the reduction in blood viscosity and, therefore, in resistance to blood flow. When peripheral resistance decreases, blood flows from arteries to veins faster and, therefore, comes back to the heart faster to be pumped again into the arteries.

Principles of Blood Flow

Part 3: Special Features of Blood Flow through Microvessels

Topic 1: Microvascular Beds [Figure 12]

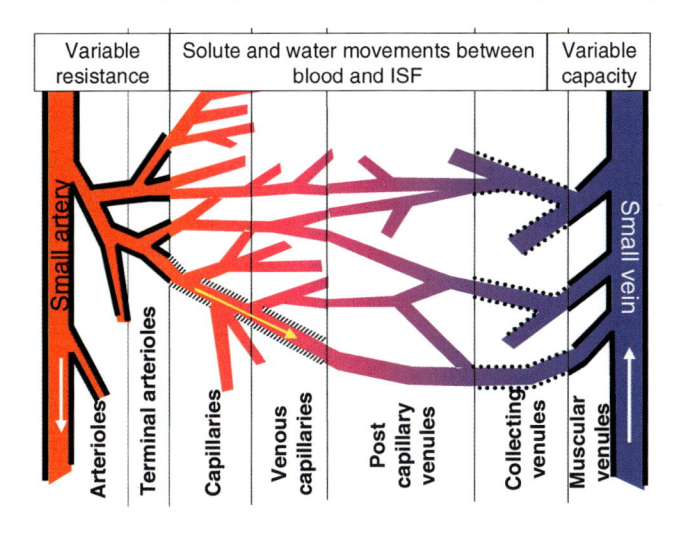

Figure 12. Microvascular terminology. Only a small fraction of the capillaries are drawn, and many of the connections are not completed. Continuous dark borders indicate continuous smooth muscle layers. Discontinuous borders indicate discontinuous smooth muscle. Vessels with no smooth muscle (capillaries, venous capillaries, and post-capillary venules) are drawn with no borders.

In addition to the names of vessels given in the figure, the yellow arrow indicates a metarteriole. Most of the capillaries in many microvascular beds arise from metarterioles rather than from true arterioles. Metarterioles have discontinuous smooth muscle. Metarterioles often constitute the arterial portion of so-called thoroughfare channels that are thought to provide a relatively low resistance to flow from small arteries to small veins.

This figure also designates the main functions of the microvessels (other than merely conducting blood).
- **Control of resistance:** Smallest arteries, arterioles, terminal arterioles, and metarterioles (these are called the precapillary resistance vessels)
- **Diffusion of materials between blood and tissue spaces:** Capillaries, venous capillaries, and post-capillary venules (these are called the exchange vessels)
- **Regulation of venous capacity:** Collecting venules, muscular venules, and smallest veins (these, together with larger veins, are called the capacity or capacitance vessels.

The network of blood vessels, with diameters of roughly 50 μm or less, which courses through tissues and connects small arteries to small veins is called the microcirculation. It consists of the smallest arteries, arterioles, terminal arterioles, metarterioles, capillaries, venous capillaries, post capillary venules, collecting venules, muscular venules, and the smallest veins. The arrangement of vessels in the microcirculation varies considerably from one tissue to another. Figure 12 illustrates an idealized arrangement.

Net movement of materials (nutrients, wastes, respiratory gases, water, etc.) between blood and extravascular tissues occurs almost exclusively across the walls of capillaries and venules. Consequently, these vessels are called exchange vessels. Flow velocity is very slow in the exchange vessels since their total cross-sectional area is very high. Transit time for a red cell passing through a capillary 0.1 mm long is, very roughly, one second.

The calibers of the smallest arteries, arterioles, and terminal arterioles are adjustable by smooth muscle contraction; therefore, the resistance to flow through the microcirculation in each tissue is adjustable. The arteriolar smooth muscle just preceding a capillary is sometimes called a precapillary sphincter, although this terminology is in decline.

Topic 2: Viscosity Decreases during Laminar Flow of Blood through Very Small Arteries and Veins

When the diameter of a vessel is only a few red cell widths, the number of concentric laminae sliding over each other is reduced to the number of red cells that can flow abreast. Most of the plasma flows in bulk behind each cell and does not shear at all. Therefore, viscosity is decreased. For reasons that are unimportant here, this phenomenon is called the sigma effect.

Topic 3: Red Cells Must Squeeze through Capillaries by Changing Shape

Figure 13

True capillaries have diameters that are considerably smaller than the diameter of a discoid red cell. However, red cells can easily be deformed. They take on a hollow bullet shape as they are squeezed through capillaries by the force of the pressure gradient. Each red cell fills nearly the entire lumen of the capillary as it slips through. Only a thin rim of plasma separates the red cell membrane from the endothelial surface. This type of flow is called plug flow.

plug flow in cap.s: 1 RBC at a time & ∆shape too!

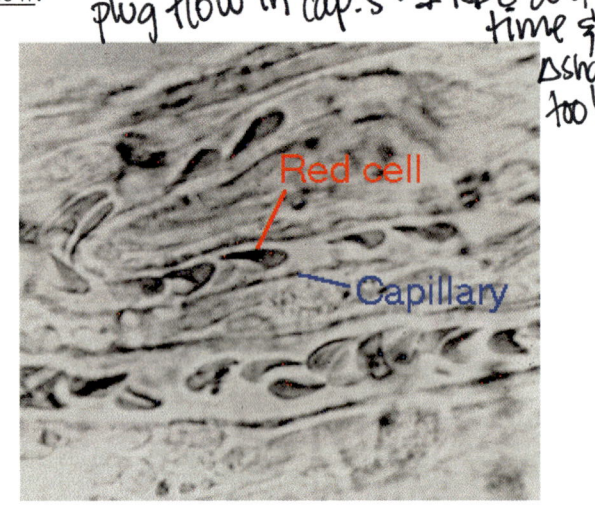

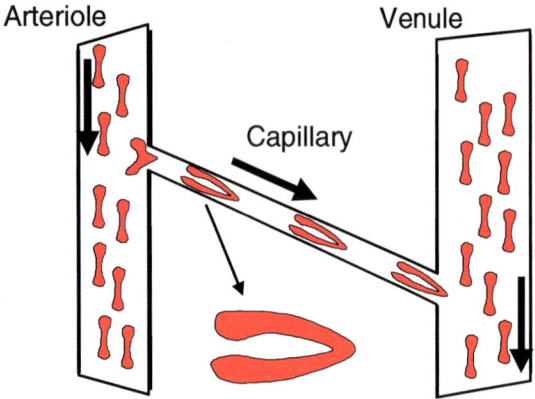

Figure 13. Flow of red blood cells through capillaries. **Top:** This is one frame from a high-speed film clip of blood flowing in microvessels of dog mesentery. Note the deformation of the red cells, especially in the capillary. [From the work of Ted Bond and M. Mason Guest, Dept. of Physiology, UTMB, Galveston, TX, 1963.] **Bottom:** Drawing of red cell cross-sections based on high-speed photography.

Flow of plasma through capillaries is largely inviscid (*i.e.* with no shearing between laminae) since it merely slides in bulk between red cells. Thus, in plug flow, a column of alternating red cells and plasma slides through the capillary. Only at the rim of this column does viscous shearing occur. For this reason, the viscosity of blood flowing through capillaries by plug flow is considerably reduced.

plug flow ⇒ ↓ viscosity in cap.s

White cells cannot readily squeeze into true capillaries. They traverse the microcirculation mainly *via* thoroughfare channels.

metarterioles

Topic 4: The Hematocrit is Low in the Microcirculation

The hematocrit is considerably lower in blood taken from the microcirculation than in blood from large arteries or veins. This situation is not fully understood, but probably results mainly from a phenomenon called plasma skimming. Remember that in arteries having diameters less than about 1 mm, red cells tend to flow preferentially in the central part of the stream (axial accumulation). Therefore, as blood flows into the microcirculation the peripheral part of the stream is mostly plasma. Branching is usually not a simple bifurcation like a symmetrical fork in the road, but more like the splitting off of an off-ramp at an acute angle to the main vessel. The blood that flows into the branch is mostly from the periphery of the main stream (the outer lane) and, therefore, has fewer red cells.

The reduced hematocrit in the microcirculation results in a further reduction in viscosity.

Topic 5: The Fahraeus-Lindqvist Effect

what are implications of ↓ viscosity?

Figure 14

The reduction of blood viscosity in the microcirculation has a name; it is called the Fahraeus-Lindqvist effect after the investigators who originally discovered it in 1930. The degree to which viscosity is reduced depends on the size of the vessel.

microcirc = ↓ viscosity

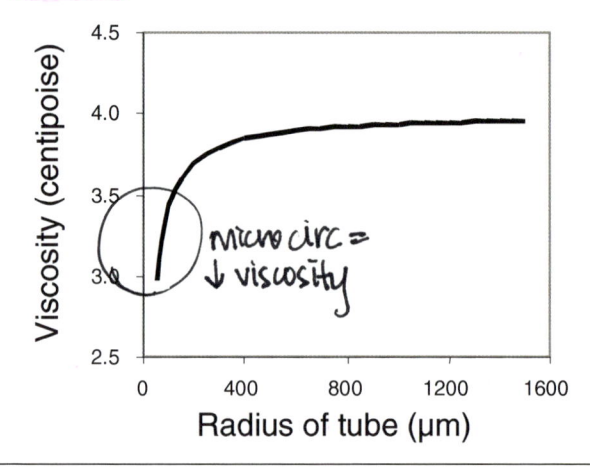

Figure 14. The Fahraeus-Lindqvist effect.

Figure 15

Because of the Fahraeus-Lindqvist effect in the microcirculation, the effective viscosity of blood flowing through vascular beds is only slightly greater than that of plasma.

Principles of Blood Flow

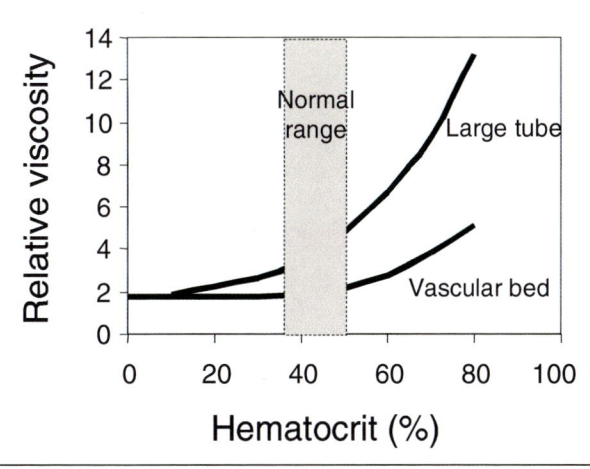

Figure 15. The effect of hematocrit on viscosity of blood flowing through either a vascular bed (dog hindlimb) or a relatively large tube.

We have discussed three mechanisms underlying the Fahraeus-Lindqvist effect:

- The sigma effect
- Plug flow
- Reduced hematocrit

(mech of F-L effect)

We have repeatedly noted that most of the total resistance to blood flow is presented by the microcirculation, especially the arterioles. Were it not for the Fahraeus-Lindqvist effect, total peripheral resistance would be much greater than it actually is, and mean arterial pressure would have to be maintained at severely hypertensive levels in order to drive blood through the microcirculation at a normal rate. Reduction of viscosity in the microcirculation is an extraordinarily important principle of blood flow. Were it not for the Fahraeus-Lindqvist effect arteries would have to be thicker and, therefore, less compliant. Loss of arterial compliance would present insurmountable obstacles to the functional stability of a recirculating hydrodynamic system.

THE WHY

means: ↓ TPR (b/c ↓ η in microc) → ↓ MAP → arteries can be more compliant

Part 4: Blood Flow through Vascular Beds

Topic 1: Pressure-Flow Relationship through Passive Vascular Beds

Recall that during laminar flow of blood through a rigid tube or system of tubes (with diameters much larger than that of red cells), the pressure-flow relationship is linear (except for anomalous viscosity at extremely low flow rates). The slope of the straight line connecting any point on this curve with the origin is equal to the reciprocal of the resistance to flow, 1/R.

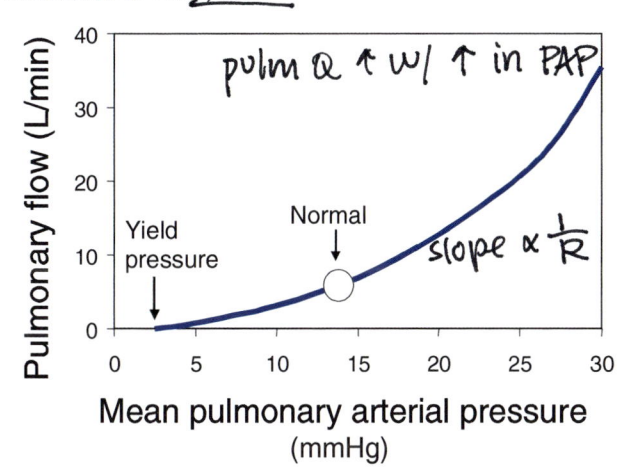

flow requires press

Figure 16. Pressure-flow curve for a passive vascular bed (pulmonary circulation).

Figure 16
Vascular beds have some interesting properties not possessed by large rigid tubes.

- Vascular beds include vessels with diameters comparable to those of blood cells. Red cells cannot flow through these vessels until rouleaux are broken up. Red cells can traverse true capillaries only after becoming elongated, uniconcave objects. These transformations require an appreciable driving pressure. Consequently, blood flow through a vascular bed remains zero until some finite driving pressure, the yield pressure, is reached.
- The yield pressure is not expected to be identical for all capillaries in a vascular bed. The least observable flow through the whole vascular bed occurs through the capillaries (and thoroughfare channels) having the largest diameters. As the driving pressure increases, flow can occur through more and more capillaries. Consequently, as driving pressure increases, resistance to flow decreases and the pressure-flow relationship gets progressively steeper. This phenomenon is often called capillary recruitment.
- Blood vessels are distensible. As the pressure difference across the wall of a blood vessel increases, its radius increases. When vessel radius increases, resistance to flow decreases. Consequently, as driving pressure increases, the

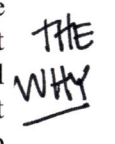

resistance through precapillary vessels, and through capillaries themselves, decreases. This effect contributes to the progressive increase in the slope of the pressure-flow curve shown in Figure 16.

Capillary recruitment and microvessel distension are important features of blood flow through the lungs. In fact, the pressure-flow relationship for the vascular bed shown in Figure 16 represents that for the pulmonary circulation. Whenever pulmonary vascular pressures increase, pulmonary vascular resistance decreases because of capillary recruitment and microvessel distension. These passive responses of the pulmonary circulation account for the fact that during exercise the percentage rise in mean pulmonary artery pressure is far less than the percentage rise in cardiac output.

Topic 2: Pressure-Flow Relationship through Reactive Vascular Beds

In most vascular beds, increased intravascular pressure, rather than causing a passive reduction in resistance to flow, results in a reactive increase in resistance to flow. Consequently, in most vascular beds the pressure-flow relationship differs in a remarkable way from the type shown in Figure 16.

Figure 17

This figure depicts the changes in blood flow through a vascular bed resulting from a sudden change in perfusion pressure (*i.e.* the difference between arterial and venous pressures). Immediately after changing perfusion pressure from a value of 100 mmHg to either higher or lower values, flow rate increases or decreases as expected, with relatively little change in resistance (dotted curve). During the next minute or so, however, flow rate tends to return toward its original value because of reactive changes in resistance to flow (solid curve). Over some range of perfusion pressures, the final steady-state flow rate is only slightly influenced by perfusion pressure. This phenomenon is called pressure-flow autoregulation. The range of perfusion pressures over which steady-state flow remains reasonably constant is called the autoregulatory range. Pressure-flow autoregulation is a property of many vascular beds, including renal, coronary, gastrointestinal, hepatic, cerebral, and skeletal muscle. The autoregulatory range varies among organs, but most maintain a rather constant rate of blood flow over a range of mean arterial pressures from about 60 to 120 mmHg. The mechanism of pressure-flow autoregulation is controversial.

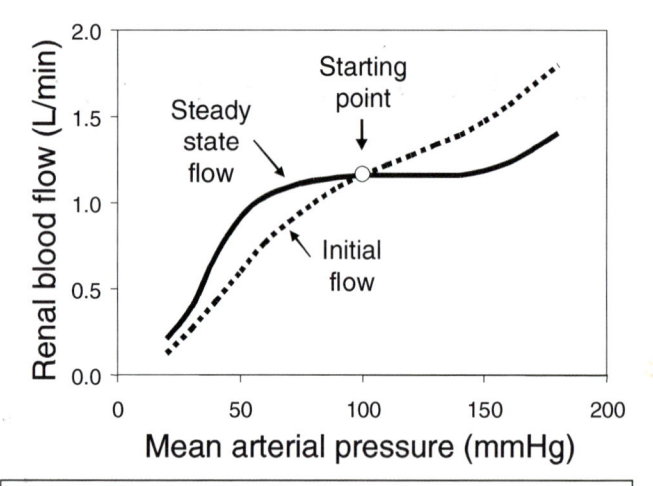

Figure 17. Pressure-flow curves for a reactive vascular bed (renal circulation). See main text for description of this experiment.

Chapter 12

Vascular Smooth Muscle

This chapter presents the physiology and a little pharmacology of vascular smooth muscle.
Part 1 describes the structure of vascular smooth muscle and the mechanism of contraction.
Part 2 discusses the membrane potential and ion channels.
Part 3 describes the mechanisms that modulate the tone of vascular smooth muscle.
Part 4 discusses a variety of specific endogenous agonists, both excitatory and inhibitory.
Part 5 categorizes vasodilator drugs according to their mechanisms of action.

Part 1: Structure and Mechanism of Contraction

Topic 1: Introduction

Smooth muscle is named for its lack of cross striations. Smooth muscle cells are very small compared to skeletal muscle cells and even small compared to cardiac muscle cells. They are very slow in their contracting and relaxing behavior – they could be called slow muscle cells.

Vascular smooth muscle ordinarily remains in a state of perpetual contraction, called tone. Adjustments in the degree of vascular muscle tone are determined by neurotransmitters, circulating hormones, nitric oxide, other endothelial factors, blood flow velocity, and wall tension. These adjustments contribute crucially to changes in TPR, arterial compliance, arterial impedance, venous compliance, venous capacity, and regional blood flows.

Smooth muscle is classically divided into two categories: multiunit and single unit. Look these up if you like, but vascular smooth muscle doesn't fit either category. Its cells are profusely connected by gap junctions, which contribute to confined regions of vascular smooth muscle (*e.g.* arterioles) acting as single units. On the other hand, single unit characteristics of smooth muscle such as propagated slow waves and myogenic automaticity (*e.g.* small intestine) are not prominent features of vascular smooth muscle.

Importance of Endothelium

Vascular smooth muscle cells are connected to underlying endothelial cells by gap junctions. They are influenced in extremely important ways by chemical and electrical events originating in endothelial cells. More of this later.

Topic 2: Vascular Walls

Figure 1
This figure illustrates the main structural features of a small muscular artery, which is the most common type of artery. The three major layers are the tunica adventitia, tunica media, and tunica intima.

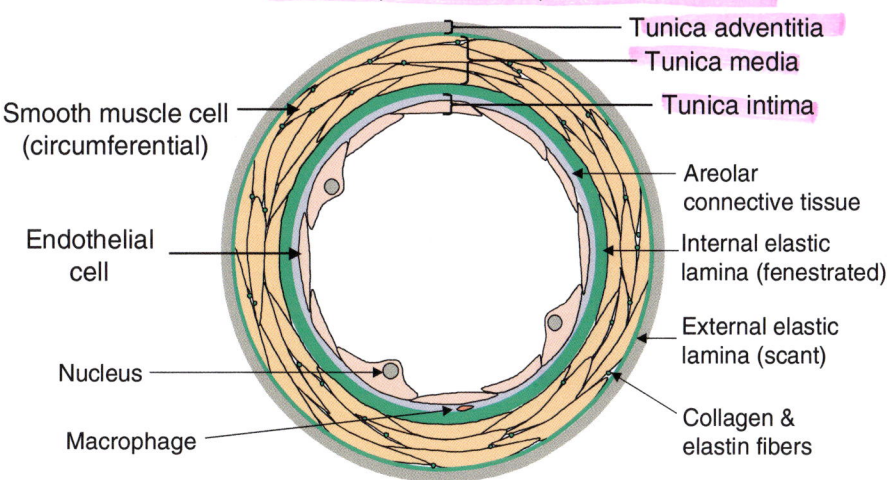

Figure 1. Diagram of a small muscular artery in cross section.

Vascular smooth muscle cells are located in the tunica media with their long axes oriented circumferentially. There is a structural progression from large arteries to capillaries. The elastic laminae, adventitia, and media become thinner and thinner until finally, in capillaries, there is only the endothelium supported by a basement membrane.

Topic 3: Microanatomy of Vascular Smooth Muscle

Myofilaments and Sarcomeres
Figure 2
In transverse section, it is obvious that vascular smooth muscle cells are packed with thin filaments. The thin filaments are composed of actin and tropomyosin (no troponin). Smooth muscle cells also have thick filaments that are composed mainly of myosin.

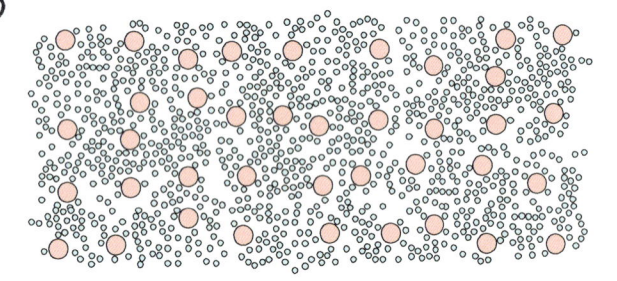

Figure 2. Diagrammatic cross section through vascular smooth muscle cell showing thick and thin filaments.

The thin filaments are extremely long, about 4.5 μm (those in striated muscle are about 1.0 μm long). The thick filaments are roughly 1.6 μm long, about the same as in striated muscle. Due to the very long thin filaments, the operating range of sarcomere lengths is especially long in vascular smooth muscle. In arteries, there are about 15 thin filaments per thick filament, somewhat less in veins. In striated muscle, the ratio is only 6:1.

Figure 3
Bundles of thin filaments terminate in structures called dense bodies. Dense bodies contain a lot

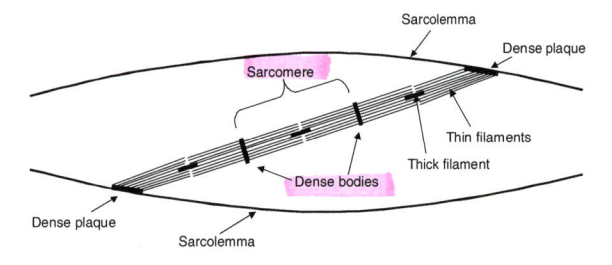

Figure 3. Diagram of a single myofibril in vascular smooth muscle.

of α actinin and are the smooth muscle counterpart of Z lines. Smooth muscle sarcomeres run from dense body to dense body. The thick filaments probably straddle the centers of sarcomeres as they do in striated muscle. Myofibrils terminate in dense plaques located along the inner surface of the sarcolemma. You cannot see cross striations in smooth muscle because the myofibrils do not parallel each other and the dense bodies are not transversely juxtaposed.

Figure 4
Thin filament bundles with associated thick filaments and dense bodies form myofibrils that traverse smooth muscle cells, but not usually along the longitudinal axis. Instead, the myofibrils run at various angles to each other, forming a crossing pattern through the cells. Therefore, the cellular mechanics of contraction, as shown in Figure 4, is somewhat different than it is in striated muscle.

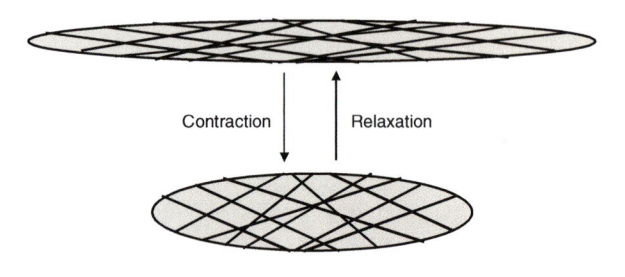

Figure 4. A diagrammatic model for contraction of a smooth muscle cell. A sampling of myofibrils is represented by the angling straight lines. As the lattice of myofibrils shortens, it gets thicker. This forces the entire cell to get shorter and thicker, maintaining constant volume.

Cytoskeleton
There is a meshwork of intermediate filaments in vascular smooth muscle that apparently holds everything together. The dense bodies are bound to the nodes of this cytoskeletal mesh.

Caveolae and Sarcoplasmic Reticulum
There are shallow invaginations all along the sarcolemma of vascular smooth muscle cells; they are called caveolae. Caveolae are the reduced counterpart of the T tubules of striated muscle. The sarcoplasmic reticulum (SR) is also reduced and is mainly located just beneath the sarcolemma in close proximity to the caveolae. There are also relatively sparse components of the SR located more internally within the cell. The SR stores Ca^{++} by virtue of an ATP-dependent Ca^{++} pump, just as in striated muscle. This pump is often called SERCA (short for SR/ER Ca-ATPase). There is no need for a more extensive system of T tubules and SR in vascular smooth muscle since fast responses are not necessary and the cells are so skinny that the time required for Ca^{++} diffusion into the interior is not a problem.

There are two different types of Ca^{++} release channels in the SR of smooth muscle. One is the ryanodine receptor responsible for Ca^{++}-induced Ca^{++} release; it is similar to the ryanodine receptor in cardiac muscle. The other is the IP_3 receptor responsible for IP_3-induced Ca^{++} release. These processes will be described in Part 3 of this chapter.

IP₃ Ca²⁺ release is diff

Topic 4: Innervation

Parasympathetic nerves do not innervate most vascular smooth muscle and we can consider parasympathetic influence on vascular bed resistances to be unimportant. An exception is in salivary glands where parasympathetic stimulation causes relaxation of vascular smooth muscle and increased blood flow.

Sympathetic nerves innervate all vascular smooth muscle (except in the lungs) and are extremely important in determining MAP, CVP, CO, and regional blood flows.

Sympathetic postganglionic nerve terminals have varicosities packed with vesicles that contain norepinephrine. This transmitter is released by exocytosis in response to action potentials. The mechanism of transmitter release will not be described here. Transmitter reuptake by sympathetic nerve endings and other mechanisms for transmitter elimination will also not be discussed. You might want to consult pharmacology textbooks for these matters.

There is no anatomic specialization on the post-synaptic smooth muscle membrane comparable to that at skeletal muscle end plates – just G-protein-linked adrenergic receptors, mainly α_1 and β_2.

Activation of α_1 receptors increases contraction of vascular smooth muscle and thus constricts blood vessels. Activation of β_2 receptors decreases contraction and thus relaxes blood vessels. The mechanisms of these responses will be described below.

Topic 5: The Mechanism of Contraction

mech = same but SLOWER

The crossbridge mechanism of contraction is essentially the same as in striated muscle (Chapter 2). The biochemical and mechanical cycles are thought to be the same – they just run slower.

Topic 6: Maintaining Tension with Low Energy Consumption

Generation of tension in smooth muscle, just as in striated muscle, requires energy commensurate with the task. But in smooth muscle, unlike in striated muscle, once the pull is completed tension can be maintained with almost no continued expenditure of energy. This amazing feature of smooth muscle is extraordinarily important for maintaining vascular tone. Almost no energy is required, and cytoplasmic Ca^{++} concentration and the degree of myosin light chain phosphorylation (described below) return almost to basal levels.

The mechanism of this so-called latch state in smooth muscle is not understood. The most prominent theory says that once the pull is accomplished the crossbridges remain in tension with little recycling. Presumably, the off rate constant between actin and S_1 is greatly reduced.

Part 2: The Membrane Potential and Ion Channels

If you think you can't remember anything about membrane potentials you might want to skim Chapter 3, Parts 3 and 4.

The resting membrane potential in vascular smooth muscle ranges between about -50 mV to -35 mV. A balance between outward currents through various potassium channels and inward currents through chloride channels, nonselective cation channels, and L-type Ca^{++} channels, establishes most of the membrane potential. A small contribution (about 10%) comes from the direct electrogenicity of the Na^+-K^+ pump.

The more important ion channels in vascular smooth muscle membranes are discussed here. Some vascular smooth muscles also have voltage-gated Na^+ channels and T-type Ca^{++} channels, but they seem to be useless since at the prevailing membrane potentials, these channels are all inactivated.

Topic 1: K^+ Channels

There are at least four important K^+ channels:

- **K_V**: Voltage-dependent K⁺ channels. K_V channels are turned on (opened) by depolarization. The resulting outward current resists further depolarization. The K_V channels are much like the delayed K⁺ channels that carry I_K in cardiac muscle where they are important in membrane repolarization during action potentials.
- **BK_Ca**: Ca⁺⁺-dependent K⁺ channels. B is for big. BK_Ca channels are turned on by increases in intracellular free Ca⁺⁺ concentration. When this happens, the resulting outward current repolarizes the membrane, thereby turning off L-type Ca⁺⁺ channels. Thus, BK_Ca channels allow the cell to resist excessive changes in intracellular free Ca⁺⁺ concentration.
- **K_ATP**: ATP-dependent K⁺ channels. K_ATP channels are turned on by decreased intracellular ATP. Thus, when O₂ or organic substrates are scarce compared to metabolic need, the membrane hyperpolarizes. *[so cell conserves E]*
- **K_IR**: Inwardly rectifying K⁺ channels. K_IR channels are turned off by depolarization. They are probably not open enough at normal membrane potentials to contribute importantly to establishing the resting potential. Their likely importance in vascular smooth muscle is that they are turned on by rises in extracellular K⁺ concentration.

Topic 2: Nonselective Cation Channels

Nonselective cation channels do not distinguish much between Na⁺, and Ca⁺⁺, but Na⁺ carries most of the inward depolarizing current since it is much more abundant in the extracellular solution. When opening of these channels increases, the resulting inward current tends to depolarize the membrane.

Topic 3: L-type Ca⁺⁺ Channels

Inward current through L-type Ca⁺⁺ channels (DHP receptors) not only contributes Ca⁺⁺ to the sarcoplasm for augmenting contraction, but also enhances membrane depolarization and can result in Ca⁺⁺ action potentials. *[Ca²⁺ used for 2 things]*

Topic 4: Chloride Channels

Inward current through chloride channels (*i.e.* outward Cl⁻ flux) contributes to the resting potential of vascular smooth muscle cells. The importance of this contribution is controversial, but it is interesting to note that the equilibrium potential for Cl⁻ (E_Cl) is about -40 mV, which is within the range of normal membrane potentials for vascular smooth muscle. Cl⁻ currents should at least resist large changes in membrane potential.

One type of Cl⁻ channel in vascular smooth muscle is opened by cytoplasmic Ca⁺⁺. Thus, when cytoplasmic Ca⁺⁺ concentration increases this channel conducts an inward depolarizing current, which opens L-type Ca⁺⁺ channels and amplifies the original rise in cytoplasmic Ca⁺⁺. Note that this effect opposes the hyperpolarizing effect of cytoplasmic Ca⁺⁺ on BK_Ca channels discussed above. *[so Ca²⁺ signals depol & repol]*

Topic 5: Action Potentials

Vascular smooth muscle cells sometimes have Ca⁺⁺ action potentials by virtue of L-type Ca⁺⁺ channels. Ca⁺⁺ action potentials increase Ca⁺⁺ entry into the sarcoplasm and, therefore, augment contraction. The importance of action potentials in most vascular smooth muscle is in question. They sometimes occur, but are probably not required for control of contraction. *[don't need AP but Ca²⁺ can induce AP]*

Part 3: Mechanisms for Modulating Tone in Vascular Smooth Muscle

Topic 1: General Principles

This is a far more complex subject than excitation-contraction coupling in striated muscle. Recall that in cardiac muscle contractility is determined by how much Ca⁺⁺ binds to troponin-C on thin filaments during each excitatory event. In smooth muscle, effects on thick filaments regulate contraction much more importantly than effects on thin filaments. Specifically, tone is regulated by phosphorylation and dephosphorylation of the regulatory myosin light chains that wrap around the stems of myosin S₁ heads. [If you need to refresh your knowledge of myofilament structure, look at Chapter 2.]

Thick Filament Regulation
Figure 5
Phosphorylation of regulatory myosin light chains increases the interaction between thick and thin filaments, making the contraction stronger.

Vascular Smooth Muscle

Dephosphorylation of regulatory myosin light chains decreases the interaction between thick and thin filaments, making the contraction weaker. Two enzymes are involved: myosin light chain kinase and myosin phosphatase.

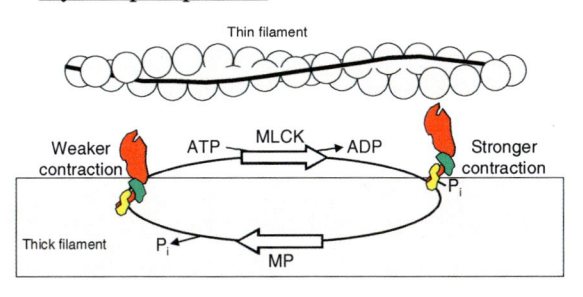

Figure 5. Thick filament regulation of tone in vascular smooth muscle.
MLCK = myosin light chain kinase
MP = myosin phosphatase
Myosin S_1 in red
Essential light chain in green
Regulatory light chain in yellow

so how do you target activity of MLCK & MP

There is always a dynamic balance between the actions of the kinase and the phosphatase on myosin light chain phosphorylation. Activation of the kinase and/or inactivation of the phosphatase strengthen contraction (increase tone). It follows, of course, that inactivation of the kinase and/or activation of the phosphatase weaken contraction. The balance between the activities of myosin light chain kinase and myosin phosphatase is the main determinant of vascular smooth muscle tone. Several pathways are involved in determining this balance; they will be described in Topics 2, 3, and 5.

Thin Filament Regulation

There is some degree of thin filament regulation in vascular smooth muscle, but it is thought to be much less important than thick filament regulation. It is not Ca^{++}-dependent. The thin filaments have no troponin. They have tropomyosin, but no troponin. However, there are other regulatory proteins bound to actin and to tropomyosin, namely caldesmon and calponin. Together with tropomyosin, caldesmon and calponin inhibit crossbridge formation, and this inhibition is reduced when these proteins are phosphorylated (more detail in Topic 4).

ppy caldesmon & calponin to ↑ contractility

Topic 2: The Ca^{++}-Calmodulin Pathway for Regulating Tone

Figure 6
Calmodulin is a cytoplasmic protein that has four binding sites for Ca^{++}. Two of these sites are always occupied. Increased cytoplasmic Ca^{++} concentration leads to more Ca^{++} binding, and when all four sites are occupied by Ca^{++}, calmodulin activates myosin light chain kinase. This tips the balance in favor of the kinase over the phosphatase with consequent increased light chain phosphorylation and increased force of contraction.

↑ IC Ca^{2+} mech ⟹ ↑ contraction

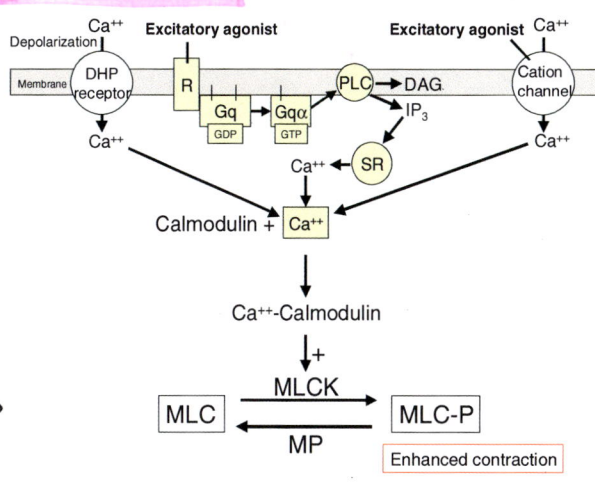

Figure 6. The Ca^{++}-calmodulin pathway for regulating tone in vascular smooth muscle. Three separate membrane mechanism feed into the final common Ca^{++}-calmodulin path. See text for description.
MLC = regulatory myosin light chain
MLC-P = phosphorylated regulatory myosin light chain
MLCK = myosin light chain kinase
MP = myosin phosphatase
R = G-protein-coupled membrane receptor
IP_3 = inositol 1,4,5 trisphosphate
DAG = diacylglycerol
PLC = phospholipase C
SR = sarcoplasmic reticulum/Ca^{++} stores

There are three general mechanisms for increasing cytoplasmic Ca^{++} concentration: 1) membrane depolarization with consequent activation of DHP receptors, 2) activation of G_q-protein-coupled membrane receptors, and 3) activation of agonist-operated cation channels.

Membrane Depolarization

Within the usual range of membrane potentials (-50 to -35 mV), DHP receptors are turned on, slight to full as the membrane depolarizes. As DHP receptors open, Ca^{++} comes in and augments contraction by the calmodulin pathway. Hyperpolarization causes relaxation. Even at -50 mV, DHP receptors are turned on enough to result in some degree of vascular smooth muscle tone. Thus, agents that depolarize the membrane increase tone and agents that hyperpolarize the membrane

↓ tone

decrease tone. This relationship is called electromechanical coupling. We will mention three examples in which electromechanical coupling apparently plays the dominant role in modulating tone.

1. **Hypoxia.** Hypoxia induces membrane hyperpolarization by opening K_{ATP} channels. The result is less Ca^{++} entry through DHP receptors and vasodilation, which helps to correct the hypoxia.

2. **Increased Extracellular K^+ Concentration.** In many tissues, heightened metabolic activity leads to significant net efflux of K^+ from cells and increased K^+ concentration in local extracellular spaces. Increased extracellular K^+ concentration promotes opening of K_{IR} channels with consequent hyperpolarization and vasodilation. This effect helps to maintain a rate of blood flow to the region commensurate with metabolic demands.

3. **Increased Extracellular Acidity.** Increased metabolic activity can also lead to increased extracellular H^+ concentration, which in turn causes hyperpolarization by augmenting the activity of potassium channels (probably mostly K_{ATP} and BK_{Ca} channels). The result is vasodilation and increased local blood flow.

What about Ca^{++}-Induced Ca^{++} Release from the SR?

Ca^{++} that comes in from the outside through DHP receptors can induce Ca^{++} release from the underlying SR through ryanodine receptors. This is Ca^{++}-induced Ca^{++} release similar to that in cardiac muscle. However, the amount of Ca^{++} entering the cytoplasm by this process seem to be rather small, and its importance for augmenting contraction in vascular smooth muscle is questionable. Most of the rise in cytoplasmic Ca^{++} concentration in response to membrane depolarization is thought to derive directly from Ca^{++} diffusion into the cells through DHP receptors.

What about Spontaneous Release of Ca^{++} from the SR?

As mentioned in Chapter 3, tiny bursts of Ca^{++} are spontaneously released from the SR through ryanodine receptors all the time. Do these "Ca^{++} sparks" increase smooth muscle tone? Probably not. In fact they may actually decrease tone by activating BK_{Ca} channels with consequent membrane hyperpolarization.

Here is an important clinical correlate. Ca^{++} channel blockers such as dihydropyridines are often used clinically to treat hypertension, angina, and heart failure. They relax vascular smooth muscle in preference to decreasing cardiac contractility. This is nice. The most important reason for this preferential effect is that L-type Ca^{++} channels (DHP receptors) have more affinity for Ca^{++} channel blockers when they are already somewhat activated by membrane depolarization. Resting membrane potentials of -50 to -35 mV for vascular smooth muscle, compared to resting membrane potentials of around -85 mV for cardiac muscle, make the difference. Vascular DHP receptors also differ slightly in primary polypeptide structure from cardiac DHP receptors, and such differences may contribute to their increased sensitivity to Ca^{++} channel blockers.

The G_q/IP_3 Pathway and the Role of the Sarcoplasmic Reticulum

There are many G-protein-coupled membrane receptors on vascular smooth muscle cells. Some of these promote contraction and others promote relaxation. The excitatory effects are mediated by G-proteins in the G_q and G_{12} classes. The inhibitory effects are mediated by G-proteins in the G_s class. The excitatory G_q pathway will be described now since it feeds directly into the Ca^{++}-calmodulin pathway (Figure 6).

When an excitatory agonist binds to its appropriate membrane receptor, G_q is activated. The α subunit of G_q (with bound GTP) activates a membrane-associated lipase called phospholipase C, which acts on a certain membrane phospholipid (phosphatidylinositol 4,5 bisphosphate) to form IP_3 (inositol 1,4,5 trisphosphate) and DAG (diacylglycerol). IP_3 diffuses in the cytoplasm to the SR. IP_3 doesn't have to diffuse very far in the cytoplasm because most of the SR lies very close to the caveolae of the sarcolemma. IP_3 binds to IP_3 receptors in the SR membranes with resulting Ca^{++} release through these receptors.

Note that there are two different types of Ca^{++} release channels in smooth muscle: ryanodine receptors (responsible for Ca^{++}-induced Ca^{++} release, and IP_3 receptors. IP_3 is by far the most important stimulator of Ca^{++} release from the SR in vascular smooth muscle.

There is often some degree of membrane depolarization associated with activation of the G_q/IP_3 pathway, which can result in activation of DHP receptors and increased Ca^{++} influx. The mechanism of this effect is not clear, nor is its importance established. Contractile responses to excitatory agonists depend predominantly on the IP₃ mechanism. Changes in membrane potential are of secondary importance. In fact, in some situations contraction can be increased with hardly any change in membrane potential. Induction of contraction without important changes in membrane potential is called pharmacomechanical coupling.

Examples of endogenous excitatory agonists that promote contraction *via* the G_q/IP₃ pathway include norepinephrine and epinephrine acting on α_1 receptors, angiotensin II acting on AT_1 receptors, vasopressin acting on V_1 receptors, and endothelin 1 acting on ET_A receptors. These agonists will be discussed more thoroughly in Part 4 of this chapter.

Agonist-Operated Cation Channels
As mentioned in Part 2, there are nonselective cation channels in the sarcolemma of vascular smooth muscle cells. At least some of these channels are directly controlled by excitatory agonists. The prime example is a certain purinergic receptor/channel called P_{2X}, which is activated by extracellular ATP. The resulting influx of Ca^{++} induces contraction by the Ca^{++}-calmodulin pathway. The concomitant influx of Na^+ along with Ca^{++} tends to depolarize the membrane a little, which might be expected to lead to further Ca^{++} influx *via* DHP receptors. However, the correlation between depolarization and contraction is not good and this pathway seems to represent pharmacomechanical coupling more than it represents electromechanical coupling.

Topic 3: The G_{12}/Rho-Kinase Pathway for Increasing Tone

Figure 7
The receptors for excitatory agonists are often linked to more than one type of G-protein. We have discussed the role of G_q. In addition, activated receptors can activate G_{12}. The alpha subunit of G_{12}, now with GTP attached instead of GDP, does a peculiar thing. It activates another G-protein called RhoA. RhoA is a small monomeric G-protein belonging to the Ras superfamily of GTP-binding proteins. It can exist either in the membrane or in the cytoplasm. Activated RhoA activates a cytoplasmic enzyme named Rho-kinase. Rho-kinase catalyzes the phosphorylation of myosin phosphatase, which reduces its activity and promotes contraction.

The above steps are all Ca^{++}-independent. Thus, for any given cytoplasmic Ca^{++} concentration, the Rho-mediated augmentation of contraction in effect increases the sensitivity of the excitatory machinery to Ca^{++}.

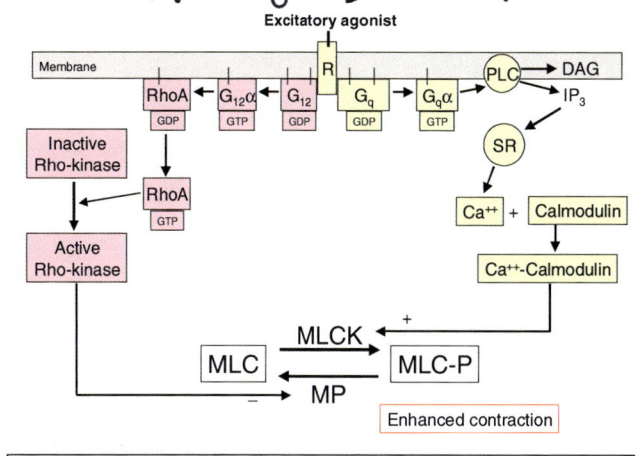

Figure 7. The G_{12}/Rho-kinase and G_q/IP₃ pathways for increasing tone in vascular smooth muscle. The G_q/IP₃ pathway is repeated here to emphasize that both pathways start from the same receptor and then run in parallel. See text for description.
MLC = regulatory myosin light chain
MLC-P = phosphorylated regulatory MLC
MLCK = myosin light chain kinase
MP = myosin phosphatase
R = G-protein-coupled membrane receptor
IP₃ = inositol 1,4,5 trisphosphate
DAG = diacylglycerol
PLC = phospholipase C
SR = sarcoplasmic reticulum/Ca^{++} stores

Other processes exist that decrease the sensitivity to Ca^{++} by decreasing the activity of myosin light chain kinase and/or increasing the activity of myosin phosphatase, but details are vague at this time.

Endogenous excitatory agonists that promote contraction partly by the Rho-kinase pathway include all of those mentioned above for the G_q/IP₃ pathway with the possible exception of angiotensin II.

Topic 4: The Thin Filament Pathway for Increasing Tone

Figure 8
Excitatory agonists, operating through G_q and phospholipase C, result in the production of IP₃ and DAG. We have already discussed the role of IP₃. What does DAG do? DAG remains in the membrane and activates a cytoplasmic enzyme called protein kinase C, which phosphorylates

various proteins that are involved in contraction. Only two of these proteins will be mentioned here – caldesmon and calponin. These proteins are bound to thin filaments. They exert an inhibitory effect on contraction, probably by influencing the position of tropomyosin along the thin filaments. Caldesmon may also compete with myosin S_1 for actin binding sites. When caldesmon and calponin are phosphorylated by protein kinase C, their inhibitory effect is diminished and the intensity of contraction is increased. This is thin filament regulation of contraction. Thin filament regulation is actually far more complex than this, but current understanding is so incomplete and foggy that further description is unwarranted.

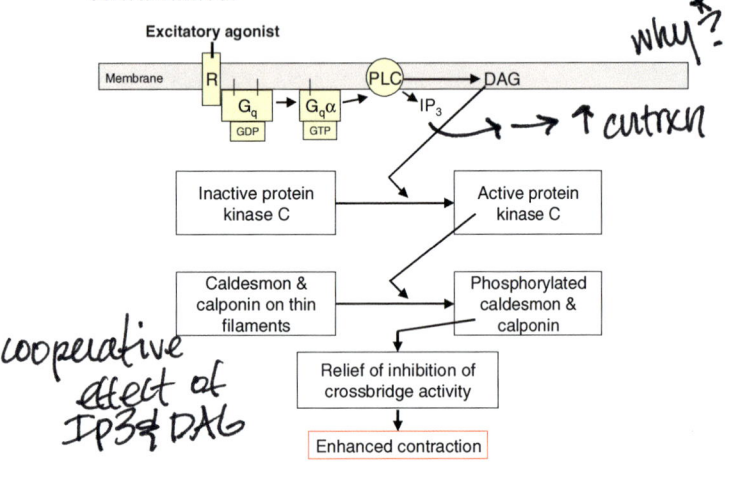

Figure 8. The thin filament pathway for increasing tone in vascular smooth muscle. See text for description.
R = G-protein-coupled membrane receptor
IP_3 = inositol 1,4,5 trisphosphate
DAG = diacylglycerol
PLC = phospholipase C

All of the endogenous excitatory agonists listed above are thought to promote contraction partly by the thin filament pathway, but not as importantly as by the G_q/IP_3 pathway, and probably not as importantly as by the Rho-kinase pathway.

Topic 5: The G_s/cGMP Pathway for Reducing Tone

Figure 9
When an inhibitory agonist binds to its membrane receptor, G_s is activated. You might remember G_s from cardiac muscle. In cardiac muscle, activated G_s has positive inotropic and chronotropic effects. In smooth muscle, however, it results in inhibition of contraction. The α subunit of G_s, with attached GTP activates membrane adenylyl cyclase and membrane guanylyl cyclase. Thus, both cAMP and cGMP are generated. cAMP activates protein kinase A (PKA) and cGMP activates protein kinase G (PKG). Both PKA and PKG phosphorylate various proteins that result in inhibition of contraction. Most notably, myosin light chain kinase is suppressed by phosphorylation and myosin phosphatase is stimulated, thereby tipping the balance toward dephosphorylation of regulatory myosin light chains and relaxation. It is likely that cGMP provides a much more important inhibitory signal than does cAMP, so we will refer to this pathway as the G_s/cGMP pathway. [Notice that myosin phosphatase is stimulated when phosphorylated by PKG even though, as mentioned above, it is inhibited when phosphorylated by Rho-kinase.]

In addition, PKG is thought to suppress L-type Ca^{++} channels and activate BK_{Ca} channels. Both of these effects tend to decrease Ca^{++} influx and, thereby, inhibit tone. PKG also inhibits RhoA (not shown in Figure 9), thereby reducing the inhibition of myosin phosphatase by Rho-kinase. This has the effect of decreasing the sensitivity to Ca^{++}.

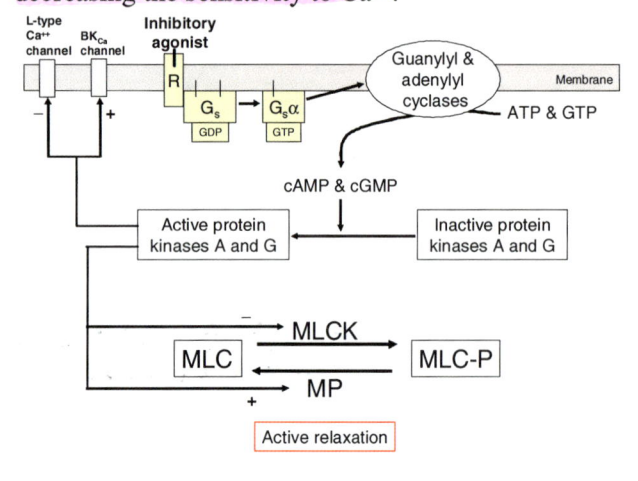

Figure 9. The G_s/cGMP pathway for decreasing tone in vascular smooth muscle. See text for description.
MLC = regulatory myosin light chain
MLC-P = phosphorylated regulatory MLC
MLCK = myosin light chain kinase
MP = myosin phosphatase
R = G-protein-coupled membrane receptor

Epinephrine acting on $β_2$ receptors, adenosine acting on A_2 receptors, and atrial natriuretic peptide all inhibit vascular smooth muscle by this pathway. In addition, nitric oxide (NO) inhibits vascular smooth muscle in the same way, except that it stimulates the pathway by activating a cytoplasmic guanylyl cyclase, bypassing the membrane events.

Part 4: Specific Endogenous Agonists

Topic 1: Excitatory Agonists

Norepinephrine and Epinephrine Acting on α_1 Adrenergic Receptors

Activated α_1 adrenergic receptors activate G_q and G_{12}. Contraction is then augmented by the Ca^{++}-calmodulin pathway (Figure 6), the G_{12}/Rho-kinase pathway (Figure 7), and the thin filament pathway (Figure 8).

While all of this is happening, the membrane depolarizes somewhat. Thus, Ca^{++} influx through DHP receptors increases, leading to a further augmentation of contraction mediated by the Ca^{++}-calmodulin pathway. It is not known how α_1 adrenergic stimulation causes membrane depolarization. Hypotheses include direct effects of norepinephrine on membrane Ca^{++} channels, K^+ channels, or nonselective cation channels.

Angiotensin II

The precursor protein, angiotensinogen, is created in the liver and secreted into blood. In blood it is converted to angiotensin I (a decapeptide) by renin, an enzyme secreted from the juxtaglomerular apparatus of the kidneys in response to sympathetic stimulation and to decreased proximal tubular delivery of Na^+. Angiotensin I is converted to angiotensin II (an octapeptide) by angiotensin converting enzyme located primarily on pulmonary endothelial cells. Angiotensin II, among many other actions, increases contraction of vascular smooth muscle. Thus, it has important effects on TPR, CO, MAP, and regional blood flows.

The mechanism of vasoconstriction in response to angiotensin II is essentially the same as that for norepinephrine – only the receptor is different (the AT_1 receptor). In addition, there is some evidence that angiotensin II does not activate the G_{12}/Rho-kinase pathway. There is usually some degree of membrane depolarization (again due to unresolved mechanisms) resulting in augmentation of contraction.

Vasopressin (Antidiuretic Hormone, ADH)

Vasoconstrictive actions of ADH are mediated by V_1 receptors. [V_2 receptors mediate the effect of ADH on renal water retention.] The post-receptor pathways are thought to be the same as for the α_1 adrenergic response.

Endothelin 1

Endothelin 1 is an extremely potent vasoconstrictor agent that is released from vascular endothelium under various circumstances. Its role in normal physiology is not understood. It has been tentatively implicated as a culprit in a wide range of cardiovascular diseases, including hypertension, heart failure, and coronary artery disease.

The signal transduction mechanism for the excitatory effect of endothelin 1 on vascular smooth muscle is similar to that for norepinephrine, angiotensin II, and vasopressin, except of course it has its own G-protein-coupled receptor in the sarcolemma (ET_A). There is an important difference however. The G_q that is activated by endothelin 1 receptors acts on Ca^{++} channels in the sarcolemma to increase Ca^{++} influx into the cell and contribute to membrane depolarization. These Ca^{++} channels are probably of the L-type (*i.e.* DHP receptors).

Topic 2: Inhibitory Agents

There are two mechanisms for decreasing tension in vascular smooth muscle, passive and active. Passive relaxation is due merely to release from stimulatory influences. For example, if norepinephrine activation of α_1 receptors decreases, smooth muscle relaxes – this is passive relaxation.

Active relaxation is more interesting. It can be the result of membrane hyperpolarization with a resulting decrease in Ca^{++} influx through DHP receptors (see Part 3, Topic 2 for inhibitory effects of hypoxia, extracellular K^+, and extracellular H^+). However, pharmacomechanical relaxation mechanisms are more important.

Epinephrine acting on β_2 receptors

At physiological concentrations, norepinephrine has almost no effect on β_2 receptors – they are activated almost entirely by epinephrine. So perhaps we should deal here only with epinephrine from the adrenal medulla. However, there is evidence that norepinephrine can be converted to epinephrine in the vicinity of postganglionic nerve endings, thus allowing for a possible effect of sympathetic nerve activity on β_2 adrenergic receptors.

The result of catecholamine activation of β_2 receptors on vascular smooth muscle is relaxation. This response operates *via* the G_s/cGMP pathway.

Nitric Oxide

Nitric oxide (NO) is generated in endothelial cells from L-arginine by the action of endothelial nitric oxide synthase (eNOS). eNOS is activated by a rise in intracellular Ca^{++} concentration. Ca^{++} influx into endothelial cells can result from the action of various agonists including acetylcholine, bradykinin, substance P, histamine, serotonin, ATP, and many others. These responses are very important in the inflammatory process. Probably the most important effector of Ca^{++} influx and NO production under normal circumstances is increased velocity of blood flow over the surface of endothelial cells.

NO diffuses from endothelial cells into nearby smooth muscle cells. It is probably also delivered to smooth muscle cells from circulating hemoglobin. Within the smooth muscle cells NO activates a cytoplasmic guanylyl cyclase by combining with its heme group. Thus, all of the G-protein-associated membrane apparatus is bypassed. Subsequent steps resulting in relaxation follow the cGMP pathway (Figure 9)

More detail about how NO contributes to regulation of regional blood flow will be presented in Chapter 16.

Bradykinin

Bradykinin is a nonapeptide (nine amino acids). It normally has no important role in regulating preload or afterload. Except for salivary glands and maybe skin, it probably has no role in regulating regional blood flows under normal healthy conditions. The import role of bradykinin is in acute inflammation. The inflammatory process is not discussed in this book, but the mechanisms of bradykinin generation and actions will be mentioned.

Figure 10

Bradykinin circulates in blood plasma as an inactive precursor called high molecular weight (HMW) kininogen. The enzyme that converts HMW kininogen to bradykinin is called kallikrein. Kallikrein also circulates in the blood as an inactive precursor called prekallikrein. Prekallikrein is converted to the active enzyme by activated Hageman factor. This same Hageman factor initiates the intrinsic leg of the blood clotting cascade. Inactive Hageman factor (factor XII) is converted to activated Hageman factor (factor XIIa) by negatively charged surfaces such as collagen and basement membrane, which are exposed to plasma by injury or certain pathological conditions. It appears that under some circumstances Hageman factor can also be activated by endothelial cell surfaces. Figure 10 illustrates this cascade.

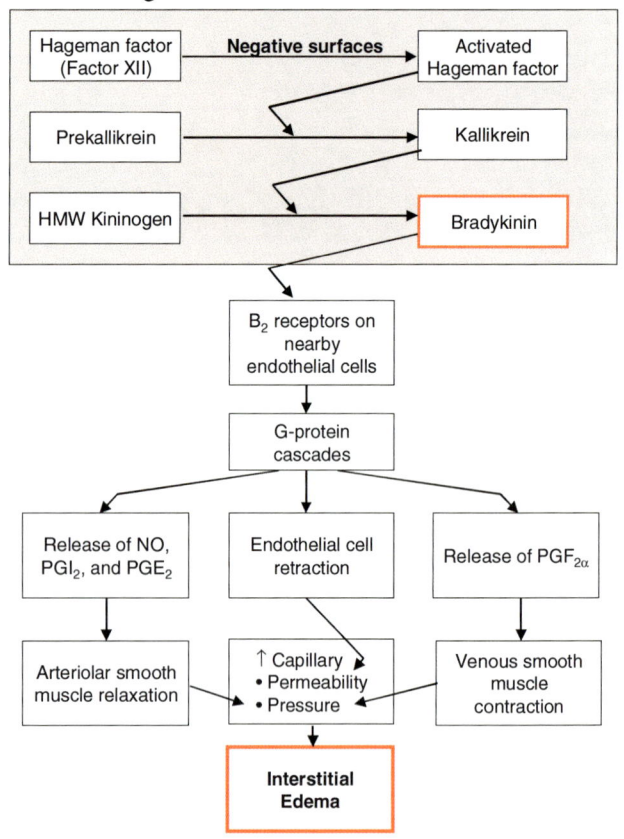

Figure 10. Generation of bradykinin and the local effects of bradykinin involved in inflammation. The gray backing indicates a negatively charged surface. [Note that the B_2 receptor is a bradykinin receptor. Try not to call it accidentally a beta 2 receptor.]
HMW = high molecular weight
NO = nitric oxide
PGI_2 = prostacyclin

It is important to realize that all of the reactions leading to the formation of bradykinin by the pathway shown in Figure 10 take place on negatively charged surfaces. Hageman factor does not generally have access to these surfaces except following some injury. Furthermore, any bradykinin that diffuses into the blood is rapidly broken down by enzymes called kininases. Thus, the action of bradykinin is ordinarily confined to the region of injury. There are two of these kininases (kininase I and kininase II). Kininase II is identical to angiotensin converting enzyme (ACE). Note that kallikrein feeds back on Hageman factor to cause further activation. Thus, a little kallikrein breeds more kallikrein and its generation is amplified.

There is an alternative pathway for localized generation of bradykinin that does not involve

Hageman factor, but we can pass on it for now. [If you want to learn more about bradykinin generation, see A.P. Kaplan, et al. Pathways for Bradykinin Formation and Inflammatory Disease, *J. Allergy Clin. Immunology*, 109: 195-209, 2002.]

Bradykinin acts on nearby endothelial cells where it activates G-protein-coupled receptors. The endothelial cells then release nitric oxide (NO) and prostaglandins (PGs) that influence nearby smooth muscle cells. The results are arteriolar dilation and venous constriction. Bradykinin also causes an increase in capillary permeability. These effects are all localized to the affected region. The increase in capillary permeability is brought about by endothelial cell retraction, which opens intercellular gaps in the endothelium (see Chapter 17, Part 3, Topic 8). All of these effects contribute to the development of interstitial edema as diagrammed in Figure 10. The mechanisms by which increased capillary blood pressure and increased capillary permeability lead to edema are discussed in Chapter 17. Bradykinin also stimulates pain fibers in the inflamed region.

In addition to bradykinin, two other kinins exist that are very closely related to bradykinin structurally and functionally. They are activated in much the same way as bradykinin, and are thought to have similar effects. The big difference is that their kininogens (low molecular weight kininogens) are located mainly in tissues, while HMW kininogen is located mainly in plasma.

There are certain situations such as severe burns in which so much bradykinin is generated in the injured area that it spills into the general circulation in sufficient quantity to have marked effects elsewhere in the body. The result can be generalized arteriolar vasodilation and increased capillary permeability. This process contributes importantly to the circulatory shock that often results from severe trauma and burns.

Remember that kininase II is identical to ACE. When ACE inhibitors are used for treating disorders such as hypertension, bradykinin may cause coughing and can even circulate in the blood in sufficient amounts to cause flushing and edema.

Atrial Natriuretic Peptide
The role of atrial natriuretic peptide (ANP) in long-term control of blood volume and mean arterial pressure will be discussed in Chapter 15. It is secreted by atrial muscle cells in response to stretch of the atrial wall. Among other things, it is a vasodilator. On vascular smooth muscle cells, it acts on G_s-protein-coupled receptors with the result that intracellular cGMP is increased and intracellular free Ca^{++} is decreased (Figure 9).

Other Vasodilatory Peptides
Other inhibitory vasoactive peptides include substance P, vasoactive intestinal peptide, calcitonin gene-related peptide (CGRP), neurotensin, and neuropeptide Y. Their roles in normal physiology are too obscure to dwell on here.

Adenosine
Adenosine is thought to be an important vasodilator in small coronary arteries and arterioles. It may also be an important arteriolar dilator in skeletal muscle. When the rate of O_2 consumption exceeds the rate of O_2 delivery (*e.g.* during myocardial ischemia or severe exercise), the rate of ATP utilization exceeds the rate of ATP generation and the concentration of AMP increases. AMP is broken down to adenosine and inorganic phosphate by an enzyme called 5' nucleotidase. Thus, when increased O_2 supply is needed, production of adenosine increases. Excess adenosine diffuses out of striated muscle cells and to nearby vascular smooth muscle cells where it activates a type of G_s-protein-coupled receptor called the adenosine A_2 receptor. Activation of A_2 receptors by adenosine, leads to smooth muscle relaxation by the Gs/cGMP pathway (Figure 9). In addition, adenosine acts on A_2 receptors on endothelial cells resulting in synthesis and release of nitric oxide. Thus, when striated muscle cells need more blood flow in order to get more O_2, resistance vessels cooperate by dilating.

Histamine
Histamine is synthesized in tissue mast cells and circulating basophils. It is stored in the secretory granules of these cells in very high concentrations (bound mainly to heparin) and released by exocytosis when these cells are activated by a variety of insults. Histamine acts locally to cause arteriolar dilation, increased capillary permeability, itching, and pain. Histamine is important in acute allergic and inflammatory responses. It probably has no role in the normal regulation of regional blood flows.

The effects of histamine are mediated by H_1, H_2, and H_3 receptors, which are all G-protein-coupled. The vascular effects involve mainly the H_1 receptors on endothelial cells leading to activation of phospholipase C and production of IP_3. The result is increased intracellular free Ca^{++} concentration which has two consequences, (1) production of NO which causes relaxation of nearby smooth muscle, and (2) endothelial cell retraction which increases endothelial permeability (especially in post-capillary venules).

Prostaglandins and Other Eicosanoids

These substances are made by endothelial cells and many other types of cells. Many of them have vasoactive properties – some cause vascular smooth muscle to contract and others cause relaxation.

They are known to be important in inflammation and some are released from endothelial cells in response to bradykinin, but no clear role has been established in normal regulation of blood flow. Their receptors on vascular smooth muscle cells are G-protein-coupled. Contraction is mediated by increased cytoplasmic Ca^{++} via the G_q/IP_3 limb of the Ca^{++}-calmodulin pathway (Figures 6 and 7). Relaxation is mediated by increased intracellular cAMP and cGMP via the G_s/cGMP pathway (Figure 9), and by decreased cytoplasmic Ca^{++}.

Endothelium-Derived Hyperpolarizing Factor

This substance can be released from endothelial cells. Its action on nearby vascular smooth muscle cells is to cause membrane hyperpolarization with consequent inhibition of contraction. Its chemical nature, stimulus for release, mechanism of action, and physiological role are not understood.

Topic 3: Summary of Endothelial Effects on Vascular Smooth Muscle

Figure 11

Many of the effects described above involve the endothelium. This figure summarizes the most relevant endothelial effects on vascular smooth muscle.

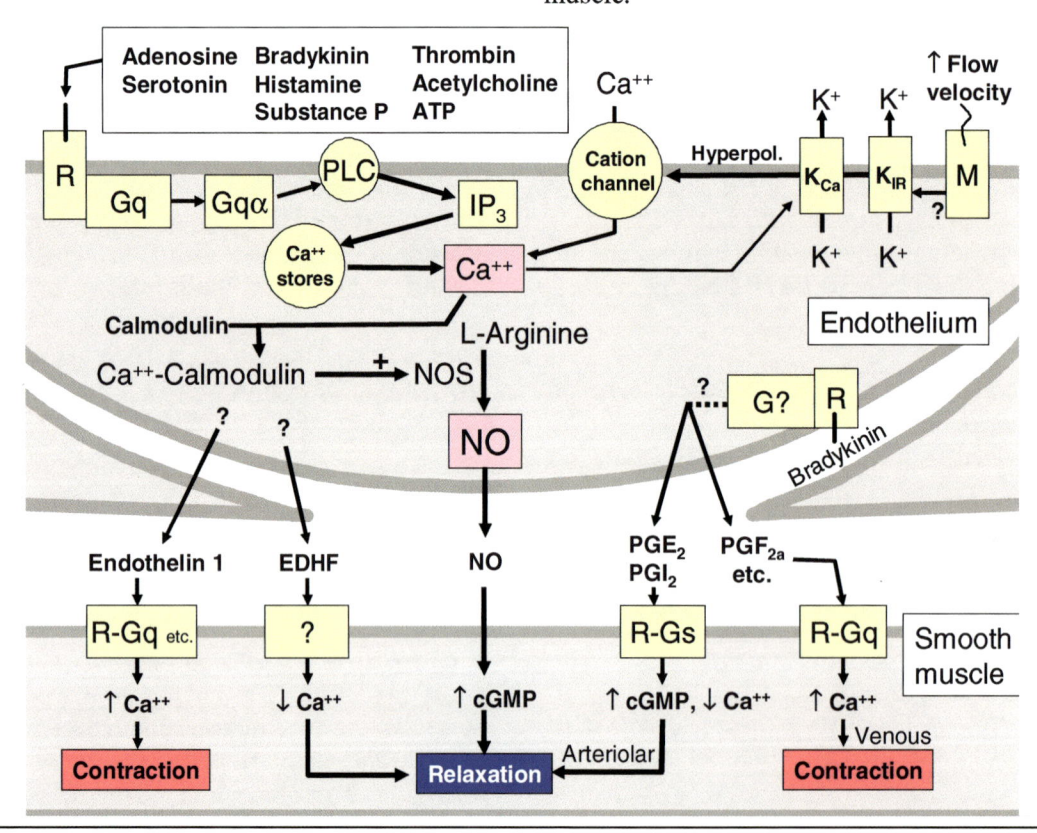

Figure 11. Some effects of endothelial cells on vascular smooth muscle. The endothelial pathways leading to increased synthesis of NO are actually much more complex than shown here.
M = mechano-receptor
NOS = nitric oxide synthase
NO = nitric oxide
EDHF = endothelial-derived hyperpolarizing factor.
R = G-protein-coupled receptor

Vascular Smooth Muscle

Here is a summary of the endogenous agonists discussed above.

	Receptors	Pathways
Excitatory Agonists		
Norepinephrine & epinephrine	α_1 adrenergic	$G_q/IP_3/Ca^{++}$/calmodulin G_q/DAG/thin filaments G_{12}/RhoA/Rho-kinase
Angiotensin II	AT_1	$G_q/IP_3/Ca^{++}$/calmodulin G_q/DAG/thin filament
Vasopressin (ADH)	V_2 (or V_1?)	$G_q/IP_3/Ca^{++}$/calmodulin G_q/DAG/thin filament G_{12}/RhoA/Rho-kinase
Endothelin 1	ET_A	$G_q/IP_3/Ca^{++}$/calmodulin G_q/DAG/thin filament G_{12}/RhoA/Rho-kinase Ca^{++} influx/depolarization
Inhibitory Agents		
Epinephrine	β_2 adrenergic	G_s/cGMP
Nitric oxide	Cytoplasmic guanylyl cyclase	cGMP
Bradykinin	B_2 on endothelial cells	See Figure 10
Atrial natriuretic peptide	?	G_s/cGMP
Adenosine	A_2	G_s/cGMP
Histamine	H_1 on endothelial cells	Nitric oxide/cGMP
Prostaglandins		G_s/cGMP
Endothelium-derived hyperpolarizing factor	?	?

Part 5: Vasodilator Drugs

Topic 1: Introduction

Vasodilator drugs are used in the treatment of hypertension, heart failure, and angina pectoris. What follows is a classification of these drugs with emphasis on mechanism of action. For pharmacological and clinical expansion of this subject, please consult pharmacology, pathophysiology, and clinical medicine textbooks.

We can divide drugs that result in vasodilation into two categories:
- Indirect vasodilators that work by inhibiting some action that causes vasoconstriction, thereby resulting in passive relaxation of vascular smooth muscle.
- Direct vasodilators that work by inducing active relaxation of vascular smooth muscle.

Topic 2: Agents that Produce Passive Relaxation (Indirect Vasodilators)

Smooth Muscle Receptor Blockers

Alpha 1 Adrenergic Blockers: Here the mechanism is obvious. If α_1 receptors on vascular smooth muscle are blocked, the main mechanism for active contraction is inhibited. Vascular smooth muscle relaxes in both resistance vessels (arterioles) and capacity vessels (veins and venules). Afterload to the heart decreases because of decreased TPR, and preload decreases due to decreased CVP. The prototype α_1 receptor blocker is prazosin, which is used in the treatment of hypertension.

Angiotensin II Receptor Blockers: Again, resistance vessels and capacity vessels are relaxed when the effect of angiotensin II on its receptor in vascular smooth muscle (AT_1 receptor) is blocked. Prime examples of AT_1 receptor blockers are losartan and valsartan. They are used for treating hypertension and heart failure.

Ca++ Channel Blockers: L-type Ca++ channel (DHP receptor) blockers inhibit activation of vascular smooth muscle brought about by depolarization. Smooth muscle in both resistance and capacity vessels can be inhibited, but resistance vessels are more sensitive. Examples are verapamil, diltiazem, and many dihydropyridines (amlodipine, nifedipine, and other -pines). These drugs are used for treating hypertension and angina pectoris.

Inhibitors of Renin Secretion and Angiotensin II Production

Beta 1 Adrenergic Blockers: These drugs are frequently used for treatment of hypertension, heart failure, and angina pectoris. They inhibit cardiac function, both heart rate and contractility, which reduces cardiac oxygen demands and MAP. Inhibiting cardiac functioning doesn't seem like a great strategy, but it seems to work. Perhaps one reason it works is that β_1 blockers also inhibit secretion of renin from the juxtaglomerular apparatus of the kidneys (see Chapter 15), thereby reducing the level of circulating angiotensin II with consequent passive relaxation of vascular smooth muscle. Examples of β_1 blockers include propranolol (also blocks β_2 receptors), metoprolol, atenolol, and many other ...olols.

ACE Inhibitors: Drugs such as captopril, enalapril, and many other -prils inhibit angiotensin converting enzyme. The result is reduced levels of circulating angiotensin II with consequent passive relaxation of both resistance and capacity vessels. ACE inhibitors are used for treating hypertension, heart failure, and angina pectoris.

Central Nervous System Adrenergic Inhibitors

Alpha 2 Agonists: These drugs inhibit sympathetic outflow from the brain. They act on α_2 receptors located mainly in presynaptic nerve endings. The result is less norepinephrine release from these nerve endings. These drugs might also have peripheral effects, but their main activity is thought to be central. The prime example of an α_2 agonist is clonidine, which is not only used as an antihypertensive drug, but also for treating anxiety, opiate withdrawal, and Tourette's syndrome.

Agents that Reduce Norepinephrine Release from Sympathetic Nerve Endings

Guanethidine: Guanethidine is the prime example of a category of drugs that inhibit norepinephrine release from postganglionic sympathetic nerve endings. It is transported into the nerve endings by the same transporter responsible for norepinephrine reuptake and is then taken up by the same transmitter vesicles that store norepinephrine, gradually replacing norepinephrine. Inhibition of norepinephrine release by guanethidine is not well understood. Guanethidine was a popular antihypertensive agent for many years, but is now seldom used because of side effects.

Reserpine: Reserpine inhibits the transport of norepinephrine into transmitter vesicles in noradrenergic nerve terminals. The vesicles become relatively depleted of norepinephrine. Diminished norepinephrine storage in transmitter vesicles leads to diminished release in response to action potentials. Reserpine is used in the treatment of hypertension.

> **Topic 3: Agents that Produce Active Relaxation (Direct Vasodilators)**

Agents that Influence the cGMP Signaling Mechanism

Nitrates and Nitrites: Examples of clinically useful nitrates and nitrites are nitroglycerin, amyl nitrite, and isosorbide dinitrate. Nitroglycerin is commonly used in the treatment of angina pectoris. These agents liberate NO in or near vascular smooth muscle cells by chemical processes that are not well understood. NO activates guanylyl cyclase, which leads to smooth muscle relaxation as discussed above. Venous smooth muscle is more sensitive to nitroglycerin than arterial muscle. The object of treatment with nitroglycerin is to provide a concentration that relaxes venous (including venular) smooth muscle without much effect on systemic arteriolar or coronary smooth muscle. The main reason that therapeutic doses of nitroglycerin relieve angina pectoris is that they decrease cardiac preload.

Na+ Nitroprusside: Na+ nitroprusside is used mainly in the treatment of hypertension. It relaxes both arterioles and veins, thereby reducing both preload and afterload. Its mechanism of action is probably the same as that of nitroglycerin and amyl nitrite (release of NO), but it is possible that it also has a direct activating effect on guanylyl cyclase.

Sildenafil: Sildenafil (Viagra) and its relatives inhibit vascular smooth muscle in the genitalia, most notably in the corpus cavernosum of the penis. The result is facilitation of penile erection. The mechanism, as currently understood, is rather simple. Viagra apparently diffuses easily across the sarcolemma without any need for a special transporter. In the cytoplasm, it inhibits the activity of a phosphodiesterase that ordinarily breaks down cGMP. Inhibition of this phosphodiesterase results in elevation of cGMP concentration in the cytoplasm with consequent inhibition of contraction by the steps illustrated in Figure 9. The cGMP phosphodiesterase in the genitalia is mainly an isoform called isoform 5, which is not common in other vascular smooth muscle. Selective action of Viagra on this particular phosphodiesterase isoform probably accounts for its relative selectivity for the genitalia.

Agents that Inhibit Ca^{++} Release from the Sarcoplasmic Reticulum

Hydralazine: The only drug in this category that is clinically useful is hydralazine. It inhibits Ca^{++} release from the SR. Hydralazine is used in the treatment of hypertension, usually along with other drugs such as β blockers and diuretics. Hydralazine inhibits arteriolar smooth muscle, but not venous smooth muscle. Thus, it reduces afterload while increasing preload. Hydralazine inhibits the action of IP$_3$ on SR IP$_3$ receptors. In addition, there is a lesser inhibitory effect on Ca^{++}-induced Ca^{++} release. It is not clear how hydralazine gets into the cell across the sarcolemma. It is also not understood why it only relaxes arteries but not veins.

Agents that Hyperpolarize the Plasma Membrane

Minoxidil and Diazoxide: These drugs are used in the treatment of hypertension. They relax arteriolar smooth muscle (not venous) by opening K$^+$ channels, thereby hyperpolarizing the plasma membrane. It is not clear which type of K$^+$ channel is most important.

Here is a summary of vasodilator drugs classed according to mechanism of action. The specific drugs listed here are those used as examples in the above discussion. Obviously, many others exist.

Indirect Vasodilators
- Smooth Muscle Receptor Blockers
    - α$_1$ adrenergic receptor blockers (prazosin et al.)
    - Angiotensin II receptor blockers (losartan, valsartan)
    - Ca^{++} channel blockers (amlodipine et al.)
- Inhibitors of Renin Secretion and Angiotensin II Production
    - β$_1$ adrenergic receptor blockers (propranolol, metoprolol, atenolol)
    - ACE inhibitors (captopril, enalapril)
- Central Nervous System Adrenergic Inhibitors
    - α$_2$ agonists (clonidine)
- Agents that Reduce Norepinephrine Release
    - Guanethidine
    - Reserpine

Direct Vasodilators
- Agents that Influence the cGMP Signaling Mechanism
    - Nitrates and nitrites (nitroglycerin, amyl nitrite, isosorbide dinitrate)
    - Na$^+$ nitroprusside
    - Sildenafil
- Agents that Inhibit Ca^{++} Release from the SR
    - Hydralazine
- Agents that Hyperpolarize the Plasma Membrane
    - Minoxidil
    - Diazoxide

Chapter 13

The Systemic Arterial System

This chapter discusses some basic physiology of the arterial system.

Part 1 explains why mean arterial pressure can be calculated simply as the product of cardiac output and total peripheral resistance, but is actually determined by the volume of blood in the arteries and compliance of the arterial tree. The ways in which the primary adjustable parameters of the system influence the distribution of blood between arteries and veins (and, therefore, mean pressures) are described.

Part 2 describes the arterial pulse and discusses the factors affecting its amplitude.

Part 3 describes variations in arterial pressures due to exercise, aging, and, hypertension.

Part 4 points out that blood flow in the large arteries is pulsatile, and mentions the importance of arterial compliance in promoting continuous flow through the microcirculation.

Part 5 deals with transmission of the pulse wave along the arterial tree.

Part 1: Mean Arterial Pressure

Topic 1: Mean Arterial Pressure can be Calculated from Cardiac Output and Total Peripheral Resistance

Mean arterial pressure is the pressure in a large artery averaged over the entire cardiac cycle. It declines only slightly with distance from the heart along the large arteries, and for this discussion can be considered the same everywhere.

On the average, the rate at which blood flows into the arterial tree (*i.e.* the cardiac output) must be exactly matched by the rate it flows out of the arteries to the veins. Therefore,

$$CO = (MAP - CVP) / TPR \quad (1)$$

CO = cardiac output
TPR = total peripheral resistance
MAP = mean arterial pressure
CVP = central venous pressure

The right hand side of this equation simply gives the average rate of flow from arteries to veins (driving pressure difference divided by resistance).

Solving Equation 1 for MAP, we get

$$MAP = CO \cdot TPR + CVP \quad (2)$$

Usually CVP is very small compared to MAP and can be ignored in Equation 2, leaving

$$MAP = CO \cdot TPR \quad (3)$$

We see that mean arterial pressure is ordinarily the product of cardiac output and total peripheral resistance. This result may seem too simple to be true; but it is approximately true, and is very useful. When CVP is elevated, as in congestive heart failure, Equation 2 should be used - but why not? It's also very simple. Note that the effect of changing CO on MAP is independent of whether a change in heart rate, contractility, blood volume, or venous capacity caused CO to change. MAP cannot tell the difference.

These equations do not directly reveal the physical factors responsible for MAP. They merely allow us to calculate the pressure difference between arteries and veins required for driving arterial outflow at exactly the same rate as inflow.

Topic 2: Mean Arterial Pressure is Determined by the Volume of Blood in the Arterial Tree

Figure 1

Arterial Compliance: The pressure within any closed, distensible container is determined by the contained volume and the elastic properties of the container walls. This relationship is generally expressed as a compliance curve. Figure 1 shows a compliance curve for the aorta. As volume increases, pressure increases. This is not surprising: a balloon would show about the same behavior. The slope of the curve at any point is called the arterial compliance.

Since MAP is normally about 90 mmHg, you can judge that a normal aorta contains an average of about 225 ml of blood. Increases or decreases in aortic blood volume would obviously result in corresponding changes in MAP. Note that over the ordinary working range of MAP, compliance remains reasonably constant. With severely elevated MAP, compliance decreases.

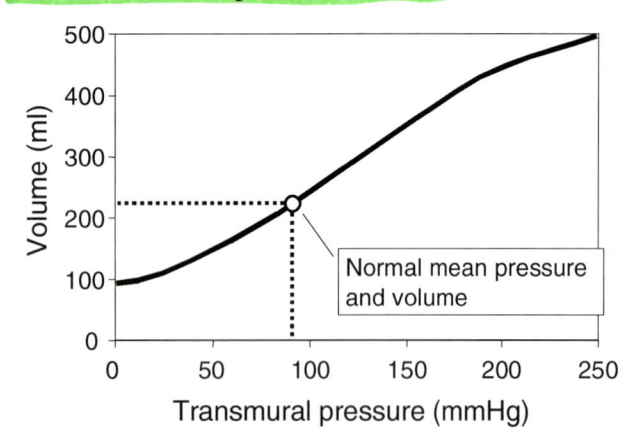

Figure 1. Compliance curve for the human aorta. Transmural pressure is the distending pressure, *i.e.* the difference in pressure between the inside of the vessel and the outside. If outside pressure is zero (*i.e.* equal to atmospheric pressure) then transmural pressure equals MAP. [Based on data of P. Hallock and J.C. Benson, *J. Clin. Invest.* 16:595, 1937.

Distensibility of the Wall: Compliance measures ease of expansion and is determined by the elastic properties of the vessel wall and by the volume of the vessel. If two vessels have identical walls but one is twice as large as the other, the larger one will have twice the compliance. Dividing compliance by volume gives the distensibility of the wall. The reciprocal of distensibility is sometimes called stiffness.

The Laplace Equation for Blood Vessels: The circumferential tension in the wall of a cylindrical container is given by the following form of the Laplace equation:

$T = P \cdot r$

  T = circumferential wall tension
  P = pressure
  r = radius of the tube

The Laplace equation tells us that the skinnier the tube, the less tension its wall must sustain for any given pressure. This is the reason that blood capillaries can contain high pressures although their walls are extremely fragile. [It is also the reason that high-pressure industrial pipes are skinny.]

Topic 3: Mean Arterial Blood Volume and Pressure are Determined by the Primary Adjustable Parameters of the System

Whenever the value of one of the primary adjustable parameters is altered, arterial and venous blood volumes change. Increased volume causes increased pressure just like pumping up an inner tube. The following adjustments all result in increased arterial blood volume and MAP:

- Increased heart rate and/or contractility. Blood is shifted from veins to arteries when the heart becomes a more effective pump.
- Increased total peripheral resistance. Blood is dammed back into the arteries. Arterial volume increases at the expense of venous volume.
- Decreased venous capacity (due to venous smooth muscle contraction or to compression of the veins). Blood is shifted (*via* the heart) from veins to arteries.
- Increased total blood volume. Pressure rises everywhere. The rise in central venous pressure results in a greater cardiac output (Starling effect) and, consequently, blood is shifted from veins to arteries.

But you already knew all this unless you just started reading here.

Pharmacological treatment of systemic arterial hypertension is aimed at one or more of the primary adjustable parameters as follows:

- Diuretics lower MAP by reducing total blood volume.
- Many antihypertensive drugs, including α_1 blockers, nitroglycerine, and nitroprusside, act, at least partly, by inhibiting venous smooth muscle, thereby increasing venous capacity.
- Many antihypertensive drugs, including α_1 blockers, Ca^{++} channel blockers, hydralazine, and nitroprusside, act, at least partly, by inhibiting smooth muscle in precapillary resistance vessels (*e.g.* arterioles), thereby reducing total peripheral resistance. Angiotensin converting enzyme (ACE) inhibitors also result in reduced tone of arteriolar smooth muscle since they decrease the rate of formation of angiotensin II.
- The therapeutic action of β_1 blockers probably depends at least partly on their ability to inhibit renin secretion from the juxtaglomerular cells in the kidneys.

For a discussion of vasodilator drugs, see Chapter 12.

The Systemic Arterial System

Part 2: The Arterial Pulse

Topic 1: The Arterial Pulse Wave

Figure 2

Since the heart is a pulsatile pump, blood enters the aorta in spurts. Each spurt immediately increases the blood pressure just beyond the aortic valve and causes distension of the ascending aorta. This pulse of increased pressure and distension rapidly moves as a wave along the arterial tree. It can be palpated over any large superficial artery. The shape of the pressure pulse in the aorta is shown in Figure 2. The maximum pressure attained is called the systolic pressure and the minimum is the diastolic pressure. The difference between systolic and diastolic pressures (*i.e.*, the amplitude of the pulse) is called the pulse pressure.

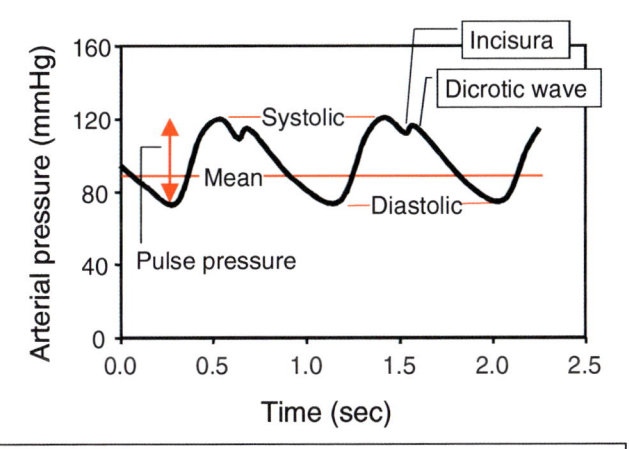

Figure 2. The aortic pressure pulse.

The mean pressure can be obtained by dividing the area under a pulse curve by the duration of the pulse. The mean pressure in the brachial artery at a heart rate of about 60-80/min is approximately equal to the diastolic pressure plus one-third the pulse pressure.

The steep ascending limb of the pulse is caused by rapid ventricular ejection. The more gradual descending limb results from run-off of blood through the microcirculation to the veins. A perturbation occurs along the descending limb. In the aorta, this perturbation consists of a sharp indentation named the incisura followed by a wave called the dicrotic wave. The incisura marks the end of ventricular systole and the beginning of ventricular diastole. The dicrotic wave is a secondary pressure pulse caused mainly by reflection of the primary pulse off the just-closed aortic valve.

Topic 2: Determinants of Pulse Pressure

The amplitude of the arterial pulse is determined by the difference between arterial inflow and outflow during the rapid ejection period. The greater the pulsatile expansion of the arterial system during each rapid ejection period, the greater is the amplitude of the pulse. The pulse pressure is also influenced by the compliance of the arterial system. For any given volume expansion during the rapid ejection period, pulse pressure increases as arterial compliance decreases. In other words, the stiffer the arterial system, the greater the pulse pressure.

Arterial expansion during the rapid ejection period is influenced by several factors, but most importantly by stroke volume. When stroke volume increases, pulse pressure increases.

Arterial expansion during rapid ejection is also influenced to some extent by the duration of the rapid ejection period. For example, when contractility increases, the rapid ejection period shortens; less time is available for peripheral run-off, and the pulse pressure increases. Changes in MAP also influence the duration of the rapid ejection period (remember the effect of afterload on the rate of rapid ejection). Afterload ↓ ejection

Figure 3

The aortic compliance curve may be helpful in visualizing how expansion of the arteries during the rapid ejection period (given by the vertical arrows) determines the pulse pressure (horizontal arrows).

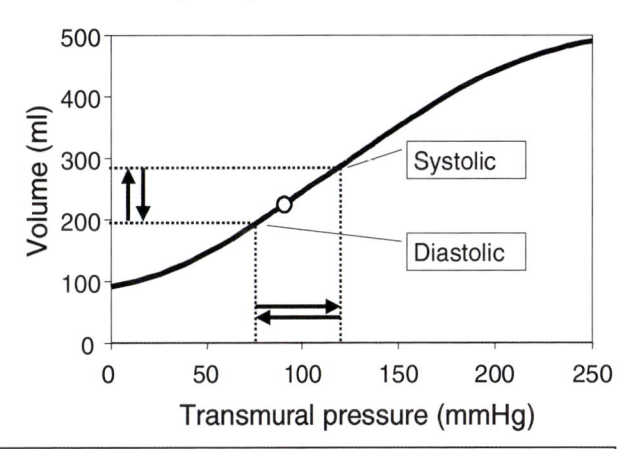

Figure 3. Aortic compliance curve. Arrows indicate the rhythmic changes in volume and pressure resulting from left ventricular pumping.

Topic 3: Systolic and Diastolic Pressures

See Figure 2 again

Systolic and diastolic pressures are determined by the mean pressure and by the amplitude of the pulsation around the mean (the pulse pressure). For any given mean pressure, as the amplitude of the pulse increases, systolic pressure goes up and diastolic pressure goes down. Analogous behavior is exhibited by a rope held out straight between two people. The rope has some mean height above the floor. If one end of the rope is rhythmically flipped above and below the mean, transverse displacement waves travel to the other end. The maximum and minimum heights are determined by the mean and the amplitude of oscillation around the mean.

Clinically, we usually report systolic and diastolic pressures, since these are the measurements made with the cuff/auscultation technique. However, it is worth keeping in mind that these quantities are secondary consequences of mean pressure and pulse pressure.

Part 3: Some Variations in Arterial Pressures

Topic 1: Effects of Exercise

The cardiovascular events occurring during vigorous exercise include:
- Reduction in total peripheral resistance (due to dilation of arterioles in active skeletal muscle)
- Increased cardiac output (mediated by increased stroke volume and increased heart rate).

Figure 4

These events have opposing effects on MAP (Equation 3). However, cardiac output increases more than peripheral resistance decreases, with the result that MAP increases. The increased stroke volume results in an increased pulse pressure. A briefer rapid ejection period (due to increased contractility and increased heart rate) contributes to this increase in pulse pressure.

Since MAP and pulse pressure both increase, the rise in systolic pressure exceeds the rise in diastolic pressure. In many forms of exercise (*e.g.* running), diastolic pressure may rise only slightly in spite of a substantial rise in MAP.

Topic 2: Effects of Aging (See Chapter 18 for more on aging)

Figure 5

This figure shows average values for systolic and diastolic pressures of normal men and women at various ages. The following observations can be made:
- Systolic, diastolic, and mean pressures all gradually increase with age
- Systolic pressure increases with age more than does diastolic pressure, so that pulse pressure gradually increases
- Systolic pressure rises faster with aging in postmenopausal women (assuming no estrogen treatment) than in men of the same ages.

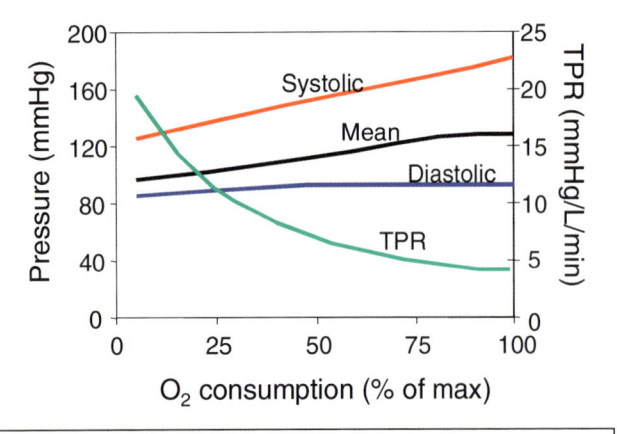

Figure 4. Effect of increasing intensity of exercise on arterial pressures and total peripheral resistance. The rate of oxygen consumption (expressed as a percent of the maximum ability to consume oxygen) is a measure of the intensity of exercise.

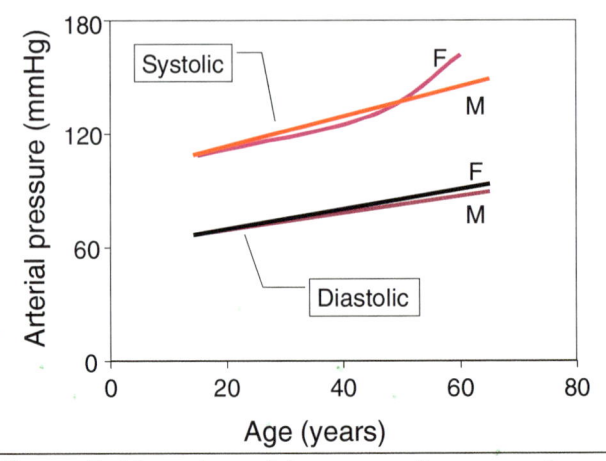

Figure 5. Normal arterial pressures for men and women as a function of age.

The Systemic Arterial System

The gradual increase in MAP is caused by a gradual increase in total peripheral resistance with aging, rather than by an increase in cardiac output. The tendency for increased TPR and MAP with age is based on population averages. Not everyone follows this tendency. In those people who develop these changes with age, the mechanisms include a decrease in β_2 adrenergic responsiveness, a decrease in release of endothelial nitric oxide, and structural changes in precapillary resistance vessels (also see Chapter 18).

Figure 6

The increased pulse pressure results from the tendency during aging (especially at rather advanced ages) for the shape of the arterial compliance curve to change. Figure 6 compares the compliance curve for a young aorta to that for an old aorta.

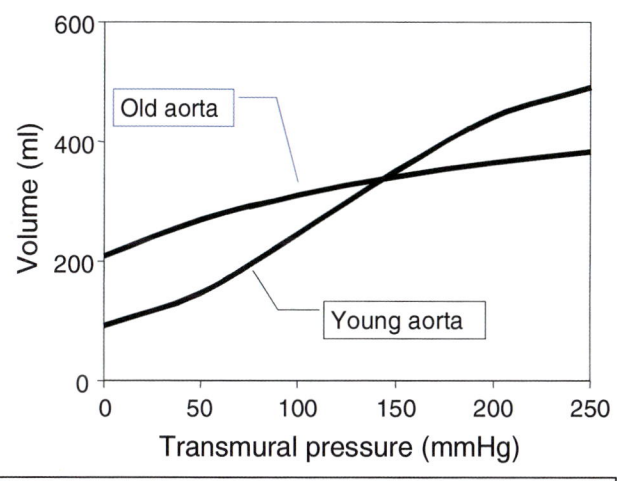

Figure 6. Compliance curves for young (about 23 years) and old (about 75 years) human aortas. [Based on data of P. Hallock and I.C. Benson, J. Clin. Invest. 16:595, 1937.]

The major differences are:
- The unstressed volume (*i.e.*, the volume at zero transmural pressure) is greater for the old aorta.
- The compliance throughout the physiological range of pressures is less for the old aorta.

As a result of decreased arterial compliance, expansion of old arteries during the rapid ejection period causes the pulse amplitude to be greater than it would be for young arteries.

Topic 3: Arterial Pressures in Systemic Hypertension

Patients with systemic arterial hypertension generally have high TPR, thus MAP is high. Often their large arteries are stiffer than normal leading to large pulse pressures. Because of the large PP, systolic pressure is elevated much more than MAP, but diastolic pressure is not elevated as much as MAP. Consequently, patients with hypertension usually have greatly elevated systolic pressure, but may have only moderately elevated diastolic pressure.

The current criterion for diagnosis of stage 1, systemic arterial hypertension is a resting diastolic pressure greater than 90 mmHg or a systolic pressure greater than 140 mmHg.

Opinion:
Assuming normal cardiac output, MAP indicates the health of small resistance vessels and PP indicates the health of large arteries. These are separate though often concurrent problems: increased MAP results from high TPR and high PP results from low arterial compliance. It would seem that MAP and PP are the metrics that should be used for patient evaluation, rather than systolic and diastolic pressures.

Part 4: Blood Flow in the Large Arteries

Topic 1: Flow in Large Arteries is Pulsatile

Blood flow in the large arteries is markedly pulsatile. In fact, flow becomes retrograde (back toward the heart) briefly during each cardiac cycle, especially in the upper aorta. Here, to some extent, the blood sloshes back and forth (mostly forth) with each cycle. Even in the larger arteries of the extremities, flow is markedly pulsatile, dropping to zero during diastole. It is not until rather small arteries are reached that forward flow becomes continuous, and not until well into the microcirculation that flow becomes essentially smooth.

Because of the very rapid changes in blood velocity in the large arteries, flow here is not entirely laminar, but rather is disturbed by brief bursts of disordered flow during systole.

Topic 2: Importance of Arterial Compliance

If the arteries were rigid tubes instead of compliant tubes and could not expand during systole, systolic pressure would be tremendously high and diastolic pressure would be zero. A volume of blood equal to the entire stroke volume would be delivered into the microcirculation during systole, but none during diastole. Flow through the capillaries, as well as through the arteries, would be extremely jerky. With compliant vessels, only a portion of the stroke volume (about one-third at resting heart rates) moves through the microcirculation during systole. The remainder (about two-thirds) distends the arteries during systole and then is gradually pushed through the microcirculation during diastole by elastic recoil of the arterial walls.

Part 5: Transmission of the Arterial Pulse Wave

Topic 1: General Characteristics

The arterial pulse wave can be pictured as a ripple traveling along the flowing stream of blood. Its velocity depends only slightly on the velocity of blood flow. Arterial pulse waves can also be likened to sound waves traveling in air. Sound waves travel much faster than the wind. Arterial pulse waves travel much faster than blood.

The velocity of the pulse wave increases as distensibility of the vessel wall decreases. Consequently, it is possible to assess the condition of the arterial tree by measuring pulse wave velocity. The arterial pulse wave normally travels at a velocity of about 3 m/s in the ascending aorta, increases to about 10 m/s in larger arterial branches, and up to 25-30 m/s in small arteries. For comparison, the mean velocity of blood flow in the aorta is under 0.5 m/s, and even less elsewhere. The progressive increase in velocity of the pulse wave is caused partly by decreasing distensibility of the arterial walls and partly by the increasing ratio of wall thickness to vessel diameter as the arterial tree is traversed.

One should not get the impression that only a short stretch of the arterial system experiences the pulse at any instant, with all the rest of the system uninvolved. The propagation velocity of the pulse is so fast relative to its duration that each wave is spread over the entire systemic arterial tree during most of its period. The smallest most distal arteries have already begun their pulsation by the time the incisura is developing at the root of the aorta.

Topic 2: Origin of the Incisura and Dicrotic Wave

At the root of the aorta, the incisura is coincident with closure of the aortic valve; at sites that are more distal, the entire wave, including the incisura, is delayed by the propagation time. The incisura results from the fact that at the moment of valve closure the column of blood in the aorta tends to continue moving forward by inertia, even though no more blood is being expelled by the left ventricle. Thus, just beyond the valve, a sharp reduction in pressure is created. This dip lasts only an instant because the flow of blood in the aorta promptly reverses its direction in response to the reversed pressure gradient. There is then a brief moment of retrograde flow in the aorta that sharply elevates the pressure at the root of the aorta thus completing the incisura.

The incisura is propagated distally as a transitory negative deflection superimposed on the primary wave. The retrograde flow in the aorta causes a rebound positive pressure at the root of the aorta that is reflected off the closed aortic valve and propagated distally as the dicrotic wave.

Topic 3: Changes in Shape of the Arterial Pulse Wave during Transmission

Figure 7

As the pulse wave travels away from the heart its shape changes. The major changes are:
- The sharp incisura is gradually smoothed out in the aorta and its name changes to the *dicrotic notch*.
- The ascending limb becomes steeper and reaches a higher systolic pressure.
- The amplitude of the dicrotic wave increases
- The diastolic pressure decreases.
- The increasing systolic and decreasing diastolic pressures lead to an increasing pulse pressure; in fact, the pulse pressure in the femoral artery may be almost twice that at the root of the aorta.

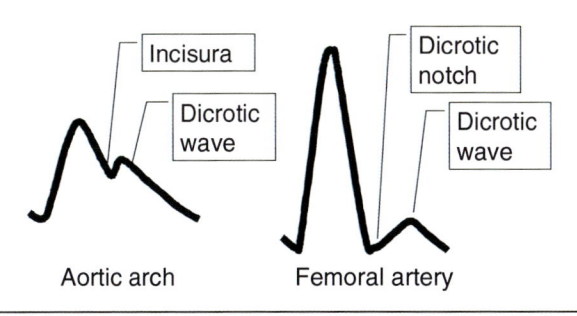

Figure 7. Shape of the arterial pulse at two different locations

The most important reasons for these changes are provided as hypertext [pulse shape].

Topic 4: Attenuation of the Arterial Pulse in the Microcirculation

Although the arterial pulse wave gradually increases in amplitude as it passes along the large arteries, it is abruptly attenuated in the precapillary resistance vessels, and is very small in the capillaries. A pulse of only about 1 mmHg normally reaches the systemic capillaries (somewhat larger in pulmonary capillaries).

Attenuation of the pulse is usually attributed to *damping* in the precapillary resistance vessels. The geometry and viscoelastic properties of these vessels are such that pressure fluctuations at the frequency of the heartbeat are not transmitted well; instead, the pulse energy is dissipated as heat. At least two other factors besides damping contribute to the abrupt attenuation of the pulse in the microcirculation. The first of these is *reflection* off the precapillary resistance barrier. That portion of the pulse energy that is reflected back toward the heart is not available for transmission into the microcirculation. The other factor is *dilution* of the pulse energy as the pulse wave enters the microcirculation, since the latter has far greater total cross-sectional area than the large arteries.

Chapter 14

The Systemic Venous System

This chapter examines the physiology of the venous system.
Part 1 looks at the compliance properties of the venous system and venous pressures.
Part 2 describes the venous pulse.
Part 3 emphasizes the importance of the venous system as a variable blood reservoir.
Part 4 describes two auxiliary pumps that aid venous return: the relatively minor respiratory pump, and the very important skeletal muscle pump.

Part 1: Venous Pressure

Topic 1: Compliance of the Venous System

Figure 1

The average pressure in the venous system is determined by the venous blood volume and the compliance properties of the veins. A reasonable value for a reclining person at rest is roughly 10 mmHg. A compliance curve for a typical large vein is shown in Figure 1; an arterial compliance curve is shown for comparison.

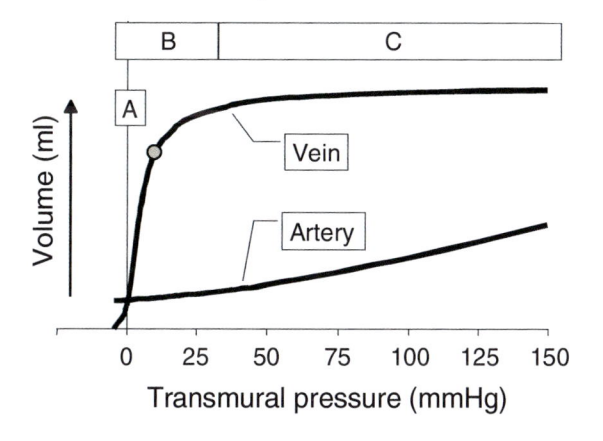

Figure 1. Compliance curve for a vein compared to that for an artery, both containing the same volume at zero transmural pressure. The dot represents mean pressure in the entire venous system at rest.
A = Pressure range in which the vein partially collapses. Compliance is very high.
B = Pressure range in which venous compliance is greater than arterial compliance.
C = Pressure range in which venous compliance is less than arterial compliance.

Figure 1 illustrates the following important features of veins:

- **Veins collapse when transmural pressure falls below zero:** If the pressure inside a vein falls just below the pressure outside of it, essentially no blood remains in the vein. It is all sucked out. This result stems from the fact that veins, unlike arteries, readily collapse. Collapse from a circular cross section to an elliptic cross section begins at a transmural pressure of roughly 6-7 mmHg. As transmural pressure is reduced further, collapse proceeds to flatter ellipses until finally, at just below zero, the vein is entirely depleted of contents.

- **Veins have a very high compliance at low pressures.** Throughout the range of transmural pressures from roughly 0-7 mmHg veins can accommodate large increases in blood volume with very small increases in pressure. In other words, over this pressure range, the compliance of veins is very large compared with that of arteries. This is because when veins are in a state of complete or partial collapse, expanding them by adding more blood does not require stretching of their walls but merely establishes a more circular cross section. Thus, to change the average pressure in the venous system by just a few mmHg requires adding or subtracting quite a lot of blood. At low venous pressure, the veins are roughly 15-20 times more compliant than are arteries at normal arterial pressures.

- The **total volume of blood that the veins can hold before their walls begin to stretch is very large.** This accounts for the fact that while the average pressure in the venous system is only about 10 mmHg, it contains at least 75% of the systemic blood volume.

- The **compliance of veins is very low at high pressures.** Further expansion of a fully rounded vein becomes progressively more difficult as the pressure increases. Just beyond full rounding, the compliance of a vein is greater than that of an artery of comparable size, but at venous transmural pressures in the approximate range of 25-50 mmHg, venous compliance becomes less than arterial compliance. At even higher transmural pressures the veins become almost completely nondistensible. Low compliance of veins at relatively high pressures is important in helping to prevent pooling of blood in the legs during standing, at which time venous hydrostatic pressures in the legs and feet may be quite high.

Topic 2: Mean Venous Volume and Pressure are determined by the Primary Adjustable Parameters of the System

The volume shifts between arteries and veins that result from readjustments in the primary adjustable parameters of the system have been described in previous chapters. Venous volume and pressure are decreased by increased heart rate, increased contractility, and increased total peripheral resistance. Increased venous capacity, or reduced blood volume result in decreased venous pressure.

Topic 3: The Venous Pressure Gradient and Central Venous Pressure

For now, we will refer to a reclining person in whom all parts of the vascular system are at approximately the same height. This restriction allows us to ignore the effects of gravity.

With a normal cardiac output of about 5-6 L/min, the pressure in collecting venules is about 13 mmHg. Average pressure in the right atrium is roughly 2 mmHg. This rather small pressure gradient is sufficient to drive blood back to the heart since the veins offer very little resistance to flow.

Most of the pressure drop from venules to right atrium occurs within the venules and small veins. There is also a small pressure drop in the large abdominal veins because these veins are often partially collapsed or compressed. Abdominal veins partially collapse whenever intra-abdominal pressure rises above intravenous pressure. Compression can occur if the intestine or the diaphragm impinges on veins. At regions of compression or collapse, resistance to flow is increased and pressure can drop a few mmHg.

When large veins are fully open, they offer almost no resistance to flow, and the pressure drop through them is negligible. This is generally true of intrathoracic veins, and it is found that venous pressures anywhere within the thorax are equal within a fraction of a mmHg. This uniform pressure in intrathoracic veins (and right atrium) is called the central venous pressure, CVP. A CVP of about 2 mmHg is normal for a reclining person.

Topic 4: Role of Negative Intrathoracic Pressure

By virtue of elastic recoil, the lungs exert a continuous inward pull on the chest wall, and the chest wall exerts a continuous outward pull on the lungs. These elastic forces result in a negative pressure in the intrathoracic space that oscillates between about -3 to -7 mmHg with breathing, and averages about -4 mmHg. Thus, the transmural pressure across the walls of intrathoracic veins and the right atrium normally averages about 6 mmHg, which is considerably greater than that for large extrathoracic veins. Consequently, the intrathoracic veins and the right atrium do not collapse. Instead, they expand with ample blood during ventricular systole to serve as a large blood reservoir that can be drawn upon by the right ventricle during diastole.

Part 2: The Venous Pulse

The left atrial pulse was described in Chapter 5. The right atrial pulse is nearly identical except that mean pressure is somewhat lower (about 2 mmHg instead of 7 mmHg). The right atrial pulse travels as a wave away from the right atrium out along the central veins. It can be detected at considerable distances from the heart.

The jugular vein (preferably the right internal jugular since it leads most directly to the right atrium) is a convenient site for observing the venous pulse. The right jugular pulse is often examined by physicians to gain information about right atrial pressure and certain aspects of right heart dynamics.

Figure 2

The waveform of a normal right jugular pulse is shown in Figure 2. The three positive waves (*a*, *c*, and *v*) and the two negative waves (*x* and *y*) are produced in essentially the same ways as their left

The Systemic Venous System

atrial counterparts described in Chapter 5.

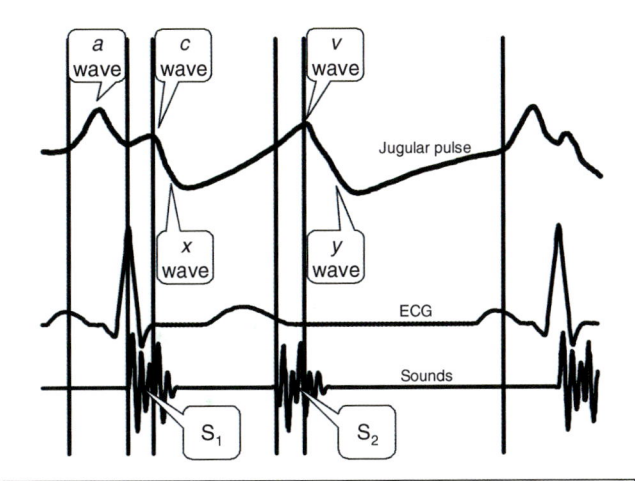

Figure 2. Waveform of the jugular pulse. ECG and heart sounds are shown for comparison. Vertical lines demarcate phases of the cardiac cycle. If you have trouble identifying the phases see Chapter 5.

- The *c* wave is caused by a small amount of blood propelled back into the right atrium before the tricuspid valve is fully closed, and by backward bulging of the tricuspid valve after it closes. In addition, the systolic pressure pulse in the nearby carotid artery is transmitted to the jugular and adds to the *c* wave (in fact, *c* stands for carotid).
- The *x* wave is caused by movement of the base of the heart toward the apex during the rapid ejection period. It represents systolic suction.
- The *v* wave is caused by atrial and central venous filling as blood circulates back to the heart during ventricular systole and the isovolumetric relaxation period. At the instant the tricuspid valve opens, blood is sucked into the right ventricle from the right atrium and right atrial pressure drops very quickly. Thus, the peak of the jugular *v* wave marks the instant of tricuspid valve opening.
- The *y* wave results from the fact that during the rapid filling period blood is sucked out of the right atrium by the recoiling right ventricle faster than it passively flows into the right atrium from the *vena cavae*. As atrial filling continues during the reduced filling period of the ventricle, atrial pressure gradually rises, thus completing the *y* wave.
- The *a* wave results from atrial contraction and is completed just prior to the onset of ventricular systole.

Mean right atrial pressure (MRAP) can be estimated from the jugular vein by noting how far up the neck the vein is distended with blood. Above the point at which transmural jugular pressure drops below zero, the jugular vein is collapsed. MRAP is estimated as the vertical distance between the point of jugular collapse and the right atrium. The subject's head and trunk can be tilted at various angles from horizontal to facilitate this measurement.

Part 3: The Venous System is a Variable Blood Reservoir

Topic 1: Effect of Sympathetic Nerve Activity on Venous Blood Volume

Figure 3

The peripheral veins are richly endowed with smooth muscle, which in turn is innervated by sympathetic nerves. Figure 3 shows the effect of increased sympathetic activity on the compliance curve for the venous system. Increased sympathetic activity, acting *via* norepinephrine and α_1 receptors, leads to constriction of the venous system so that for any pressure the system contains less blood (*i.e.* venous capacity is reduced).

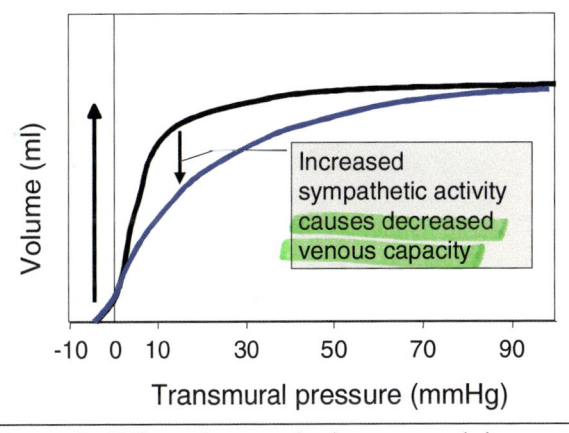

Figure 3. Effect of sympathetic nerve activity on the venous compliance curve.

Topic 2: The Reservoir Function of the Venous System

Figure 4

Since the volume of blood contained in veins is large and variable, the venous system is a blood reservoir. Figure 4 shows results of an experiment that demonstrates shifting of fluid out of leg veins in response to sympathetic nerve stimulation.

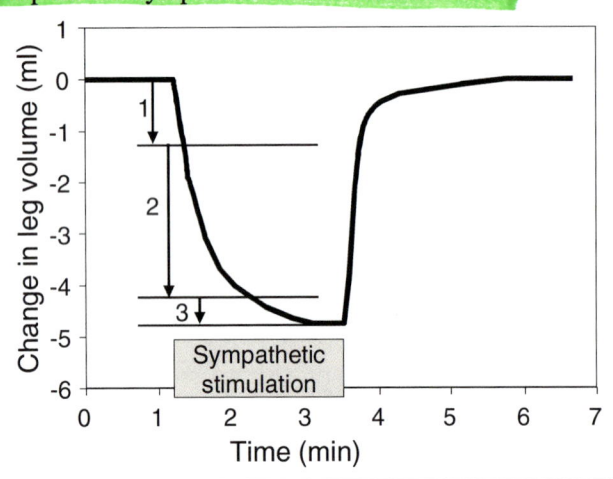

Figure 4. Effect of sympathetic nerve stimulation on leg volume. Steps 1, 2, and 3 correspond to the three mechanisms of blood mobilization described in the text. The data are from experiments on cats by S. Melander, *Acta Physiol. Scand.* 50 (Suppl. 176): 1-86, 1960.

There are three components to the decrease in fluid volume (measured as a change in total leg volume).
1. The first component results from the fact that when arteriolar resistance increases, flow rate into small veins momentarily becomes less than flow rate out. The walls of the veins passively recoil to contain the reduced volume.
2. The second component results from sympathetic excitation of vascular smooth muscle in the walls of the veins themselves. Blood is squeezed out of the leg toward the heart.
3. The third, and slowest, component of volume decrease results from the fact that when arterioles constrict, the pressure in capillaries and venules goes down. When this happens, the balance of pressures normally maintained between capillary/venule blood and tissue spaces is upset, and a slow net movement of extravascular fluid into the capillary/venule blood takes place. This fluid flows out of the leg as blood. The mobilization of extravascular fluid augments the reservoir function of the veins themselves.

A maximum of about one-third of the total blood volume in the leg can be shifted out of the veins.

Topic 3: Role of the Venous Reservoir in Exercise

In certain special circumstances, shifting of blood from veins to other parts of the circulation is particularly important. Two of these circumstances will be mentioned here. The first is exercise.

During vigorous exercise, the arterioles in active skeletal muscle dilate. There can be a considerable drop in total peripheral resistance and a large increase in blood flow through the active muscles. Decreased total peripheral resistance promotes an increased volume of blood in the veins, and if the capacity of the venous system were not diminished during vigorous exercise, the venous volume would rise. The increased venous blood volume would be at the expense of arterial blood volume and MAP would decrease. This would be self-defeating, since the decrease in MAP would tend to decrease blood flow through active muscles.

Fortunately, during vigorous exercise, there is increased sympathetic activity to veins and they constrict. Venous constriction during exercise is probably essential to attain the necessary increases in MAP and CO (although there is currently some controversy about the importance of this effect). Venous constriction is greatly aided by compression of the veins by contracting skeletal muscle, which will be discussed below.

Topic 4: Role of the Venous Reservoir in Hypovolemia

The second special circumstance to be mentioned here is hemorrhage. Following severe hemorrhage (say 25% of total blood volume) there is a problem keeping the mean arterial pressure high enough to keep blood flowing through vital organs fast enough. Arterioles in many organs constrict and this helps support MAP; but more to the present point, veins constrict, and an appreciable fraction of the remaining blood is shifted to the arterial side.

Venous-to-arterial shifting of blood supports MAP and helps keep the circulation going at a rate consistent with life; it can be regarded as an autotransfusion. The reflex pathways involved in this response are discussed in Chapter 15.

Part 4: Venous Pumps

Topic 1: The Respiratory Pump

During quiet breathing, intrathoracic pressure drops to about -7 mmHg during inspiration and rises to about -3 mmHg during expiration. Therefore, with each inspiration, the central veins expand and blood is sucked into them from the extrathoracic veins. During expiration, blood is squeezed out of the thoracic veins. The volume of blood sucked into the thorax during inspiration is greater than the volume squeezed back out during expiration. This discrepancy probably results from the fact that during inspiration, the right ventricle passively expands and its stroke volume increases by the Starling effect. Thus, some of the blood sucked into the thorax during inspiration is pumped onward by the heart and is not available to be squeezed out of the thorax during expiration.

This mechanism provides a minor auxiliary pump that aids venous return.

Topic 2: Venous Compression during Exercise and the Skeletal Muscle Pump

When a skeletal muscle contracts it compresses intramuscular veins, forcing blood from these veins back toward the heart. The blood is squeezed toward the heart by this action rather than back through the microcirculation because it takes the path of least resistance. When the skeletal muscle relaxes, its intramuscular veins refill with blood from the microcirculation. The venous valves prevent refilling from the more central veins. Rhythmic contraction-relaxation cycles keep pumping blood onward toward the heart. During strenuous running, this action of the leg and thigh muscles keeps the average pressure in the small intramuscular veins less than that in the femoral veins.

Thus, the skeletal muscle pump actually performs work on the blood and can be regarded as a booster pump in series with the heart. It has been estimated that during strenuous running the skeletal muscle pump in the legs and thighs provides almost one-third of the total power required to keep blood circulating, with the heart providing the remaining two-thirds!

In addition to the effectiveness of this mechanism as a booster pump, it also helps reduce total venous volume. When venous volume is reduced, arterial volume and pressure are increased. Thus, the skeletal muscle pump helps shift blood from veins to arteries. The increased MAP resulting from this shift increases the flow rate through the microcirculation and, therefore, in the steady state, increases cardiac output. Many authors refer to rhythmic venocompression, and to venoconstriction, as mechanisms for increasing the volume of "circulating" blood. This is misleading, since the blood involved was already circulating. The important thing accomplished is a shift in volume from venous to arterial sides and an increase in cardiac output.

Selected References for Chapter 14

- C.G. Caro, T.J. Pedley, R.C. Schroter, and W.A. Seed, *The Mechanics of the Circulation*, Oxford University Press, 1978, Chapter 14: The Systemic Veins, p. 434-475.
- G.A. Brecher, *Venous Return*, Grune & Stratton, 1956.

Chapter 15

Neuro-Humoral-Renal Control of the Circulation

You already know that mean arterial pressure (MAP), central venous pressure (CVP) and cardiac output (CO) are determined by the primary adjustable parameters of the cardiovascular system: heart rate, cardiac contractility, total peripheral resistance, venous capacity, and total blood volume. In this chapter, we will examine the mechanisms that control these global variables.

Part 1 will discuss the baroreceptor reflexes
Part 2 will treat the control of renal NaCl and water output
Part 3 will describe the mechanisms for long-term control of blood volume, MAP, and CVP
Part 4 will deal with the responses to acute hypovolemia
Part 5 will describe other cardiovascular situations and responses

It is assumed that you are already familiar with the anatomy and general functioning of the autonomic nervous system. A considerable amount of renal physiology must be mentioned in this chapter, but details of renal mechanisms are omitted. Some previous knowledge of renal anatomy and physiology would be helpful, but should not be essential.

Part 1: The Baroreceptor Reflexes

Topic 1: The Baroreceptors

Arterial Baroreceptors
Large arteries possess in their walls sensory nerve endings that are mechanically stimulated by stretch. As a large artery is expanded by an increase in blood pressure, these nerve endings are excited and generate action potentials at increased frequency. Since circumferential stretch is caused by increased blood pressure, these stretch receptors monitor arterial pressure. They are called arterial baroreceptors (baro = pressure).

Reduction of MAP below normal decreases the frequency of action potential firing. This is possible because the baroreceptors are tonically active at normal resting MAP.

Figure 1
Many of the arterial baroreceptors are clustered in the arch of the aorta and the carotid sinuses. The carotid sinuses are slightly bulbous regions where the internal carotid arteries branch off from the common carotid arteries.

Stimulation of the arterial baroreceptors by increased MAP initiates baroreceptor reflexes that attempt to return MAP back down to its previous value. Reduced baroreceptor activity resulting from decreased MAP initiates baroreceptor reflexes that attempt to return MAP back up to its previous value. Thus, the baroreceptor reflexes are negative feedback mechanisms that resist changes in MAP.

The arterial baroreceptors are not only sensitive to MAP, but also to the rate of change of MAP. Consequently, the rate of baroreceptor firing is increased by an increase in pulse pressure or heart rate and decreased by a decrease in pulse pressure or heart rate.

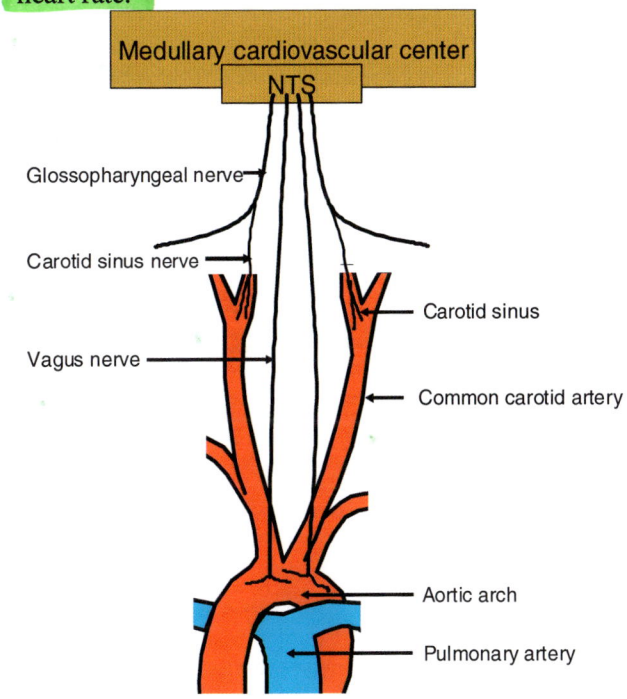

Figure 1. Arterial baroreceptors and their afferent nerves. NTS is the nucleus tractus solitarius.

Figure 2

This figure shows the effect of arterial pressure on the frequency of baroreceptor discharge. Note that the frequency is considerably higher when arterial pressure is pulsatile (normal situation) than when it is steady (experimental situation).

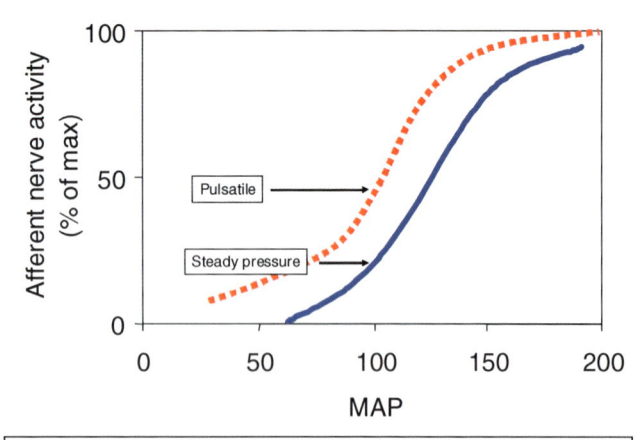

Figure 2. Stimulus-response relationship for arterial baroreceptors.

Cardiopulmonary Baroreceptors

There also are stretch receptors in the atria, ventricles, pulmonary artery, and pulmonary veins. They are called cardiopulmonary baroreceptors. They sense preload (an oversimplification, but a useful concept for now). For example, the right atrial baroreceptors sense CVP. Since preload is strongly influenced by blood volume, the cardiopulmonary baroreceptors detect changes in blood volume and are often called volume receptors. They are thought to be importantly involved in the long-term control of blood volume. The cardiopulmonary baroreceptors also assist the arterial baroreceptors in correcting changes in MAP.

[Note: The traditional view is that the cardiopulmonary baroreceptors regulate MAP by long-term effects on blood volume, but have little role in short-term control. According to this view, the arterial baroreceptors carry the burden for short-term control of MAP, but have nothing to do with long-term control. There is no evidence to support this concept. Current evidence shows that no distinct division of labor exists. The arterial and cardiopulmonary baroreceptors are both involved in short-term control and are both involved in long-term control.]

Topic 2: Afferents

See Figure 1 again
Afferent nerve fibers from baroreceptors in the carotid sinuses feed into the glossopharyngeal nerves and then into the medulla oblongata *via* the nucleus tractus solitarius (NTS). Afferent nerve fibers from baroreceptors in the aortic arch and the cardiopulmonary regions feed into the vagus nerves and again into the medulla oblongata *via* the NTS.

Topic 3: The Cardiovascular Center of the Medulla Oblongata

There is a diffuse neuronal network (often called "center") in the medulla oblongata that receives information from a variety of sources relevant to the cardiovascular system. These sources include the arterial baroreceptors, the cardiopulmonary baroreceptors, "exercise receptors" from skeletal muscle, peripheral and central $H^+/CO_2/O_2$ receptors (called chemoreceptors), the hypothalamus, the area postrema in the floor of the fourth ventricle, and the cerebral cortex. This medullary cardiovascular center integrates all incoming information, and then generates appropriate output. Output from the medullary cardiovascular center involves the autonomic nervous system, and a pathway to the hypothalamus that modulates the secretion of antidiuretic hormone (ADH) from the posterior pituitary gland.

Topic 4: Efferent Activity

Increased input from peripheral baroreceptors to the medullary cardiovascular center, due to increased MAP and CVP, results in decreased sympathetic activity, increased parasympathetic activity to the heart, and decreased secretion of ADH.

Sympathetic tracts leave the medulla and descend in the spinal cord. These tracts synapse with sympathetic preganglionic fibers in the intermediolateral cell columns. Synapses with postganglionic sympathetic fibers are in the paravertebral and prevertebral sympathetic ganglia. Postganglionic sympathetic fibers go to the effector organs, which (for cardiovascular control) are principally the heart, blood vessels, adrenal medullae, and kidneys.

Parasympathetic preganglionic fibers leave the medulla oblongata mainly from the nucleus ambiguous. Synapses with postganglionic parasympathetic fibers are within the effector organs. The only important effector organ in this regard is the heart (mainly the SA and AV nodes).

ADH is a nonapeptide (9 amino acids). It is also

Neuro-Humoral-Renal Control of the Circulation

called vasopressin. ADH is synthesized in certain neurons of the paraventricular and supraoptic nuclei of the hypothalamus. It is transported down the axons of these neurons and stored in their nerve endings, which lie in the posterior pituitary gland. When these hypothalamic neurons are excited, action potentials travel to their terminals, which then release ADH into capillary blood. Secretion of ADH results mainly from increased osmolarity of blood plasma (there are osmoreceptors in the hypothalamus) and decreased stretch of arterial and cardiopulmonary baroreceptors. The main target organs for ADH are blood vessels and the kidneys.

Topic 5: Effects

The principal effector organs for the baroreceptor reflexes are the heart, precapillary resistance vessels (let's just call them arterioles), veins, the adrenal medullae, and the kidneys.

Heart

Sympathetic postganglionic neurons release norepinephrine, which activates β_1 receptors on P cells of the SA node and AV node. It also activates β_1 receptors on working myocytes of the atria and ventricles. The prime results are increased heart rate and increased contractility. Less important results are increased conduction velocity, decreased action potential duration, and decreased contraction duration. [Mechanisms are discussed in Chapter 4.] Consequently, increased sympathetic activity to the heart tends to increase CO and MAP, but reduces CVP. Decreased sympathetic activity does the opposite.

Parasympathetic postganglionic neurons release acetylcholine, which activates muscarinic receptors on P cells of the SA node and AV node. The result is decreased heart rate and decreased conduction velocity through the AV node. [Mechanisms are discussed in Chapter 4.] Consequently, increased parasympathetic activity to the heart tends to reduce CO and MAP while increasing CVP. Decreased parasympathetic activity does the opposite.

Acetylcholine can also activate muscarinic receptors on atrial and ventricular myocytes, thereby reducing contractility. This negative inotropic effect may have some physiological importance for the atria but not for the ventricles since parasympathetic innervation of the ventricles is extremely sparse. Pharmacological doses of muscarinic agonists can have a large negative inotropic effect on the ventricles, but this would probably happen only in an experimental situation.

Arterioles

Sympathetic postganglionic neurons release norepinephrine, which activates α_1 receptors on smooth muscle cells of arterioles. The resulting vasoconstriction increases TPR and, therefore, tends to increase MAP and reduce CVP. Reduced sympathetic activity to arterioles inhibits smooth muscle tone and, therefore, reduces TPR and MAP while increasing CVP.

When arterioles constrict, pressure in the capillaries and venules decreases. When this happens, water from the interstitial spaces shifts into blood and becomes blood plasma. Blood volume increases and, therefore, arterial volume and MAP increase.

There are no important parasympathetic effects on arterioles in most tissues.

Veins

Sympathetic postganglionic neurons release norepinephrine, which activates α_1 receptors on venous smooth muscle. The resulting venous constriction increases CVP (preload to the heart) and, therefore, increases CO and MAP. Reduced sympathetic activity to veins inhibits their tone and, therefore, tends to reduce CVP, CO, and MAP.

There are no important parasympathetic effects on veins.

Adrenal Medullae

Sympathetic preganglionic fibers innervate the adrenal medullae. Their nerve endings release acetylcholine that activates nicotinic receptors on adrenal medullary cells causing secretion of epinephrine (and a lesser amount of norepinephrine). These hormones circulate in the blood and act on β_1 receptors in the heart to increase heart rate and contractility. Circulating norepinephrine also acts on α_1 receptors in arterioles to increase TPR, and on α_1 receptors in veins to decrease venous capacity. Thus, increased sympathetic activity to the adrenal medullae tends to increase CO and MAP. Decreased sympathetic activity to the adrenal medullae has the opposite effect.

Epinephrine (but not norepinephrine) also activates β_2 adrenergic receptors. In skeletal muscle, the result is relaxation of arteriolar smooth muscle and increased blood flow. This effect is thought to have importance in promoting muscle blood flow during the early stages of the fight or flight response and in pre-exercise anticipation, but is probably not important in regulating MAP.

Kidneys
The effects of sympathetic nerve activity on the kidneys will be discussed in Part 2 of this chapter.

Topic 6: Resetting

Adaptation of Baroreceptors
Figure 3
If an increase in MAP is maintained for as little as 10 minutes during exercise, the sensitivity of arterial baroreceptors decreases as shown in the figure. The consequence of this adaptation (also called resetting) is that the arterial baroreceptor reflexes allow MAP to rise to a level appropriate for the intensity of exercise and yet still dampen transient fluctuations in MAP. The cardiopulmonary baroreceptors also rapidly adapt to any maintained CVP (minutes to hours). The mechanism of rapid adaptation is not understood.

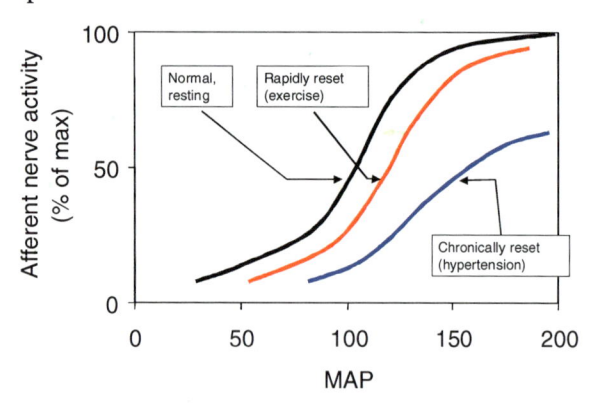

Figure 3. Adaptation of arterial baroreceptors.

During chronic hypertension, the arterial baroreceptors adapt in proportion to the severity of the hypertension. Consequently, the arterial baroreceptors do not resist pathological hypertension, nor do they cause hypertension. What they do is attenuate transient fluctuations in MAP at any chronic level of MAP.

Resetting of the Medullary Cardiovascular Center
Resetting is not entirely a matter of peripheral adaptation. The "gain" of the medullary cardiovascular center is also changed. For example, during a sustained increase in MAP (endurance exercise, chronic hypertension), increased baroreceptor input to the cardiovascular center is not taken as seriously as it ordinarily is and the reflex reduction in sympathetic output is diminished.

Topic 7: Physiological Roles of the Baroreceptor Reflexes

Short-Term Control of MAP
The term short-term control refers to baroreceptor reflex responses that are effective within seconds. These reflexes are not only fast, but they are also very effective. They attenuate the fluctuations in MAP that occur in response to ordinary daily activities such as postural changes, walking, light exercise, eating, defecation, and moderate excitement. Short-term control of MAP involves neural reflexes that go directly to the heart and blood vessels.

Figure 4
Here is a histogram showing the relative frequency of any given MAP over a 24 hr period. In this example, MAP ranges from about 70 to 125 mmHg and averages 90 mmHg. After denervation of the arterial baroreceptors (actual experiments done on dogs) the 24 hr average MAP remains nearly the same, but the range increases greatly.

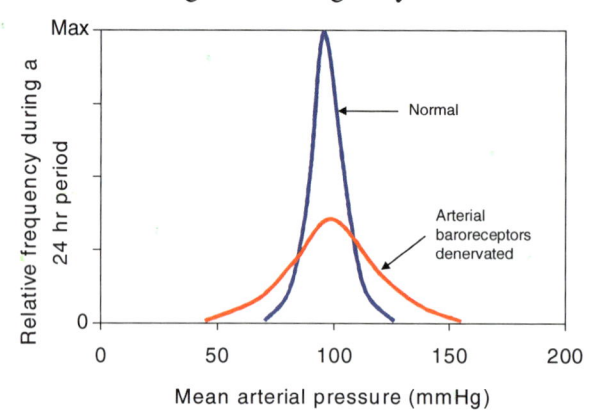

Figure 4. Relative frequency of MAP values over a 24 hr period in normal dogs and in dogs with all arterial baroreceptors denervated.

When both the arterial baroreceptors and cardiopulmonary baroreceptors are denervated, the intraday fluctuations in MAP become even greater than they are when only the arterial baroreceptors are denervated (data not shown). This observation provides evidence that the cardiopulmonary baroreceptor reflexes supplement the arterial baroreceptor reflexes in the short-term control of MAP.

Trace the Fast Baroreceptor Reflexes

Figure 5

Let's use, as an example, suddenly standing from a reclining posture. The immediate effects and the compensatory effects on CO were discussed in Chapter 8. It would be appropriate at this point for you to review that discussion and the accompanying Guyton diagrams.

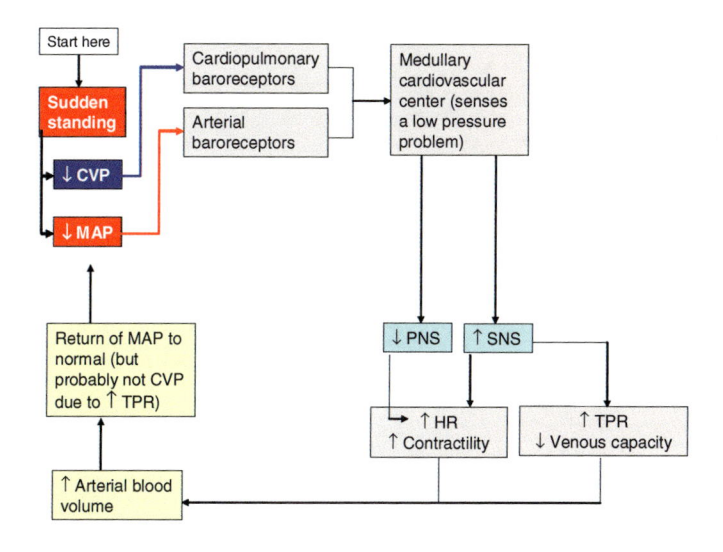

Figure 5. Fast reflex responses to decreased MAP and CVP due, for example, to standing up.

Upon standing (without exercise), MAP and CVP both decrease due to the effects of gravity on the distribution of blood. Consequently, stimulation of arterial and cardiopulmonary baroreceptors decreases and they decrease their firing rate. The medullary cardiovascular center receives this negative input, interprets it as a low-pressure problem, and increases its sympathetic output. It also decreases its parasympathetic output to the heart. Consequently, heart rate, cardiac contractility, and TPR all increase while venous capacity decreases. All these effects tend to increase MAP up to the level that is normal for a standing posture (*i.e.* a little higher than in the reclining posture).

The compensatory increase in TPR tends to decrease CVP while the decrease in venous capacity tends to increase CVP. The overall result is that CVP decreases a little upon standing even after compensatory mechanisms have elevated MAP to its normal value (see Figure 9 in Chapter 8). Thus, a low-pressure signal from the cardiopulmonary baroreceptors to the medullary cardiovascular center continues after standing up, and helps to maintain normal MAP.

If we were to start with an increase in MAP and CVP resulting from a postural change or onset of some ordinary activity, the result would be the opposite of all the above effects.

The fast baroreceptor reflexes start in less than a second following a sudden change in cardiovascular pressures, and are well established within a few seconds. In addition, the kidneys change their rate of urine output, which eventually changes blood volume. The renal response begins promptly, but takes minutes to hours to be effective, and is involved with long-term control of MAP.

Long-Term Control of Blood Volume and MAP

Long-term control of MAP involves effects of baroreceptors on the kidneys that regulate total blood volume. Therefore, before discussing long-term control we must describe the control of renal NaCl and water output. This will be done in Part 2 of this chapter. Long-term control of MAP will then be discussed in Part 3.

Intermediate Control of MAP

Certain hormonal mechanisms involved in control of MAP, principally those involving actions of ADH and angiotensin II on blood vessels, are slower than direct neural reflexes but faster than control of blood volume by renal mechanisms. These processes will be discussed in connection with responses to acute hypovolemia in Part 4 of this chapter.

Part 2: Control of Renal NaCl and Water Output

Topic 1: Introduction

The difference between water intake and water loss determines changes in total body water. Water intake, while somewhat controlled by the thirst mechanism, tends to be fortuitous. Tight regulation of total body water and, therefore, of total blood volume is a renal function. The kidneys excrete NaCl and water at whatever rate is necessary to maintain total body NaCl and water, and blood volume reasonably constant. Total blood volume is a major determinant of arterial blood volume and of venous blood volume. Therefore, it is a major determinant of MAP and CVP.

The rate of renal NaCl and water excretion is controlled by:
- MAP
- The sympathetic nervous system
- Humoral mechanisms, namely the renin-angiotensin-aldosterone system, antidiuretic hormone (ADH), and atrial natriuretic peptide (ANP)

Only general features of renal physiology related to salt and water balance will be discussed here. Details of the various transport processes and control mechanisms will be omitted.

Topic 2: The Effect of MAP on Urine Output

The rate at which the kidneys excrete Na$^+$ and water is the difference between the rate that Na$^+$ and water are filtered out of blood across the glomerular capillaries and the rate that they are reabsorbed back into blood by the renal tubules (proximal tubules, loops of Henle, distal tubules, and collecting ducts). Increased MAP causes increased glomerular filtration rate (GFR) and decreased proximal tubular reabsorption of Na$^+$ and water. Therefore, when MAP increases, urinary output of both Na$^+$ and water increases. These phenomena are called pressure diuresis and pressure natriuresis.

Figure 6

This figure illustrates pressure diuresis. As MAP increases, the rate of urine output increases. The curve for pressure natriuresis (not shown) is essentially identical to the curve for pressure diuresis. The short horizontal line in the figure represents average daily water intake as percent of normal. Since over a period of a few days average water output must equal average water intake, the system operates where the intake line crosses the pressure diuresis curve (renal function curve), and that coordinate is called the operating point.

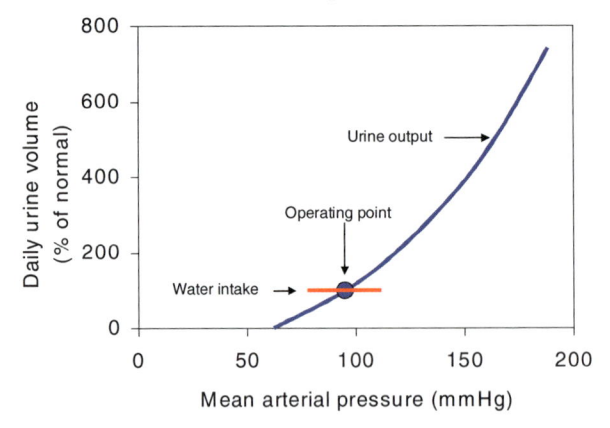

Figure 6. Pressure diuresis. This is sometimes called the renal function curve.

If a large amount of salt and water are ingested (let's say in roughly isotonic proportions), blood volume and MAP increase producing a pressure diuresis/natriuresis. As long as this is just an acute event, pressure diuresis/natriuresis can eliminate the excess salt and water, returning MAP to normal within an hour or so. Neuro-humoral mechanisms normally contribute to the speed of this compensation by causing adjustments in the various renal settings that help control GFR and tubular reabsorption. But even without these adjustments, pressure diuresis/natriuresis could eventually handle the problem.

Figure 7

Now let us consider a very different situation in which large amounts of salt and water are ingested daily for an indefinite time (*i.e.* the average American high salt diet containing about 3.5 g of Na$^+$ per day). If average daily salt and water intake increase and all renal properties remain constant, the operating point shifts upward (more urine) and to the right (higher MAP). Pressure diuresis-natriuresis cannot correct this situation. In order to maintain normal MAP, renal properties must change in response to changes in salt and water intake. The renal function curve must be shifted to the left.

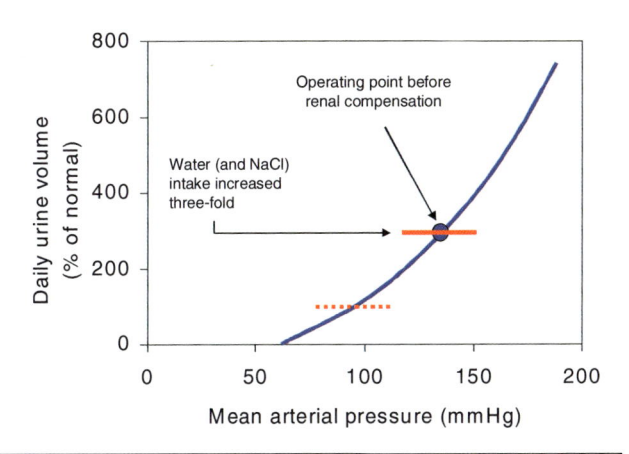

Neuro-Humoral-Renal Control of the Circulation

Figure 7. Renal function curve showing that without changes in renal properties, chronically increased salt and water consumption causes chronically increased MAP.

Topic 3: Adjustments in Renal Function

Figure 8

In this figure, the renal function curve has shifted to the left, making it easier to get rid of excess salt and water. Now, in spite of continued excessive salt and water intake, the operating point lies at a normal MAP

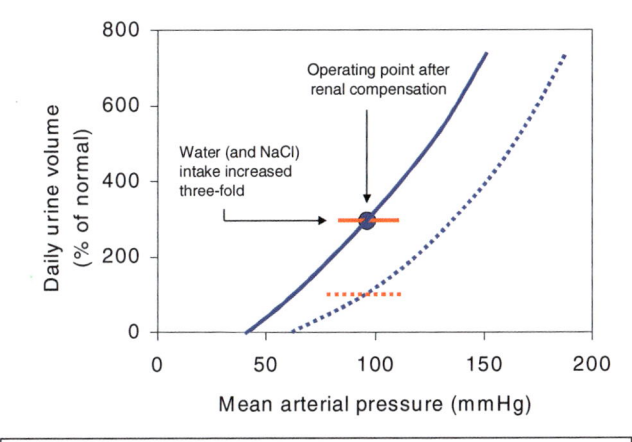

Figure 8. Several renal variables are adjusted in response to increased total body salt and water content. These adjustments shift the renal function curve to the left, returning MAP toward normal.

Several adjustable variables of renal function can shift the renal function curve to the left (to get rid of salt and water) or to the right (to conserve salt and water). These variables include the resistances of the glomerular afferent and efferent arterioles, the efficacy of Na^+ reabsorption by the renal tubules, and the permeability of the collecting duct epithelium to water. These variables are adjusted by neurohumoral mechanisms that are activated in response to changes in MAP, CVP, Na^+ delivery to the macula densa, and blood osmolarity.

Topic 4: Neural Regulation of Renal NaCl and Water Excretion

Increased sympathetic nerve activity to the kidneys, reflexly caused by decreased MAP and/or CVP, results in decreased urine formation and, therefore, tends to increase total blood volume and return MAP and CVP toward their original values. This effect is complex and involves at least the following three mechanisms:

1. **Sympathetic Effect on Glomerular Filtration Rate (GFR):** Increased sympathetic activity to the renal glomeruli reduces GFR. The result is decreased urine output and, therefore, increased blood volume, CVP, CO, and MAP.

2. **Sympathetic Effect on Proximal Tubular Reabsorption of Water:** Increased sympathetic activity to the absorptive cells of the proximal tubules in the kidneys induces increased proximal tubular reabsorption of NaCl and water. Again, the consequence is decreased urine output, and, therefore, increased blood volume, CVP, CO, and MAP.

3. **Sympathetic Effect on Renin Secretion by the Juxtaglomerular Apparatus:** Increased sympathetic activity to the kidneys induces secretion of renin from juxtaglomerular cells into blood. Renin sets off a sequence of events involving angiotensin and aldosterone that results in decreased urine output and, therefore, increased blood volume, CVP, CO, and MAP. This sequence of events will be described in more detail in the next topic.

Topic 5: The Renin-Angiotensin-Aldosterone System

Figure 9

Renin is a proteolytic enzyme that is secreted from the juxtaglomerular cells of the kidneys. Juxtaglomerular cells are specialized smooth muscle cells located mainly in the arterioles leading to each glomerulus (the afferent arterioles). A loop of distal tubule lies adjacent to each afferent arteriole. In this loop is located a group of specialized epithelial cells called the macula densa. The macula densa senses Na^+ concentration in the fluid flowing through the distal tubules and appropriately signals the adjacent juxtaglomerular cells to increase or decrease their secretion of renin. The combination of juxtaglomerular cells and macula densa is called the juxtaglomerular apparatus.

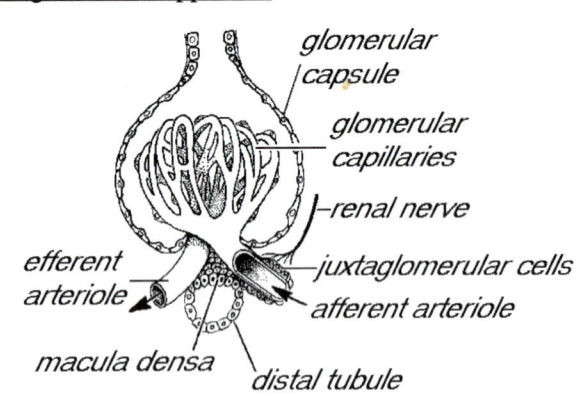

Figure 9. The juxtaglomerular apparatus.
Drawing by Dr. Donald Stubbs
The University of Texas Medical Branch
Dept. of Physiology & Biophysics
Galveston, TX

Renin is secreted from juxtaglomerular cells in response to the following stimuli:
- Increased sympathetic nerve activity with norepinephrine acting on β_1 receptors
- Decreased blood pressure in the afferent arteriole [thus afferent arterioles are baroreceptors]
- Decreased distal tubular delivery of Na^+ to the macula densa, resulting from decreased glomerular filtration rate (GFR) and/or increased proximal tubular reabsorption of Na^+

Angiotensinogen is a protein that circulates in blood all the time. In the general circulation, renin (secreted from the juxtaglomerular cells) catalyzes the conversion of angiotensinogen to angiotensin I.

As blood flows through the lungs, angiotensin I (a decapeptide) is converted to angiotensin II (an octapeptide). Angiotensin-converting enzyme (ACE) catalyzes this reaction. ACE is located mainly on the surface of pulmonary capillary endothelial cells.

Angiotensin II has many major effects, all of which tend to increase MAP:
- It stimulates general vasoconstriction. TPR is increased and venous capacity is slightly reduced. Both of these effects shift blood from veins to arteries and, therefore, increase MAP.
- It decreases GFR. Urine output is reduced and, consequently, total blood volume and MAP are increased.
- It increases proximal tubular reabsorption of NaCl and water. A greater fraction of the glomerular filtrate is reabsorbed. This effect tends to increase total blood volume and MAP. Increased proximal tubular reabsorption of NaCl, together with decreased GFR, result in decreased delivery of Na^+ to the macula densa and, therefore, even more secretion of renin from the juxtaglomerular cells.
- It stimulates secretion of aldosterone from the adrenal cortex. Aldosterone is the most important of the adrenal mineralocorticoid hormones. Aldosterone augments NaCl and water reabsorption from the distal tubules of the kidneys, an effect that results in increased blood volume and MAP.
- It stimulates angiotensin receptors in the area postrema of the brain (a region in the floor of the fourth ventricle that is unprotected by the blood-brain barrier). Activation of these receptors results in increased activity of the sympathetic nervous system (via the medullary cardiovascular center), which increases renin secretion from juxtaglomerular cells. This positive feedback loop strongly conserves body water.
- It enhances the sense of thirst.
- It induces ADH release from the posterior pituitary.

Topic 6: ADH (Vasopressin)

As described earlier, decreased baroreceptor input to the medullary cardiovascular network and increased osmolarity of blood plasma both promote the secretion of antidiuretic hormone (ADH, vasopressin) from the posterior pituitary gland. ADH has three major effects:
- It decreases urine output. It does this by increasing the permeability of renal collecting ducts to water so that more water is reabsorbed. When more ADH is secreted from the posterior pituitary, less urine is excreted. Total blood volume, arterial blood volume, and MAP increase.
- It promotes contraction of vascular smooth muscle. When more ADH is secreted from the posterior pituitary, TPR increases and venous capacity decreases. The result is increased arterial blood volume and MAP.
- It activates ADH receptors in the area postrema that result (via the medullary cardiovascular

center) in decreased sympathetic activity. Decreased sympathetic activity to the kidneys results in increased Na$^+$ excretion, thereby helping to correct the osmolarity problem.

Topic 7: Atrial Natriuretic Peptide

Distension of the atria (increased preload to the ventricles) promotes secretion of a small protein called atrial natriuretic peptide (ANP). This hormone is stored in atrial myocyte granules that are readily visible in histological specimens. Circulating ANP:
- Increases GFR (due to relaxation of afferent and efferent arterioles)
- Reduces NaCl and water reabsorption by the collecting ducts
- Inhibits renin secretion from the juxtaglomerular apparatus
- Inhibits aldosterone secretion from the adrenal cortex
- Inhibits ADH secretion from the posterior pituitary
- Inhibits the action of ADH on the distal tubules

Thus, ANP counteracts the renin-angiotensin-aldosterone system and the ADH system. The result is increased NaCl and water excretion in the urine. Urine volume increases at the expense of total blood volume. Consequently, arterial blood volume and MAP decrease.

Part 3: Long Term Control of Blood Volume, MAP, and CVP

Topic 1: In the Long Term, MAP is Controlled by Regulation of Total Blood Volume

Changes in MAP result from changes in arterial blood volume. Short-term fluctuations in arterial blood volume and pressure that support ordinary daily activities (including exercise) are caused mainly by adjustments in heart rate, contractility, TPR, and venous capacity. However, in the long term, adjustments in total blood volume determine arterial blood volume and, therefore, MAP. Adjustments in total blood volume are accomplished mainly by the kidneys in concert with control of total body Na$^+$. Increased extracellular Na$^+$ results in an increase in both interstitial and blood volume while decreased extracellular Na$^+$ has the opposite effect. The kidneys normally respond to variations in salt and water intake to keep total body Na$^+$ and water reasonably constant, and, in the process, keep MAP reasonably constant. The average daily rate of Na$^+$ and water output by the kidneys must exactly equal the average daily rate of Na$^+$ and water intake (adjusted for sweat, feces, and insensible water loss from skin and lungs).

The neurohumoral processes controlling renal salt and water excretion were discussed in Part 2 of this chapter, but how do they all work together and what are their relative importances? This very hard question presently cannot be given an entirely satisfactory answer. Clues come from an important line of experimentation involving salt and water loading in animals. One variation of these experiments is to give rats a diet extremely rich in NaCl (commonly 8% by weight). Eating this stuff kicks in the thirst mechanism. Water intake increases enormously so that total salt and water intake is almost isotonic. Amazingly, these animals do not get hypertensive. Readjustments in renal properties shift the renal function curve to the left sufficiently for renal salt and water output to match intake with only a minor increase in MAP.

Now this experiment is done again, but with one or more of the potential compensatory mechanisms inactivated. If hypertension results, then that potential compensatory mechanism is implicated as having a role in long-term control of MAP. For example, after denervation of the arterial baroreceptors, salt and water loading results in hypertension. After eliminating the effects of decreased sympathetic activity, salt and water loading results in a far more severe hypertension. Eliminating the effects of decreased angiotensin II and ADH also results in severe hypertension in salt-loaded animals. [Interested readers might want to look at a review by J.W. Osborn (*Clinical and Experimental Pharmacology and Physiology*, 24:109-115, 1997.]

Topic 2: A Model for Long-Term Control of MAP and CVP

Figure 10

Here is a model for long-term control of MAP and CVP. It is not the intention here to discuss the etiology of essential hypertension, but many possibilities clearly exist. It is best to study this model one path at a time, but it is also important to realize how interrelated the various paths are. Begin at the *Start* sign.

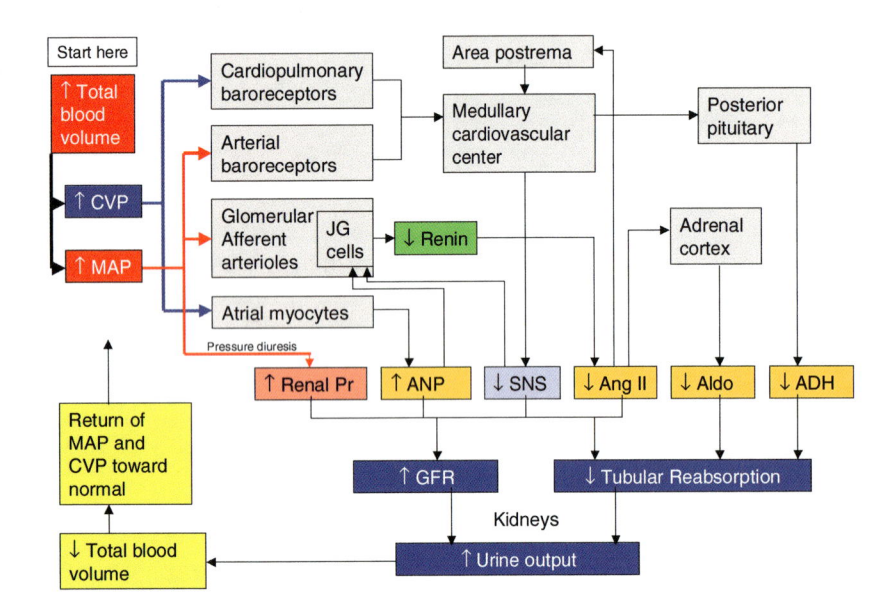

Figure 10. Long-term control of MAP and CVP – responses to increased salt and water load.
Renal Pr = renal pressure
ANP = atrial natriuretic peptide
SNS = sympathetic nervous system
AngII = angiotensin II
Aldo = aldosterone
GFR = glomerular filtration rate.

First, trace the path involving glomerular afferent arterioles.
- Increased MAP, by increasing pressure in the glomerular afferent arterioles, leads to decreased renin secretion from JG cells.
- This leads to decreased circulating angiotensin II.
- This causes increased urinary output of NaCl and water by increasing GFR and decreasing tubular reabsorption.
- This causes decreased blood volume and return of MAP and CVP toward normal.

Next, look at the loop from decreased angiotensin II all the way back to a further decrease in angiotensin II.
- Decreased angiotensin II (*via* the area postrema and the medullary cardiovascular center) results in decreased sympathetic activity.
- The loop continues to the JG cells and decreased renin.
- Then on to decreased angiotensin II.
- This positive feedback loop should greatly augment urinary output of Na^+ and water.

Now trace the path involving atrial myocytes.
- Increased CVP (resulting from increased total blood volume) stretches atrial myocytes.
- This leads to increased secretion of ANP.
- Circulating ANP acts directly on the kidneys to increase GFR and decrease tubular reabsorption.
- ANP also reduces renin secretion from the juxtaglomerular cells.
- This results in reduced formation of angiotensin II.
- Consequently, sympathetic nerve activity, and aldosterone secretion are reduced.
- ANP has several other effects (not indicated in the figure but mentioned earlier) that help shut down the renin-angiotensin-aldosterone system and the ADH system.

Now consider the arterial and cardiopulmonary baroreceptors.
- When MAP and CVP are increased, reflexes operating through the medullary cardiovascular center cause decreased sympathetic activity and decreased secretion of ADH from the posterior pituitary.
- Decreased sympathetic activity directly increases GFR and decreases tubular reabsorption.
- Decreased sympathetic activity also suppresses the renin-angiotensin-aldosterone system by reducing renin secretion from the JG cells.

An interesting question arises regarding arterial and cardiopulmonary baroreceptors. Renal responses cause gradual changes in total blood volume, but arterial and cardiopulmonary baroreceptors adapt rapidly to any prevailing pressure. How can a rapidly adapting mechanism control a sluggish response?
- Arterial baroreceptors: One suggestion is that tonic activity from the arterial baroreceptors, although relatively unresponsive to changes in MAP, is necessary for the medullary cardiovascular center to respond properly to

influences from the area postrema.
- Cardiopulmonary baroreceptors: The only suggestion here is that the cardiopulmonary baroreceptors must not adapt completely. An error signal must be maintained for as long as cardiac preload is aberrant, although this has not yet been proved.

A comment about ADH is necessary. The model indicates that a decrease in ADH results from increased total blood volume. However, when salt loading is the initiator of the rise in blood volume, there is a tendency for blood osmolarity to increase. Stimulation of hypothalamic osmoreceptors by increased blood osmolarity results in increased ADH in an attempt to promote water conservation by the kidneys and return osmolarity to normal. There is often a fight between baroreceptors and osmoreceptors for control of ADH secretion. Osmoreceptors ordinarily win and blood osmolarity is controlled. However, during severe hypotension (*e.g.* hemorrhagic shock), baroreceptors win and secretion of ADH increases, thereby helping to conserve blood volume even if blood osmolarity decreases.

The Medullary Cardiovascular Center is the Final Arbiter

It is up to the medullary cardiovascular center to evaluate all inputs and determine just the right outputs to the sympathetic nervous system and posterior pituitary to cope effectively with deviations in MAP and CVP.

Topic 3: Are the Adjustments to High Salt and Water Loads Perfect?

The answer is no, at least not in most humans. This conclusion is based on the so-called DASH-Sodium study published in the New England Journal of Medicine (NEJM 344:3-10, 2001). DASH stands for Dietary Approaches to Stop Hypertension. This report demonstrates that when people were put on diets containing only 1.2 g of Na^+ per day their arterial pressures dropped several mmHg compared to those who were put on the American average of 3.5 g per day. This happened whether the subjects were normal or hypertensive. For details and advice about NaCl intake, see the article in NEJM and the accompanying editorial. The conclusion here is that renal compensation for changes in salt and water intake is not complete, even in most normal people.

Part 4: Responses to Acute Hypovolemia (Hemorrhage)

Topic 1: Renal Responses

The renal responses to decreased total blood volume, total body Na^+, MAP, and CVP are, of course, just the opposite of the ones shown in Figure 10. All the directional arrows are simply turned upside down.

The effects of the renal responses are slow. They are well suited for matching Na^+ and water output to long-term Na^+ and water intake as explained earlier. They are also important for gradually returning total body Na^+ and water back to normal following a sublethal hemorrhage. However, rapid responses to sudden blood loss are required to prevent acute cardiovascular collapse.

Topic 2: Rapid Responses

Figure 11
Rapid responses involve adjustments in all the cardiovascular control parameters: heart rate, contractility, TPR, venous capacity, and total blood volume. The receptors and neurohumoral mediators are mostly the same as they are for renal responses, but the target organs are different. The target organs for fast responses are the heart, arteriolar smooth muscle, and venous smooth muscle. Most of these responses shift blood from the systemic veins to systemic arteries.

The fastest of these responses (within seconds) is the increase in sympathetic nervous activity, leading directly to increases in heart rate, contractility, TPR, and venoconstriction. Part of the effect of increased sympathetic activity is due to the release of catecholamines from the adrenal medulla. The responses involving angiotensin II and ADH are somewhat slower.

Check out the path from decreased MAP to decreased capillary pressure. The result of decreased capillary (and venular) pressure is net movement of fluid from interstitial spaces to blood (transcapillary refill, autotransfusion). Transcapillary refill is more gradual than the above neurohumoral responses but is a very important compensation for acute blood loss. Arteriolar constriction contributes to decreased capillary pressure, although the latter path is not indicated in the figure.

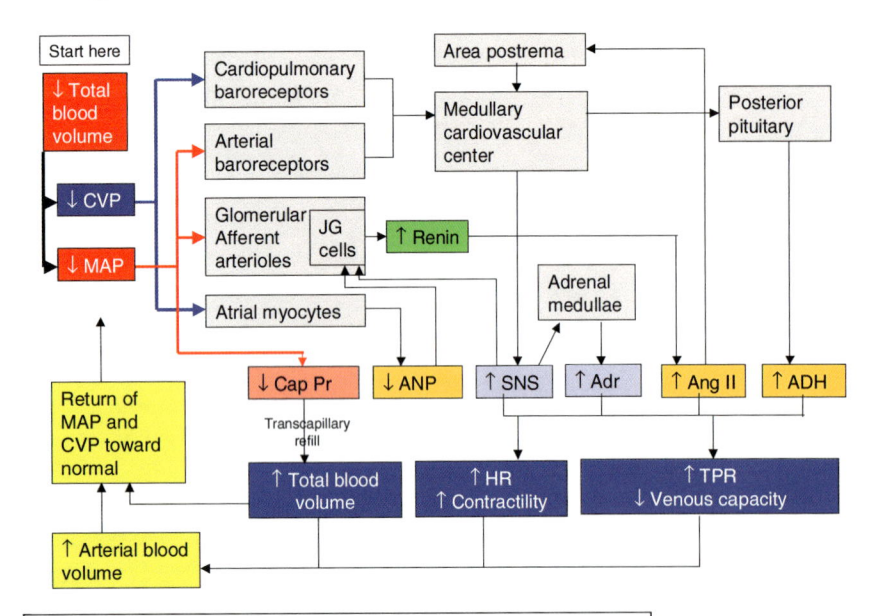

Figure 11. Fast and semi-fast responses to blood loss.
CapPr = capillary pressure
ANP = atrial natriuretic peptide
SNS = sympathetic nervous system
Adr = adrenal medullary hormones (epinephrine and norepinephrine)
AngII = angiotensin II.

Another response that is slower than the neural reflexes but much faster than renal compensation involves secretion of glucose from the liver (not depicted in the figure). Circulating epinephrine stimulates glycogenolysis and glucose output from the liver. The concentration of glucose rises in blood and interstitial spaces. The resulting increased extracellular osmolarity draws water out of cells, thereby helping to restore blood volume. Animals depleted of hepatic glycogen by fasting compensate less effectively following hemorrhage because their livers cannot secrete glucose.

Severe hypovolemia kicks in two additional rapid responses that are not shown in the figure. These responses are:

- **Peripheral Chemoreceptor Reflexes:** There are cell aggregates near the carotid sinuses and along the aortic arch that sense pH and the partial pressure of O_2. When stimulated by sufficiently low PO_2 or pH, or by high PCO_2, these chemoreceptors send impulses to the medullary cardiovascular center that reflexly increase sympathetic activity. The peripheral chemoreceptor reflexes are not involved in ordinary control of cardiovascular functions. However, during severe hypovolemia, decreased blood flow to these receptors can result in significant local hypoxia. In addition, during hypovolemia the pH of blood tends to decrease. The combination of decreased pH and decreased local PO_2 stimulates the peripheral chemoreceptors. The resulting increase in sympathetic activity augments the baro-receptor reflexes.

- **The Central Ischemic Response:** When MAP drops below about 60 mmHg (i.e. below the brain's autoregulatory range) the brain becomes ischemic (inadequately perfused with blood). Ischemia of the medullary cardiovascular center quickly results in a profound increase in sympathetic activity, which can significantly augment the baroreceptor reflexes. The central ischemic response is thought to be the strongest natural activator of the sympathetic nervous system.

The peripheral chemoreceptor reflexes and the central ischemic response are emergency measures that help combat acute hypovolemia.

Topic 3: How Effective are the Responses?

While donating a unit of blood in the blood bank (500 ml), your MAP drops several mmHg but then, over the subsequent hour or two, gradually returns to normal. It would return to normal even without drinking liquids, although this speeds the process. A unit of blood for a 70 kg person is roughly 10% of total blood volume. We can similarly cope with sudden blood loss due to trauma if it doesn't exceed roughly 20% of total blood volume.

The initial drop in MAP would be much more profound were it not for the fast baroreceptor reflexes that increase sympathetic activity to the heart, arterioles, and veins. In fact, a sudden 20% blood loss would usually be lethal without baroreceptor responses.

The gradual return to normal MAP results initially

from the vasoconstricting effects of angiotensin II and ADH, and from transcapillary refill.

Even after normal MAP is attained, arterial baroreceptor reflexes continue to participate since they are activated by reduced pulse pressure. The drop in pulse pressure results from reduced left ventricular stroke volume due to increased heart rate and decreased preload. Decreased preload is the consequence of reduced blood volume and increased TPR.

With blood loss greater than about 10% of total blood volume, decreased preload causes decreased cardiac output in spite of an increase in heart rate. With 10-20% blood loss, the decrease in cardiac output may last for hours – long after MAP has returned to normal.

During the subsequent day or so, increased water intake and decreased water excretion return everything to normal. Complete, spontaneous recovery of MAP and cardiac output usually occurs with initial drops in MAP to as little as 45 mmHg.

The brain and coronary circulations do not participate in reflex vasoconstriction. On the contrary, as MAP falls, the phenomenon of pressure-flow autoregulation in these vascular beds maintains reasonably normal blood flow until MAP drops below about 60 mmHg.

Sudden loss of more than 30% of total blood volume can cause an abrupt drop in MAP to less than 45 mmHg. When MAP drops this much it does not usually return spontaneously to normal in spite of intense activation of all the mechanisms discussed above. This degree of hemorrhage, however, is usually not fatal, unless accompanied by trauma or dehydration.

When 40-50% of the blood is lost, there is a valiant reflexive effort to return MAP to normal, but it fails. MAP gradually declines and then suddenly drops to death. Survival is dependent upon resuscitation measures, principally prompt intravenous replacement of the lost fluid.

When MAP drops below some ill-defined value, roughly 20-30 mmHg acutely or 40-50 mmHg for an extended period, resuscitation measures generally fail.

Topic 4: Circulatory Shock

Global inadequacy of blood flow to the organs of the body so that their metabolic needs are not met is called circulatory shock. Etiologies include:
- Primary cardiac insufficiency (cardiogenic shock)
- Profound decrease in TPR and increase in venous capacity (neurogenic shock, anaphylactic shock)
- Hypovolemia (hemorrhagic shock, burn shock, intestinal obstruction, dehydration)
- Sepsis

When a tissue is not perfused adequately with blood, its rate of anaerobic metabolism increases as its rate of aerobic metabolism decreases. Consequently, lactic acid is produced in cells and leaks into interstitial spaces and blood. Local tissue acidosis and general blood acidosis develop. The degree of acidosis is a measure of the degree of shock.

The responses to blood loss were described in the previous topic of this chapter. With this information, you will not be surprised to learn that we consider circulatory shock to present in three stages. These stages are:

The Nonprogressive Stage
If MAP remains above about 45 mmHg, the situation usually does not get progressively worse. Instead, spontaneous recovery sets in and is usually complete. However, even after MAP returns to normal, decreased cardiac output, increased heart rate, decreased pulse pressure, acidosis, tachypnia (rapid breathing), and perhaps weakness and malaise are telltale signs that shock still exists.

The Progressive Stage
Various degradative processes take place during severe shock. Metabolic run-down of tissues because of hypoxia is involved. Strength of vascular smooth muscle wanes and it becomes harder to maintain arteriolar and venous tone. Ischemia of the intestinal tract results in endotoxin transfer from gram-negative gut bacteria into blood. Endotoxin results in release of certain cytokines that can cause a systemic inflammatory response and compromise various cardiovascular functions. Substances such as bradykinin and histamine can cause increased capillary permeability so that fluid leaks down its pressure gradient from blood to interstitial spaces, exacerbating the hypovolemia. A

substance called myocardial depressant factor is released from some unknown location and reduces cardiac contractility. Another substance that circulates during shock causes generalized membrane depolarization, cell swelling; and, therefore, further loss of blood volume. We call it *circulating depolarizing factor (CDF)*. It probably contributes to dysfunction in many tissues.

These destructive effects fight against the compensations discussed above. With an initial drop in MAP to below 45 mmHg, the struggle cannot often succeed and shock progresses to multiple organ failure and finally to death unless it is reversed by effective resuscitation. This is the progressive stage.

The good news is that effective resuscitation is possible by bolstering the body's natural responses with prompt intravenous infusion of isotonic "crystalloid" or "colloid" solutions. The solutes in a crystalloid replacement solution are low molecular weight salts. Colloid replacement fluids contain, in addition, large molecular weight solutes such as plasma proteins or starch derivatives.

Lactated Ringer's, an isotonic crystalloid solution, is the standard replacement fluid for hypovolemic shock in the United States. However, since it contains no colloids and, therefore, has no colloid osmotic pressure (oncotic pressure), it quickly distributes throughout the entire extracellular space. About 2 to 6 times the volume of blood loss must be administered to restore vascular volume. When more efficient or more rapid resuscitation is required, colloid solutions such as Hespan are useful. Another approach to provide rapid resuscitation is to give a small bolus infusion of very hypertonic saline to draw water out of cells osmotically.

The Irreversible Stage

If the drop in MAP is extremely severe (below roughly 30 mmHg acutely or 40-50 mmHg sustained), irreversible shock may occur. The most vigorous attempts at fluid replacement often fail. Severe and prolonged ischemia of the medullary cardiovascular center finally shuts down sympathetic outflow and vascular smooth muscle relaxes. Blood shifts from arteries to veins. Fluid runs out of the vascular system into interstitial spaces and on into the cells of the body. This is the irreversible stage.

Part 5: Other Cardiovascular Situations and Responses

Topic 1: Exercise

During sustained dynamic exercise, the arterial baroreceptors, cardiopulmonary baroreceptors, and the medullary cardiovascular center quickly accommodate to the situation. They no longer force MAP and CO to remain at the resting norm. Instead, they let MAP and CO rise to meet the needs of exercise. During exercise:

- Increased sympathetic activity and decreased parasympathetic activity increase heart rate.
- Increased sympathetic activity increases cardiac contractility.
- Increased sympathetic activity increases peripheral resistance in non-active skeletal muscle, splanchnic organs, kidneys, and skin. [Peripheral resistance decreases in active skeletal muscle during dynamic exercise in spite of increased sympathetic activity due to local mechanisms that are discussed in Chapter 16.]

How is sympathetic activity adjusted during exercise to change MAP and CO by just the right amounts to support particular intensities and durations of exercise? We cannot give an entirely satisfactory answer to this question. One suggestion, for which there is some evidence, is that whenever higher centers command motor neurons to activate skeletal muscle, there is a proportionate command to the medullary cardiovascular center that increases sympathetic activity. This mechanism for matching cardiovascular responses to the intensity of exercise is called central command. In addition, there are receptors within skeletal muscle that send impulses to the medullary cardiovascular center in proportion to the intensity of exercise, again increasing sympathetic activity. We don't know what stimuli in exercising muscle excite these "exercise receptors." Candidates include decreased PO_2, increased PCO_2, decreased pH, and stretch.

Topic 2: Postural changes

The reflex compensations to changes in posture were discussed in Chapter 8.

Topic 3: Bed Rest and Space Flight

Prolonged bed rest, even for a healthy person, has important cardiovascular consequences. After only a few days of continuous horizontal existence, orthostatic hypotension becomes apparent upon standing. The subject gets woozy and may faint due to a sudden drop in MAP. There are two causes of post-bed-rest orthostatic hypotension: decreased total blood volume and decreased reactivity of the baroreceptor reflexes.

- **Decreased total blood volume:** Upon changing from a standing to a horizontal posture, blood redistributes such that less is in the legs and more is in the thorax. [See the discussion of postural effects in Chapter 8 for a more detailed description.]. Consequently, CVP increases and, in turn, CO and MAP increase. Cardiopulmonary and arterial baroreceptor reflexes gradually reduce blood volume over a period of several days utilizing the mechanisms described earlier in this chapter, thereby returning CVP and MAP to normal.
- **Decreased reactivity of the baroreceptor reflexes:** Blunting of the baroreceptor reflexes during continuous bed rest is not well understood, but is probably akin to disuse atrophy of skeletal muscle – use it or lose it.

Owing to the absence of gravity during space flight, blood redistributes very much as it does during bed rest with less in the legs and more in the thorax. Blood volume decreases and the baroreceptor reflexes are weakened. Upon return to earth, most astronauts have a difficult time with orthostatic hypotension.

Topic 4: Emotional Responses

Fight or Flight Reaction
Sudden fright, extreme excitement, or rage elicits general and massive sympathetic activity that abruptly raises MAP, CVP, and CO. This response is usually called the fight or flight reaction. It is also called the alerting or alarm reaction. It enhances our ability to cope with the precipitating situation. Many other organs of the body are involved in the fight or flight reaction but details are beyond the scope of this text.

Vasovagal Faint (neurcardiogenic syncope)
Some people are afflicted with a response to certain emotional stimuli that causes decreased sympathetic activity to the heart and blood vessels, and a profound increase in parasympathetic activity to the heart. The result is a large decrease in TPR and a dramatic drop in heart rate. Both of these effects cause MAP to plummet. Cerebral blood flow drops. Unless a horizontal posture is taken immediately, the victim faints. Sometimes even a horizontal posture doesn't prevent fainting.

A common stimulus is an intravenous injection or just the sight of an oncoming syringe with needle. Another is the sight of blood, especially one's own. An injury or a pain that is perceived as being ominous can induce the vasovagal response. Merely listening to a lecture about some horrible disease can induce the reflex in certain individuals. Some young people reject careers related to medicine because they are afflicted with the vasovagal response.

The vasovagal response originates in the cerebral cortex and reaches the medullary cardiovascular center *via* the anterior hypothalamus. It has no apparent beneficial qualities. It seems to be unrelated to the individual's physical strength, emotional stability, intelligence, or resolve to resist.

Physicians should be aware that when a patient faints, the vasovagal response might be the cause rather than some more profound disease. Dentists should be alert to the possibility of vasovagal faint and, when it happens, should promptly put the patient in a horizontal position.

Blushing
Many people respond to certain kinds of embarrassment by selective reduction of sympathetic activity only to the skin, especially of the face and neck. The resulting cutaneous hyperemia (blushing) can be readily observed in light-skinned individuals. The blushing response originates in the cerebral cortex and passes to the medullary cardiovascular center *via* the hypothalamus.

Topic 5: The Diving Reflex

When aquatic mammals (whales, dolphins, *etc.*) dive, their heart rate decreases dramatically due to increased parasympathetic activity. In addition, blood flow through most organs (except brain and heart) markedly decreases due to increased sympathetic activity to resistance vessels. Thus, most tissues use little oxygen and the dive can be prolonged. It is hard to think of any other situation in which parasympathetic activity to the heart and sympathetic activity elsewhere are both increased at the same time.

For unclear reasons, we humans have a rudimentary diving reflex. If we put our face in water (especially if it is cold), heart rate decreases and TPR increases. People with supraventricular tachycardias can sometimes take advantage of the diving reflex. Immersing the face in water is one of various "vagogenic" maneuvers that can sometimes convert a supraventricular tachycardia to a normal sinus rhythm by inhibiting SA node rhythmicity and inhibiting impulse conduction through the AV node. Other vagogenic maneuvers include massage of the carotid sinuses and the Valsalva maneuver.

Topic 6: The Valsalva Maneuver

The Valsalva maneuver is a forced expiration against a closed glottis. It causes increased intrathoracic pressure. Blowing up a balloon, certain weight-lifting exertions, straining at stool, etc. can increase intrathoracic pressure enough to cause marked cardiovascular responses.

The first thing that happens during a Valsalva maneuver is an increase in MAP. This is caused by increased intrathoracic pressure squeezing down on intrathoracic arteries. Increased intrathoracic pressure also squeezes down on intrathoracic veins and, therefore, reduces venous return, preload to the heart, CO, and, consequently, MAP. So MAP rises for a few heartbeats, but then falls. If the maneuver is maintained too long, the subject might faint. If the maneuver is stopped after about 10 sec, CO increases greatly and elevates MAP and pulse pressure to such an extent that arterial baroreceptors are strongly stimulated. Parasympathetic activity to the heart markedly increases, thereby suppressing the SA and AV nodes. Thus, the Valsalva maneuver can be useful in managing supraventricular tachycardias. It can also be useful for testing the effectiveness of the arterial baroreceptor reflexes in cases of suspected disorders of the autonomic nervous system.

Topic 7: The Cushing Reflex

Any abnormal increase in intracranial pressure squeezes down on cerebral blood vessels, thereby decreasing cerebral blood flow. When this happens a reflex is initiated that increases general sympathetic activity and, therefore, MAP. This is called the Cushing reflex. The Cushing reflex has emergency value since the resulting increase in MAP increases cerebral blood flow and protects against cerebral ischemia. Increased intracranial pressure can result from growth of brain tumors or from intracranial bleeding (*e.g.* from trauma) since the cranium is a rigid, closed container.

The Cushing reflex probably involves the same receptors and pathways that are involved in the central ischemic response (described in Part 4 of this chapter).

Topic 8: The Bainbridge Reflex

When CVP is increased by rapid intravenous infusion of blood plasma or Ringer's solution, an unusual type of cardiopulmonary baroreceptor reflex is initiated that decreases parasympathetic activity to the heart and, therefore, increases heart rate. Thus, the increase in CVP is minimized. This effect, called the Bainbridge reflex, is seen at normal heart rates. If heart rate is already high (*e.g.* in hypovolemia), the response to intravenous infusion is usually a reduction of heart rate due to increased stimulation of arterial and cardiopulmonary baroreceptors. The Bainbridge reflex probably has a role in helping to match cardiac output with venous return, at least in some circumstances. It must be admitted, however, that we do not really know its importance in normal physiology.

Topic 9: The Bezold-Jarisch Reflex

Injection of veratridine (a neurotoxin) into coronary arteries induces a reflex that powerfully increases parasympathetic activity and produces a profound bradycardia. Cardiac output and, therefore, MAP plummet. This phenomenon was discovered well over a century ago and is called the Bezold-Jarisch reflex. Substances that are more physiologically relevant than veratridine, such as bradykinin, can elicit it. The receptors are located mainly in the posterior wall of the left ventricle.

Myocardial infarctions are occasionally associated with profound bradycardia (more often with tachycardia). The reason for mentioning the Bezold-Jarisch reflex here is that it has been implicated in the occasional bradycardia that follows infarctions of the left ventricular posterior wall.

Topic 10: Effect of the Respiratory Cycle on Vascular Pressures

During inspiration, MAP and CVP decline. During expiration they rise.

Arterial
The cycle in MAP is usually a little out of phase with the respiratory cycle, but minimal pressure occurs sometime during inspiration and maximal pressure occurs sometime during expiration. Systolic and diastolic pressures change in proportion to the change in MAP. The normal difference between minimal and maximal systolic pressures during the respiratory cycle is very roughly 5 mmHg.

The medullary cardiovascular center varies its activation of the sympathetic nervous system in synchrony with the respiratory cycle. More sympathetic activity is delivered to the heart and blood vessels during inspiration and less during expiration. Parasympathetic activity to the heart also cycles with the respiratory cycle (decreased during inspiration and increased during expiration), thereby contributing to an increase in heart rate during inspiration and a decrease during expiration, a feature called sinus arrhythmia.

These cycles of autonomic nervous activity by themselves would be expected to increase arterial pressure during inspiration and decrease it during expiration, and this is exactly what happens in anesthetized animals with open chests. The resulting waves in arterial pressure are called Traube-Hering waves.

In normal people with closed chests, effects of intrathoracic mechanics on left ventricular stroke volume override Traube-Hering waves. There are two common explanations.
1. During inspiration, intrathoracic pressure drops several mmHg. Consequently, the heart and all intrathoracic blood vessels, including those in the lungs, distend with more blood. Pooling of blood in the lungs temporarily decreases return of blood to the left ventricle. Left ventricular stroke volume decreases and this results in a decrease in MAP. During expiration, intrathoracic pressure increases, squeezing down on the heart and all intrathoracic blood vessels. Blood is displaced from the lungs into the left ventricle. Left ventricular stroke volume and, therefore, MAP increase.
2. During inspiration, venous return to the right heart increases. As the right ventricle swells with more blood, the interventricular septum bulges to the left and impinges upon left ventricular filling. Consequently, left ventricular stroke volume declines during inspiration and recovers during expiration.

Presumably, the effects of intrathoracic mechanics on arterial pressures during the respiratory cycle would be far more pronounced were it not for the counteracting effects of the cycle in autonomic activity.

Venous
The drop in CVP during inspiration and rise during expiration are probably entirely mechanical. The decline of intrathoracic pressure during inspiration expands the heart and all intrathoracic blood vessels. Therefore, intrathoracic blood pressures decline. The reverse occurs during expiration.

Clinical Correlates

Pulsus Paradoxus
In certain cardiac disorders, the variation in arterial pressures with the respiratory cycle is exaggerated. Instead of a 5 mmHg swing in systolic pressure, there can be as much as a 50 mmHg swing. If the swing is greater than 10 mmHg, it is called pulsus paradoxus (clearly a misnomer since the crest in the arterial pressure wave still occurs during expiration and the trough during inspiration). Pulsus paradoxus is commonly observed in cardiac tamponade.

Kussmaul's Sign
In some cardiac disorders, principally constrictive pericarditis, CVP (usually assessed by estimating pressure in the right jugular vein) increases during inspiration and decreases during expiration, just the opposite of the normal cycle. This abnormality is called Kussmaul's sign.

The mechanical explanations of pulsus paradoxus and Kussmaul's sign are very interesting but complex, and will not be tackled here.

Topic 11: Mayer Waves

Sometimes there are rhythmic fluctuations in arterial pressures that are slower but have greater amplitude than those due to respiration (rarely as much as 40 mmHg). These cycles are called Mayer waves. They are apparently due to continuous overshooting of the arterial baroreceptor reflexes. Some house thermostats have a similar problem – it gets too hot, then too cold, etc. I don't know any physiological importance of Mayer waves, but their presence might affect the accuracy of arterial pressure measurements. Always measure arterial pressures more than once.

Selected References for Chapter 15

- J.W. Osborn, The sympathetic nervous system and long-term regulation of arterial pressure: what are the critical questions? *Clinical and Experimental Pharmacology and Physiology* 24: 68-71, 1997.
- P.B. Raven, J.T. Potts, and X. Shi, Baroreflex regulation of blood pressure during dynamic exercise, *Exercise and Sport Sciences Reviews* 25: 365-389, 1997.
- H.W. Reinhardt and E. Seeliger, Toward an integrative concept of control of total body sodium. *News Physiol. Sci.* 15: 319-325, 2000.

Chapter 16

Control of Regional Blood Flow

This chapter describes the mechanisms employed for control of regional blood flow. Control of blood flow in three specific regions, the brain, skeletal muscle, and myocardium are discussed to illustrate how these mechanisms operate.

Part 1 describes the principles and mechanisms for control of regional blood flow.
Part 2 discusses control of the cerebral circulation.
Part 3 discusses control of skeletal muscle circulation.
Part 4 discusses coronary blood flow

Part 1: Principles and Mechanisms for Control of Regional Blood Flow

Topic 1: Active Hyperemia and Oxygen Delivery

Active Hyperemia
Most tissues, and regions within tissues, have the ability to capture precisely the rate of blood flow necessary to meet metabolic demands for oxygen. If the rate of oxygen consumption increases, the rate of blood flow increases. This happy relationship is called active hyperemia. It is also called metabolic hyperemia. It can also be called metabolic autoregulation. It is caused by dilation of pre-capillary resistance vessels.

A Closely Related Phenomenon – Hypoxic Vasodilation
If O_2 delivery decreases due to reduced partial pressure of oxygen in arterial blood (PaO_2), precapillary resistance vessels dilate and the rate of blood flow increases. [There is an important exception to this principle – the pulmonary circulation. In the lungs hypoxia (especially in the alveoli) causes vasoconstriction.]

Oxygen Extraction from Blood
In addition to active hyperemia, increased metabolic activity also results in a greater amount of oxygen extracted by the tissue from each milliliter of blood. A steeper oxygen concentration gradient from blood plasma to mitochondria accounts partly for this phenomenon. Capillary recruitment caused by dilation of terminal arterioles also contributes to increased oxygen extraction. Increased O_2 delivery to mitochondria is the product of increased blood flow (active hyperemia) and increased O_2 extraction.

Topic 2: Other Influences on Regional Blood Flow

Besides active hyperemia, you need to remember two other important influences on regional blood flow: pressure-flow autoregulation and control of MAP (see Chapter 11, Part 4).

Pressure-Flow Autoregulation
Most organs, while in a basal metabolic state, maintain for themselves a reasonably constant rate of blood flow during normal variations of mean arterial pressure. This phenomenon is called pressure-flow autoregulation.

Participation in Control of Mean Arterial Pressure
Control of mean arterial pressure involves adjustments in blood flow through many vascular beds. These adjustments are accomplished by sympathetic nervous activity and circulating hormones.

Active hyperemia works in concert with pressure-flow autoregulation and global control. In many tissues (*e.g.* cardiac muscle, active skeletal muscle, and brain), active hyperemia dominates. For example, during global sympathetic activation, norepinephrine activates α_1 receptors on coronary smooth muscle, which is expected to cause vasoconstriction. However, simultaneous activation of β_1 receptors on P cells of the SA node and working myocardial cells causes increased heart rate and contractility. The resulting increase in metabolic rate induces active hyperemia. The direct effect of norepinephrine on the coronaries is overridden and coronary blood flow increases.

The following topics describe the mechanisms of active hyperemia.

Topic 3: Vasodilation Mediated by Substances Released from Tissue Cells

Figure 1

Increased O_2 consumption leads to increased release of various chemicals from the metabolically active cells, including CO_2, H^+, K^+, and adenosine. These chemicals can cause relaxation of vascular smooth muscle. Thus, they are called vasodilator metabolites. According to one popular model of active hyperemia, the local effect of vasodilator metabolites on nearby precapillary resistance vessels contributes importantly to active hyperemia. The increase in local blood flow together with capillary recruitment washes out excesses in these chemicals. The imbalance between O_2 consumption and O_2 delivery is corrected and all is well. Unfortunately, we do not yet know how important this mechanism is compared to the other mechanisms described below.

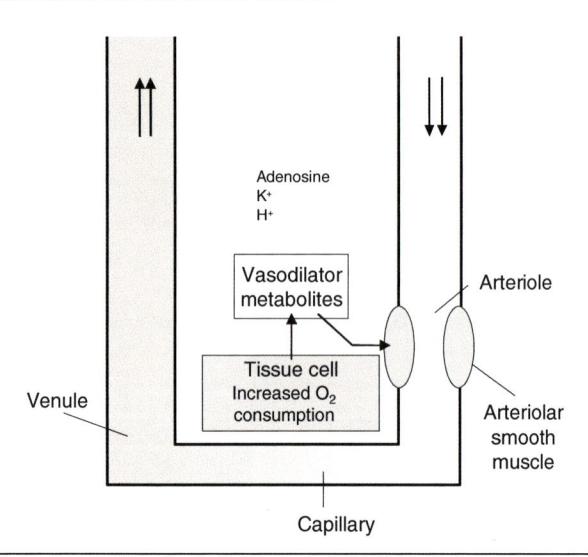

Figure 1. The vasodilator metabolite model for control of regional blood flow. Substances such as H^+, K^+, and adenosine, released from actively metabolizing cells, relax smooth muscle of nearby precapillary resistance vessels. Consequently, local blood flow increases.

Adenosine is probably the most promising candidate vasodilator metabolite. If O_2 consumption exceeds O_2 delivery, ATP production is diminished and adenosine accumulates in the cells because of the action of 5' nucleotidase on AMP. Some of this extra adenosine leaks into the interstitial spaces. At nearby smooth muscle cells, adenosine activates a G_s-protein cascade that results in relaxation by the mechanism shown in Figure 9 of Chapter 12. It also acts on endothelial cells to promote release of nitric oxide.

Topic 4: Vasodilation Mediated by ATP-Dependent K^+ Channels in Vascular Smooth Muscle

Figure 2

An O_2 consumption/delivery imbalance in a tissue can lead to decreased O_2 supply to the vasculature within that tissue. Decreased O_2 supply to smooth muscle cells in precapillary resistance vessels can lead to decreased ATP within those cells and consequent opening of ATP-dependent K^+ channels (K_{ATP} channels). When this happens, the plasma membrane hyperpolarizes. Membrane hyperpolarization reduces smooth muscle tone, precapillary resistance vessels dilate, and blood flow increases. The relative importance of this mechanism has not been determined.

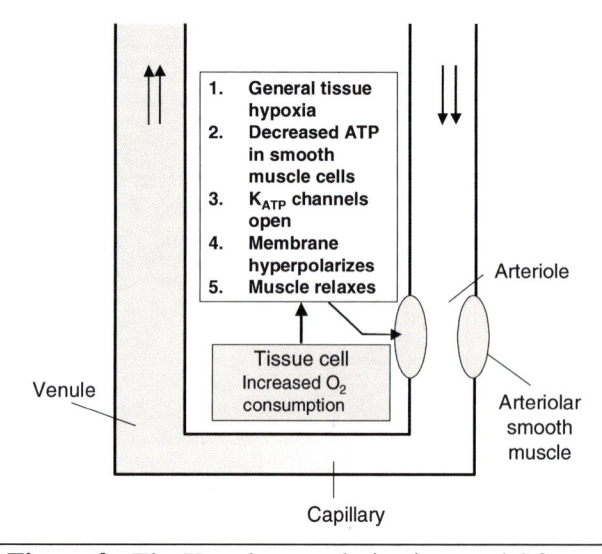

Figure 2. The K_{ATP}-hyperpolarization model for control of regional blood flow. See text for clarification.

Topic 5: Vasodilation Mediated by Nitric Oxide

Endothelial cells generate nitric oxide (NO) from L-arginine. The reaction is catalyzed by endothelial nitric oxide synthase eNOS. eNOS is activated by increased intracellular free Ca^{++} concentration. NO diffuses from endothelial cells to nearby smooth muscle cells where it activates cytoplasmic guanylyl cyclase. The resulting cGMP activates protein kinase G whose resulting phosphorylations cause smooth muscle relaxation. Continuous release of NO from endothelial cells tends to keep precapillary resistance vessels always more relaxed than they otherwise would be.

Effect of Shear Rate on NO Release
Figure 3

In addition to its continuous release, NO production by endothelial cells is dependent on the rate of blood flow. Increased shear rate at the surface of endothelial cells causes membrane hyperpolarization which drives Ca^{++} influx through nonselective cation channels (Figure 11, Chapter 12). The resulting increase in intracellular Ca^{++} concentration activates eNOS. Thus, an increase in blood flow resulting from exercise and from release of vasodilator metabolites can augment itself by shear-induced NO release.

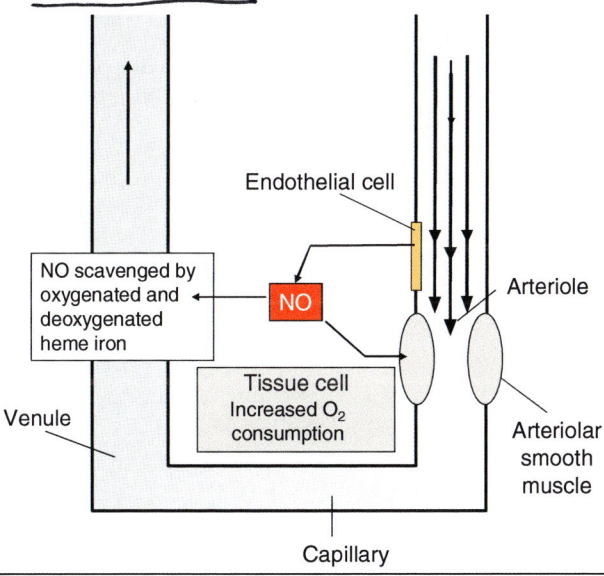

Figure 3. The nitric oxide model for control of regional blood flow. Nitric oxide (NO) is slowly released all the time from endothelial cells and helps keep vascular smooth muscle relatively relaxed. Increased flow rate, resulting from exercise and local metabolites stimulates shear-sensitive channels on the membranes of endothelial cells resulting in increased Ca^{++} influx and increased NO synthesis and release. NO relaxes smooth muscle in nearby precapillary resistance vessels. Consequently, increased local flow is amplified.

Various humoral agents can increase production of NO from endothelial cells (by raising intracellular Ca^{++}); these include adenosine, acetylcholine, bradykinin, substance P, histamine, serotonin, ATP, and many others. Many of these responses are probably not important for active hyperemia, but many of them are very important for the hyperemia of inflammation.

Scavenging of Nitric Oxide

The lifetime of free NO is brief. It quickly reacts with oxygen and water to form a variety of oxides and nitrates, some of which can be toxic. Even more quickly, it binds to the heme iron of oxygenated hemoglobin. It is then very rapidly converted to nitrate (NO_3^-) by a dioxygenation reaction. The nitrate is then released and is harmless. In this way, heme iron scavenges NO.

Some NO also binds to deoxygenated heme iron and is either converted to nitrite (NO_2^-) or is transferred to a cysteine residue on globin to form S-nitroso-hemoglobin.

The relative importance of these two pathways for NO scavenging (oxygenated vs. deoxygenated Hb) is highly controversial.

There is evidence that heme can convert NO_2^- back to NO in relatively hypoxic conditions and this may contribute to increased blood flow and O_2 delivery as needed. There is also evidence that S-nitroso-hemoglobin can release NO when PO_2 falls, further contributing to metabolic autoregulation.

Prompt scavenging of NO by heme iron prevents dangerous buildup of NO in tissues. It also helps to localize the effects of locally released NO. It also protects NO from spontaneous reaction with oxygen and water.

If NO were scavenged too fast by Hb, total peripheral resistance would be too high. In fact, this is a serious problem in developing blood substitutes based on Hb derivatives. These are called hemoglobin-based oxygen carriers, HBOCs. Such blood substitutes may carry and release O_2 just fine, but they result in unacceptable increases in peripheral resistance, and so far have been disappointing for treating hypovolemia in spite of a tremendous amount of research effort and money. Too much NO scavenging is thought to be the main problem, although a relative deficit of the Fahraeus-Lindqvist effect may contribute since it depends on the presence of red blood cells (Chapter 11, Part 3).

When Hb is sequestered in red cells, it scavenges NO more slowly than when it is dissolved in plasma, thereby allowing the vasodilatory effect of NO to be maintained at appropriate levels. It is not clear how this works. It has been proposed that there is actually a diffusion barrier around red cells that slows entry of NO.

Atherosclerosis and NO
There is strong evidence that atherosclerotic arteries and arterioles fail to release NO properly. Many stimuli that normally cause vasodilation no longer do so in atherosclerotic arteries, and may even cause vasoconstriction. In people with severe coronary atherosclerosis, failure of NO-induced coronary vasodilation during periods of increased myocardial oxygen consumption may contribute to myocardial ischemia and angina pectoris.

Just a Thought
As you know, drugs that block L-type Ca^{++} channels, such as dyhydropyridines, are used to inhibit smooth muscle in precapillary resistance vessels. What if Ca^{++} influx into endothelial cells were mediated by L-type Ca^{++} channels? Ca^{++} channel blockers would then be expected to inhibit nitric oxide release from endothelial cells and, therefore, be far less effective as vasodilators. It has recently been found that the increase in endothelial cell Ca^{++} that triggers NO production in response to bradykinin and substance P does not depend on L-type Ca^{++} channels. If this were also true of other stimulators of NO production such as shear rate, it would imply that dihydropyridines could directly inhibit vascular smooth muscle by blocking L-type Ca^{++} channels without interfering with the normal production of NO. This would be a nice arrangement.

Topic 6: Reactive Hyperemia

Here's an experiment you can try on yourself (at your own risk). Tie a tourniquet around your upper arm to prevent arterial inflow and keep the pressure on for about a minute or until it starts to hurt. Then release the tourniquet and watch the color of the arm. While the tourniquet was producing ischemia, the arm probably became very pale or even blue. After release of the tourniquet, the arm should have become quite pink. The latter response represents greatly increased blood flow to the arm after release of the tourniquet. This phenomenon is called reactive hyperemia. It can be explained by the buildup of vasodilator metabolites.

Update on the Role of Nitric Oxide in Cardiovascular Physiology

There are three types of nitric oxide synthase: endothelial (eNOS), neuronal (nNOS) and inducible (iNOS). Both eNOS and nNOS are present, not only in endothelia and brain respectively, but also in cardiac muscle and vascular smooth muscle. There is strong evidence that eNOS and nNOS play important roles in cardiovascular physiology besides the classical role of eNOS generating NO for vasodilation as described above. Synthesis of NO by eNOS and nNOS can be stimulated by mechanical forces: by shear at the surface of endothelial cells due to flowing blood, and by stretch of cardiac myocytes.

Inotropic Effects
Nitric oxide is a positive inotropic agent at low concentrations but a negative inotropic agent at high concentrations.

Chronotropic Effect
Nitric oxide has a negative chronotropic effect that is at least partly due to an augmentation of parasympathetic action on the SA node.

Lusitropic Effect and Duration of Contraction
Nitric oxide is a positive lusitropic agent, *i.e.* it increases the rate of ventricular relaxation. Consequently, it tends to reduce the duration of systole.

The Starling Effect
The length-tension relationship for cardiac muscle was described in Chapter 4. Over the working range, the slope of this relationship is very steep compared to that of skeletal muscle. It now seems likely that NO release induced by stretch of the sarcomeres is involved in this response, perhaps by increasing Ca^{++} release from the sarcoplasmic reticulum or perhaps by increasing sensitivity of the myofilaments to Ca^{++}. Thus, NO might contribute to the Starling effect (increased stroke volume with increased preload); however, it is not clear just how import this NO effect is.

The Anrep Effect

In addition to the immediate effect of stretching sarcomeres on the subsequent force of contraction and velocity of shortening, there is a more gradual positive inotropic effect over the next couple of minutes. This effect results in the ability of the heart to gradually restore its stroke volume in the face of an increase in afterload, *i.e.* the Anrep Effect mentioned in Chapter 7. NO produced by eNOS and nNOS may be involved in this gradual increase in contractility

Cardiac and Vascular Remodeling

Nitric oxide seems to be involved in concentric and eccentric remodeling of the heart resulting from chronic pressure or volume overload respectively (see Chapter 10). It is also apparently involved in the outward remodeling of arteries resulting from chronic partial obstruction. These effects are thought to be initiated by mechanical forces (shear and stretch) causing activation of eNOS and nNOS.

[The above effects of nitric oxide and roles of eNOS and nNOS have been extensively reviewed by J.L. Balligand *et al.* in *Physiological Reviews*, 89:481-534, 2009. Unfortunately, it is very hard to evaluate the importance of these effects.]

Relationship to Dystrophin and Muscular Dystrophy

The dystroglycan/dystrophin complex of striated muscle was described in Chapter 2 (see Figure 13 in that chapter). A group of protein subunits called syntrophins is attached to dystrophin. It turns out that nNOS is attached to α–syntrophin. Absence of dystrophin (as in Duchenne muscular dystrophy) apparently results in absence of nNOS in the cortical dystroglycan/dystrophin complex. It is possible that a deficiency in nitric oxide contributes to the cardiomyopathy of muscular dystrophy. [D.P. Judge, *et al.*, *Am. J. Cardiovasc. Drugs*, 11:287-294, 2011.]

Part 2: Control of Cerebral Blood Flow

Topic 1: Adequate Blood Flow to the Brain must be Maintained at Any Expense

Figure 4

The brain requires a continuous supply of oxygen and glucose. Its stores of glycogen and its ability to perform anaerobic metabolism are minimal. Unconsciousness occurs after only about 7 sec of complete ischemia (neck tourniquet in human volunteers). Irreversible brain damage occurs after a few minutes of oxygen deprivation. Most other organs put up with anoxia for much longer periods. It is extraordinarily important, therefore, that adequate cerebral blood flow be maintained in all circumstances and at any expense.

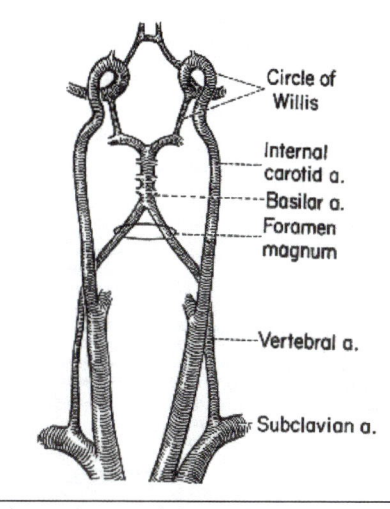

Figure 4. Main arterial supply to the brain and the circle of Willis.
Drawing by Dr. Donald Stubbs
The University of Texas Medical Branch
Dept. of Neuroscience and Cell Biology
Galveston, TX

Topic 2: Pressure-Flow Autoregulation

The cerebral circulation performs pressure-flow autoregulation as effectively as any organ in the body. Flow is nearly constant over a wide range of mean arterial pressures. Thus, increased MAP during exercise doesn't materially increase cerebral blood flow and decreased MAP during moderate hypotensive episodes doesn't dangerously decrease cerebral blood flow. During serious circulatory shock, with a mean arterial pressure of only 60 or 70 mmHg, cerebral blood flow is essentially uncompromised. The mechanism of cerebral pressure-flow autoregulation might be myogenic (maintenance of constant arteriolar wall tension). It might also involve local vasodilator metabolites and circulating nitric oxide. The relative contributions of the various mechanisms for regional control are not understood.

The autoregulatory range automatically resets when MAP changes over an extended period. For example, at a normal MAP of about 90 mmHg, the autoregulatory range for cerebral blood flow is about 60 to 120 mmHg. During chronic hypertension with an MAP of 120 mmHg, cerebral blood flow autoregulates between about 90 and 150 mmHg.

Topic 3: Lack of Participation in Control of MAP

The cerebral circulation does not participate in control of MAP. It would be crazy, wouldn't it, if constriction of cerebral arterioles shut down cerebral blood flow to help support arterial pressure during exercise or when an upright posture is taken? We would be fainting all the time. Instead, cerebral blood flow remains nearly constant during exercise or postural changes. During hypovolemic shock, blood flow through most organs is decreased due to arteriolar vasoconstriction resulting from sympathetic nerve activity and circulating vasoconstrictor agents. Not so for the cerebral circulation. It is essentially immune from these influences. This is good since the main purpose of the physiological compensations during shock is to protect blood flow to the brain (and heart).

Sympathetic nerves do innervate cerebral arterioles (although α_1 adrenergic receptors are sparsely distributed). The function of sympathetic activity to cerebral arterioles is speculated to be protection of cerebral capillaries from excessive pressure during exercise and other situations in which MAP is increased.

Topic 4: Active Hyperemia

Total oxygen consumption by the brain remains nearly constant under normal circumstances. Accordingly, total cerebral blood flow remains nearly constant. However, the brain is not a homogeneous organ. Its localities perform different functions that change in relative intensity with time. Variations in regional neural activity result in marked variations in local oxygen consumption and, therefore, in local blood flow. The likely mechanisms of local active hyperemia in the brain include release of vasodilator metabolites, locally released nitric oxide, and circulating nitric oxide.

Topic 5: Effects of Blood CO_2 and O_2

Figure 5
Changes in the partial pressure of CO_2 in arterial blood ($PaCO_2$) have profound effects on total cerebral blood flow. As $PaCO_2$ increases, cerebral blood flow increases as shown in Figure 5. Normal $PaCO_2$ is at the steepest part of the curve. This phenomenon is not due to a direct effect of CO_2 on cerebral arterioles. Rather, cerebral arteriolar smooth muscle is very sensitive to changes in H^+ concentration. As $PaCO_2$ increases, the H^+ ion concentration increases in the walls of cerebral arterioles due to the reactions: $CO_2 + H_2O \leftrightarrow H_2CO_3 \leftrightarrow H^+ + HCO_3^-$.

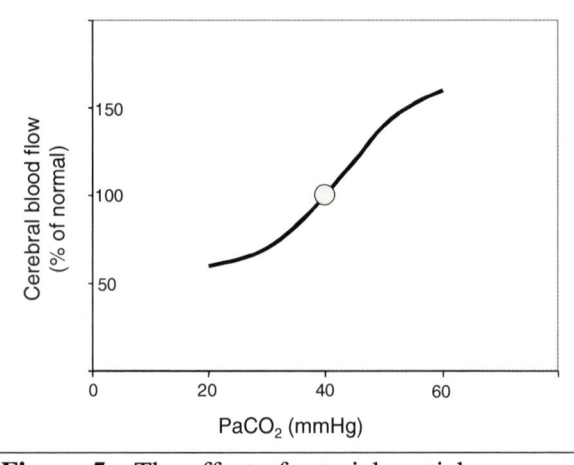

Figure 5. The effect of arterial partial pressure of CO_2 ($PaCO_2$) on total cerebral blood flow. Normal $PaCO_2$ is indicated by the dot and is at about the steepest part of the curve.

The usefulness of this response to $PaCO_2$ is not entirely clear, but it supports the idea that local active hyperemia in the brain may importantly involve local interstitial H⁺ concentration. This makes sense because neuronal activity is sharply depressed by increased H⁺ ion concentration (decreased pH) and, therefore, it is very important for the brain to control local H⁺ concentration.

The vasoconstricting effect of low PaCO₂ can be dramatically illustrated by hyperventilation. Try it if you want, at your own risk. Puff in and out for a few seconds and you will feel woozy – the result of hypocapnic cerebral vasoconstriction.

If the partial pressure of oxygen in arterial blood decreases, cerebral blood flow increases. This response simply represents the usual hypoxic vasodilation characteristic of most tissues.

Part 3: Control of Skeletal Muscle Blood Flow

Topic 1: Preliminaries

Figure 6
This figure illustrates that an anastomosing system of capillaries lies in close proximity to each skeletal muscle fiber with the long axis of the capillary network paralleling that of the muscle fibers.

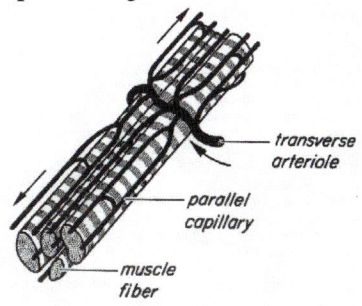

Figure 6. The microcirculation in skeletal muscle. Drawing by Dr. Donald Stubbs.

Resting skeletal muscle is good at pressure-flow autoregulation. It also participates importantly in the control of MAP by adjustments in flow resistance mediated by sympathetic nerve activity to precapillary resistance vessels (norepinephrine acting on α₁ adrenergic receptors). The intramuscle veins participate to a lesser degree in control of MAP by adjustments in venous capacity mediated by sympathetic nerve activity.

Topic 2: Active Hyperemia and Oxygen Delivery

Blood flow increases in exercising muscle commensurate with the increase in metabolic rate. Intense exercise can result in a 20-fold increase in blood flow through active muscles! No other tissue comes close to this degree of active hyperemia. We can assume that all of the potential mechanisms for active hyperemia described in Part 1 of this chapter participate: local vasodilator metabolites, ATP-dependent K⁺ channels in vascular smooth muscle, nitric oxide released locally from endothelial cells, and circulating nitric oxide released from hemoglobin.

During exercise, sympathetic nerve activity to skeletal muscle increases. In those muscles not vigorously participating, increased sympathetic activity results in increased resistance to flow which helps support mean arterial pressure. In the active muscles, however, the vasocontrictive effects of sympathetic nerve activity are overwhelmed by the local responses to increased metabolic rate, and active hyperemia dominates. In those types of exercise that involve large masses of skeletal muscle such as running, swimming, wrestling, etc., total peripheral resistance can drop to as little as one third its value at rest in spite of greatly increased global sympathetic activity.

The increase in O₂ delivery to mitochondria during exercise is considerably greater than the increase in blood flow. This difference is due to increased O₂ extraction. In resting skeletal muscle, venous blood is about 75% saturated with O₂. In intensely exercising skeletal muscle, O₂ saturation in venous blood can be as little as 10%. Thus, O₂ extraction can increase about 3.6-fold and O₂ delivery to mitochondria can increase as much as 70-fold. Increased O₂ extraction during exercise results from an increased PO₂ gradient between red cells and mitochondria (which leads to faster diffusion), and from capillary recruitment due to relaxation of terminal arterioles. Capillary recruitment during exercise can be considerable since, in resting skeletal muscle, blood flows through only a small fraction of the capillaries.

There is another contribution to increased O₂ delivery during exercise. In exercising muscle, blood PCO₂, H⁺ concentration, and temperature all increase. These changes all promote O₂ release from hemoglobin.

Topic 3: Epinephrine-Induced Arteriolar Dilation

Increased sympathetic activity during exercise or emotional excitement increases secretion of epinephrine from the adrenal medulla. Circulating epinephrine activates α_1 receptors on vascular smooth muscle in various tissues. Consequent arteriolar constriction helps support mean arterial pressure. At low concentration, however, epinephrine has a greater effect on β_2 receptors than on α_1 receptors. In skeletal muscle, activation of β_2 receptors on arteriolar smooth muscle by low concentrations of epinephrine results in arteriolar vasodilation and increased blood flow. This effect probably contributes to muscle hyperemia at initiation of the fight or flight response and during pre-exercise anticipation. As the concentration of epinephrine increases, its effect on α_1 receptors becomes significant and contributes to vasoconstriction in non-exercising skeletal muscle as well as splanchnic organs, skin, and kidneys.

Topic 4: Phasic Flow during Contraction-Relaxation Cycles and the Skeletal Muscle Pump

When muscles contract they squeeze down on their blood vessels. Blood is forced from intramuscle veins into bigger veins. Inflow to veins from arteries is reduced or even stopped altogether. During relaxation, arterial inflow picks up again. During rhythmic contraction-relaxation cycles, most arterial inflow occurs during relaxation and most venous outflow occurs during contraction. Venous valves prevent return of blood from larger veins to smaller veins during relaxation. Thus, rhythmically contracting skeletal muscle actively pumps blood toward the heart as described in Chapter 14.

Part 4: Coronary Blood Flow

Topic 1: The Cardiac Vasculature

Figure 7
This figure identifies the major coronary arteries. They lie on the epicardial surface of the heart. The left and right coronary arteries come off the root of the aorta just beyond the cusps of the aortic valve. The left coronary artery divides into the left anterior descending artery (LAD) and the left circumflex artery, which together carry roughly 60% of total coronary blood flow. The right coronary artery carries the rest. The left coronary artery supplies mainly the left side of the heart and the right coronary artery supplies mainly the right, but there is considerable overlap, especially in the posterior myocardium.

From the main epicardial arteries, smaller arteries dive into the myocardium and subdivide into a complex anastomosing microvascular network. As usual, arterioles provide most of the variable resistance to flow. Capillaries and venules are the exchange vessels. Most of the small veins return to the epicardial surface and converge into larger epicardial veins.

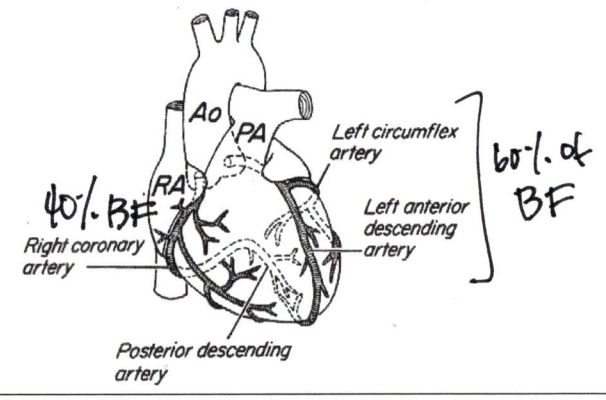

Figure 7. The major coronary arteries. Drawing by Dr. Donald Stubbs.

Figure 8
About 75% of cardiac venous blood enters the coronary sinus, which feeds, into the right atrium. A smaller volume of venous blood flows from the right ventricular myocardium to the right atrium through epicardial vessels called anterior cardiac veins. In addition, some venous blood from the myocardium flows directly into all four cardiac chambers via short tributaries, some of which are called thebesian veins (there are other names too, but they are not important here).

Control of Regional Blood Flow

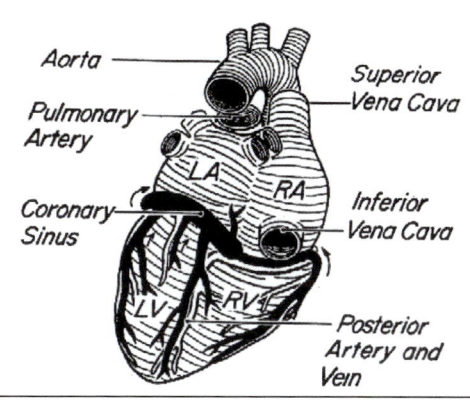

Figure 8. The major veins on the posterior surface of the heart. Drawing by Dr. Donald Stubbs.

Figure 9
There is roughly one capillary for each cardiomyocyte.

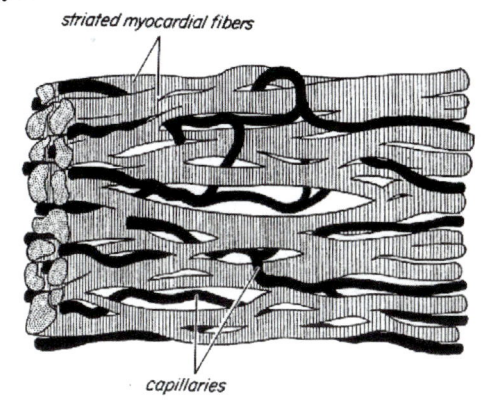

Figure 9. Arrangement of capillary network in myocardium. Drawing by Dr. Donald Stubbs.

Figure 10

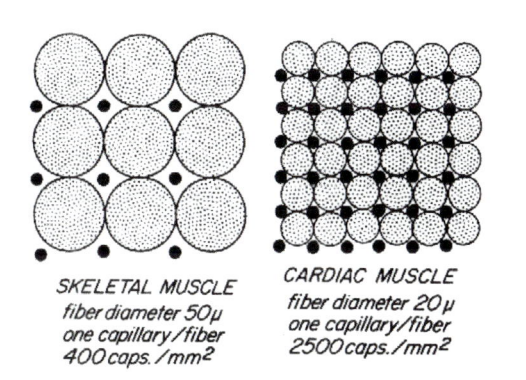

Figure 10. This drawing of cross-sections through skeletal and cardiac muscle shows relative capillary densities. Large stippled circles are muscle fibers and small solid circles are capillaries. Drawing by Dr. Donald Stubbs.

Since cardiac myocytes are much skinnier than skeletal muscle myocytes, but each is provided with about one capillary, the oxygen source (red cells) is much closer to the average mitochondrion in cardiac muscle than it is in skeletal muscle. Thus, oxygen transfer from red cells to mitochondria is faster in cardiac muscle.

Topic 2: Adequate Blood Flow to the Heart Must be Maintained at Any Expense

Therefore, just like the brain:
- Pressure-flow autoregulation is well developed.
- There is complete lack of participation in the neuro-humoral control of MAP during postural changes, exercise, and hypovolemia.
- Metabolic autoregulation is supreme.

Topic 3: Metabolic Autoregulation of Coronary Blood Flow

Increased demand for oxygen causes increased coronary blood flow. The factors that lead to increased myocardial demand for oxygen were discussed in Chapter 9. The mechanisms of metabolic autoregulation in the heart include all those discussed above: local vasodilator metabolites, ATP-dependent K^+ channels in vascular smooth muscle, nitric oxide released locally from endothelial cells, and circulating nitric oxide released from hemoglobin. Special importance is usually ascribed to the vasodilator, adenosine, which is released from hypoxic cardiac muscle cells. Adenosine may well be the most important vasodilator metabolite in the heart, but there is probably no reason to rank its importance above the nitric oxide mechanisms.

Topic 4: Oxygen Delivery

Figure 11
Increased oxygen delivery to metabolizing cells is the product of increased blood flow and increased oxygen extraction. In cardiac muscle, we have a unique situation. Even at rest, oxygen extraction is nearly as large as it ever can be, about 70%. So much oxygen is removed from hemoglobin as blood passes though the cardiac vessels that cardiac venous blood is nearly black. Increased oxygen delivery to cardiomyocytes, therefore, is almost entirely due to increased blood flow (metabolic hyperemia) rather than increased oxygen extraction

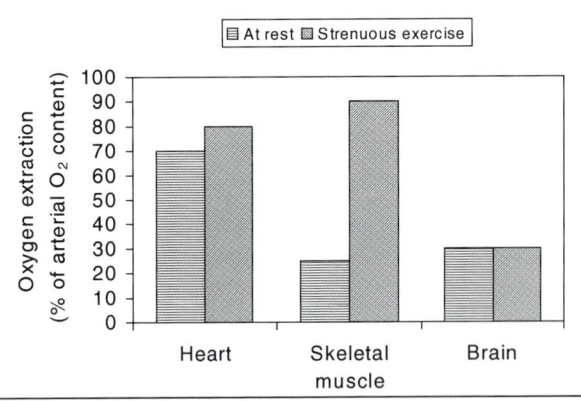

Figure 11. Oxygen extraction from blood by heart, skeletal muscle, and brain at rest and during strenuous exercise.

It is interesting to compare oxygen extraction by myocardium to that of various other tissues. During strenuous exercise, oxygen consumption increases tremendously in both cardiac and skeletal muscle. In the heart, increased O_2 extraction contributes only moderately to increased O_2 supply; most must be provided by increased blood flow. This contrasts with skeletal muscle in which there is a large increase in O_2 extraction during exercise.

Topic 5: Coronary Blood Flow Oscillates with the Cardiac Cycle

The driving force for coronary blood flow is the pressure in the root of the aorta, which rises during the rapid ejection period and falls during the rest of the cardiac cycle. If the heart were like the brain, which doesn't contract rhythmically, coronary flow would rise during the rapid ejection period and fall the rest of the time. But remember that when muscle contracts, it squeezes down on its blood vessels. Therefore, during myocardial contraction arterial inflow is impeded while venous outflow is augmented. This effect is especially pronounced in the left ventricle compared to the weaker right ventricle and atria.

Figure 12

This figure shows the variations in coronary inflow during the cardiac cycle. During the early part of systole (isovolumetric contraction period and first part of the rapid ejection period), coronary inflow is abruptly decreased. This effect is so pronounced in the left ventricle that left coronary flow actually goes back toward the aorta for an instant. Then, as aortic pressure rises during the rapid ejection period, there is a large spurt of arterial inflow. This spurt is followed by decreased inflow as aortic pressure decreases during the reduced ejection period. But myocardial relaxation progresses during the reduced ejection period until, finally, decreased resistance causes increased flow in spite of decreasing aortic pressure. Thus, there is a second spurt of coronary inflow during the final moments of systole and early part of diastole. This second spurt gradually subsides during diastole as aortic pressure subsides.

In the left ventricle, about 75% of coronary inflow occurs during diastole. This proportion is considerably less in the right ventricle. Venous outflow from all chambers of the heart is much greater during systole than during diastole.

There is one other important point. The squeezing effect of systole on left ventricular coronary inflow is more important in the endocardial myocardium than in the epicardial myocardium (presumably because intraventricular pressure becomes much higher than intrathoracic pressure during systole). This effect may contribute to the fact that myocardial infarctions are far more common in myocardium near the endocardial surface than near the epicardial surface.

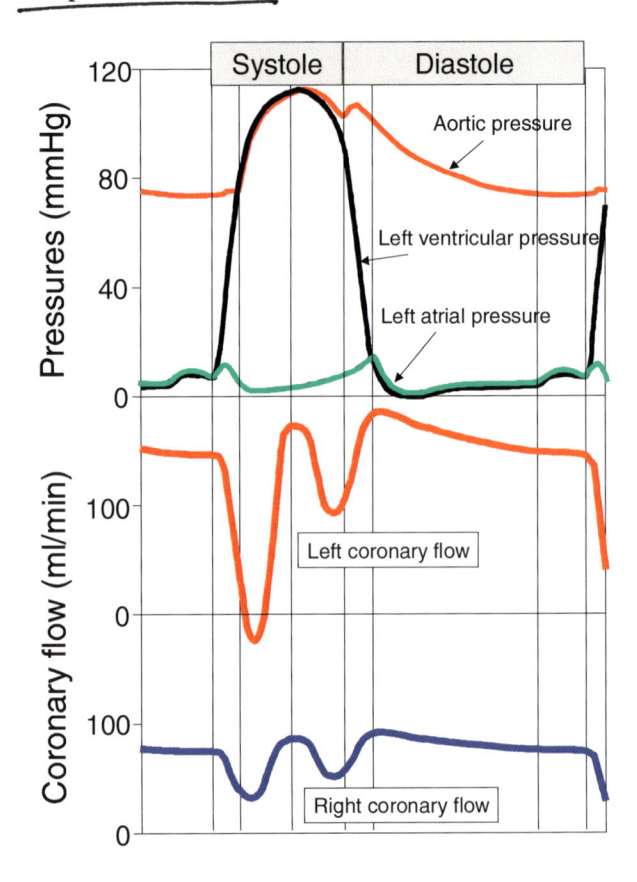

Figure 12. Variation in coronary arterial inflow during the cardiac cycle.

Topic 6: Coronary Collaterals and Angiogenesis

Look at a tree sometime. There are no connections between branches except where they arise from larger branches. A collateral is a vessel that connects one vascular branch to another, side by side. Normally, almost no collateral vessels exist in the human heart.

However, if atherosclerosis gradually occludes a main coronary artery or one of its branches, collaterals develop that connect vessels of nearby, normally perfused branches to vessels of the occluded branch. These collaterals develop at all levels of the microcirculation: small arteries, arterioles, capillaries, venules, and small veins. Collateralization during progressive occlusion of a coronary branch can save from death the cardiomyocytes that are normally dependent on the occluded branch. Repeated, brief episodes of coronary occlusion also induce collateralization.

The process by which new vessels are generated is called angiogenesis. Angiogenesis generally results in an increased number of capillaries in the affected region – called capillarization. The main stimulus for angiogenesis in the heart is probably hypoxia in and around the ischemic vascular tree (endothelial cells, smooth muscle cells, and tissue cells). Increased velocity of blood flow and increased wall tension in nearby, normally perfused vascular branches may also be important stimuli. Increased flow velocity and wall tension in a normal branch is expected when a parallel branch is occluded since the occlusion tends to increase upstream pressure.

Angiogenesis starts with breakdown of the basement membrane due to release of proteases from the endothelium and/or tissue cells. This is followed by mitosis of endothelial and smooth muscle cells and their migration and modeling into tubes that connect to nearby preexisting vessels. Many growth factors and transcription factors (such as a very important one called hypoxia-inducible factor, HIF) are involved, but details would take us beyond the scope of this chapter.

One more important point: Physiological hypertrophy of the heart due to endurance training (see Chapter 10) is associated with increased capillarization and probably collateralization, so that the ratio of capillaries to myocyte mass actually increases and the distance between capillaries and myocyte mitochondria decreases. Unfortunately, this is not the case with pathological hypertrophy due to continuous pressure overload and the capillary/myocyte mass ratio decreases.

Chapter 17

Transvascular Movements of Solutes and Water

Here we describe the processes involved in solute and water transfer between blood plasma and interstitial spaces.
Part 1 describes the exchange vessels.
Part 2 discusses diffusion of solutes.
Part 3 discusses osmosis and reverse osmosis across exchange vessel walls.
Part 4 briefly discusses the physiology of the lymphatic system.
Part 5 briefly discusses the blood-brain barrier.

Part 1: The Exchange Vessels

Topic 1: Microvascular Networks and Transvascular Exchange

The general architecture of microvascular networks was discussed in Chapter 11, Part 3. The terminology of micro vessels was also presented. These matters should be reviewed. The emphasis there was on blood flow. Here we discuss the movement of materials across vessel walls between blood and interstitial spaces.

Profuse branching generally provides a complex microvascular network around each tissue cell. Primary substrates for metabolism diffuse from blood to cells and metabolic products diffuse from cells to blood. Small electrolytes equilibrate between blood plasma and interstitial fluid. Substances transported by absorptive or secretory epithelia diffuse into the blood. Circulating signaling molecules diffuse out of the blood. In addition, fluid continuously percolates by bulk flow between blood plasma and the interstitial spaces. These processes are called transvascular exchange and the vessels across which these processes take place are called the exchange vessels.

Topic 2: Which Vessels are the Exchange Vessels?

Traditionally, the capillaries are the exchange vessels. In reality, using modern terminology, the capillaries, venous capillaries, and post-capillary venules are the major exchange vessels. These microvessels have no smooth muscle and consist only of a thin endothelium with supporting basement membrane. Metarterioles and collecting venules have discontinuous smooth muscle and contribute slightly to transvascular exchange.

An appreciable amount of oxygen diffuses from small arteries and arterioles to the counter-flowing blood in venules and small veins, thereby short circuiting most of the metabolizing cells. This phenomenon promotes the release of nitric oxide from hemoglobin and may be important in the control of regional blood flow (see Chapter 16, Part 1). Carbon dioxide diffuses in the opposite direction, from venules to arterioles, and helps to unload O_2 from hemoglobin by the Bohr Effect. [Note: Increased partial pressure of CO_2 in red cells decreases the affinity of hemoglobin for O_2. This is called the Bohr Effect.]

Topic 3: Endothelial Structure and Pathways for Transport

Based on structural and functional criteria we divide the endothelia of exchange vessels into three general categories: continuous, fenestrated, and discontinuous. The continuous endothelia are further divided into continuous-tight and continuous-leaky.

Figure 1
Continuous-Leaky Endothelia
This is the kind of exchange vessel endothelium present in skeletal muscle, cardiac muscle, and many other locations in the body. A monolayer of endothelial cells is wrapped into a thin tube that is covered on the outside by a basement membrane. The cells are very thin – roughly 0.3 μm. Their nuclei bulge into the lumen. The endothelial cells are connected to each other by tight junctions (*zonula occludens*). There are many small invaginations of the plasma membrane (caveolae) and many endocytotic vesicles in the cytoplasm.

In continuous-leaky endothelia, the tight junctions between cells are very permeable to small molecules and probably do not actually make a continuous seal all the way around each cell. They provide transendothelial pathways with pore diameters of roughly 4-5 nm through which small molecules, ions, and water can readily diffuse. However, they are rather impermeable to plasma proteins.

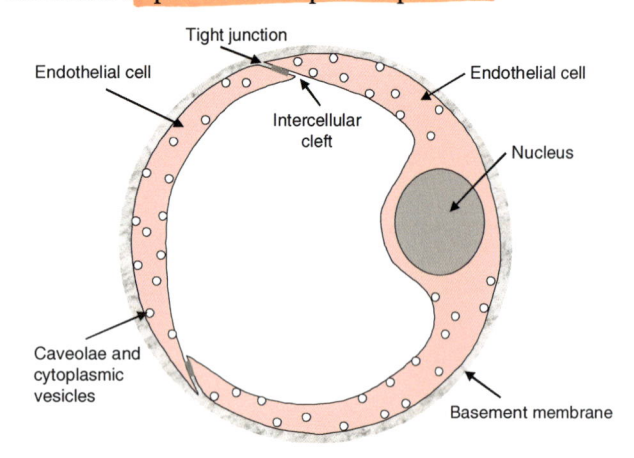

Figure 1. Diagram of a continuous-leaky endothelium. Essential features are:
- Tight junctions and intercellular clefts that are very permeable to small molecules and ions.
- Many caveolae and cytoplasmic vesicles apparently undergoing transcytosis.

Mechanisms for transport across continuous-leaky endothelia:
- Diffusion between cells
  Small molecules, ions, and water can rapidly diffuse through the intercellular clefts, the tight junctions offering little resistance.
- Diffusion through cells
  Molecules that are soluble in both water and lipid can diffuse across the plasma membranes of endothelial cells. Such molecules include O_2, CO_2, ethanol, and various other drugs. Water can also, to some degree, take this path. The surface area available for this kind of transport far exceeds that available for diffusion between cells. Therefore, transendothelial diffusion of O_2 and CO_2 can be quite rapid.
- Transcytosis
  Proteins that are too large to diffuse through intercellular pores can sometimes be slowly transported from blood to interstitial space by transcytosis. This process involves swallowing by endocytosis at the luminal membrane (caveolae), transcellular vesicular transport (endocytotic vesicles), and regurgitation by exocytosis at the outer membrane (caveolae again).

Figure 2
Continuous-Tight Endothelia
This type of endothelium is located exclusively in the brain. The structure is similar to that of continuous-leaky endothelia except that the tight junctions are not leaky. They are nearly impermeable. They have essentially no pores through which small molecules, ions, and water can diffuse. In addition, the endothelial cells have very few caveolae and endocytotic vesicles, so transcytosis is minimal.

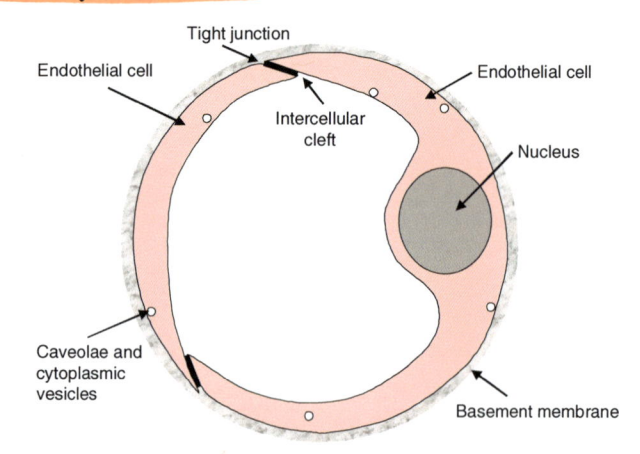

Figure 2. Diagram of a continuous-tight endothelium. Essential features are:
- Nearly impermeable tight junctions.
- Near absence of caveolae and cytoplasmic vesicles.

Mechanisms for transport across continuous-tight endothelia:
- Diffusion through cells
  Again, molecules like O_2, CO_2, H_2O, and certain drugs can diffuse through the cell membranes and, therefore, diffuse rapidly cross the endothelial cells.
- Mediated transport
  Endothelial cells of cerebral exchange vessels possess, in their plasma membranes, many proteins that catalyze the transport of small molecules and ions. These processes will be discussed in Part 5 of this chapter - *The Blood-Brain Barrier*.

Figure 3
Fenestrated Endothelia
These are the endothelia of exchange vessels in small intestinal villi, kidneys, and endocrine glands. They are like continuous-leaky endothelia with an important addition – they have many holes (fenestrations, windows) that penetrate an extremely thinned out cytoplasm. These holes are often regularly spaced in dense arrays. Fenestrated

Transvascular Movements of Solutes and Water

endothelia are far more permeable to small molecules, ions, and water than are continuous-leaky endothelia.

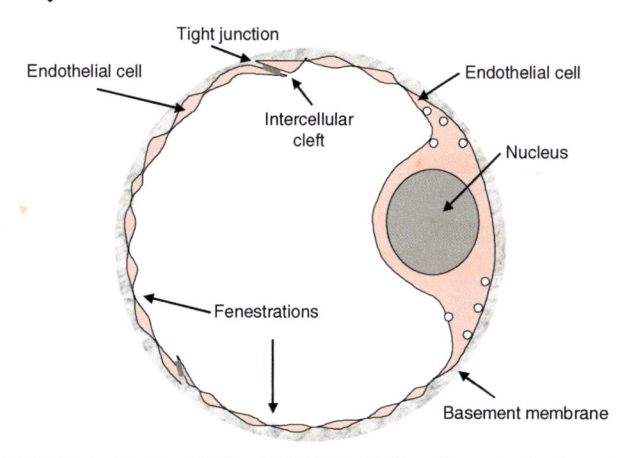

Figure 3. Diagram of a fenestrated endothelium. Essential features are:
- Many fenestrations that are very permeable to small molecules and ions.
- Tight junctions and intercellular clefts that are very permeable to small molecules and ions.
- Caveolae and cytoplasmic vesicles apparently undergoing transcytosis.

In most tissues having a fenestrated endothelium, each fenestration is spanned by a thin diaphragm separating the blood and interstitial spaces. The nature of these diaphragms is not well understood, but they are very permeable to small molecules, ions, and water.

Mechanisms for transport across fenestrated endothelia:
- Diffusion between cells
- Diffusion through cells
- Diffusion through fenestrations
- Transcytosis

Figure 4
Discontinuous Endothelia (Sinusoids)

In liver, spleen, and bone marrow, the exchange vessels are very large and are called sinusoids. There is little or no basement membrane. The endothelial cells of sinusoids are not joined to each other by tight junctions. Instead, there are large intercellular gaps. There are also very large scattered fenestrations that have no diaphragms. Proteins and lipoprotein particles can rapidly move through the intercellular gaps and fenestrations of sinusoidal endothelia.

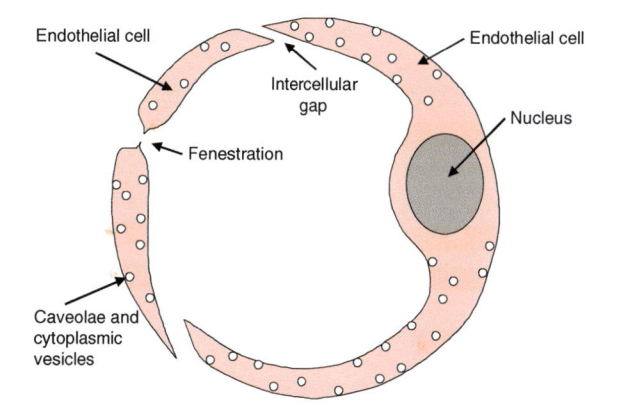

Figure 4. Diagram of a discontinuous endothelium. Essential features are:
- Large intercellular gaps with no tight junctions
- Scattered large fenestrations.
- Caveolae and cytoplasmic vesicles apparently undergoing transcytosis.
- Little or no basement membrane.

Mechanisms for transport across discontinuous endothelia:
- Diffusion and flow through intercellular gaps and fenestrations are the main transport mechanisms for large and small molecules and ions.
- Transcytosis probably contributes slightly to transport of macromolecules.
- Diffusion through the cell membranes contributes to O_2 and CO_2 exchange.

Part 2: Transendothelial Diffusion of Solutes

Topic 1: Principles of Diffusion

The classic equation for diffusion across a membrane is:

$$\frac{dS}{dt} = \frac{D\,A\,\beta}{w}(C_{s1} - C_{s2})$$

In this equation
- dS/dt is the rate of diffusion of substance S from side 1 to side 2 across a membrane
- D is the diffusion coefficient of the substance in the membrane
- A is the area of the membrane
- β is the relative solubility of S in the membrane compared to that in water
- w is the thickness of the membrane
- C_{s1} and C_{s2} are the concentrations of the substance in the aqueous solutions on sides 1 and 2 of the membrane respectively

This equation is derived from Fick's First Law of Diffusion for the special case of diffusion across a membrane.

The obvious conclusions from this equation are that the rate of diffusion across a membrane increases as
- the diffusion coefficient of S in the membrane increases
- the area of the membrane increases
- the solubility of S in the membrane increases
- the concentration drop from side 1 to side 2 increases
- the thickness of the membrane decreases

The diffusion coefficient is a function of molecular size: the smaller the molecule, the larger is its diffusion coefficient.

For a substance that is lipid soluble enough to diffuse mainly through the cell membranes, β is the ratio of lipid solubility to that of water solubility. For a substance that diffuses mainly through aqueous pores, β is the porosity of the endothelium (*i.e.* the ratio of intercellular pore area to total endothelial area).

Of course, movement of substances between blood and tissue cells requires diffusion across a number of layers in series including the endothelium, the basement membrane, and interstitial connective tissue. The above principles apply qualitatively to the entire sandwich.

There is another important principle of diffusion that was originally quantified by Albert Einstein. The average time required for molecules to diffuse any particular distance is proportional to the square of the distance and inversely proportional to the diffusion coefficient. Since the distance is squared, it is a very important factor. For example, if D = 1.0 x 10^{-5} cm^2/sec (approximately D for glucose in water at 37° C), the average molecule travels 1.0 μm in 0.5 msec, but to travel 100 μm requires 5 sec. To go 1.0 cm takes the average molecule nearly 14 hours, and 10.0 cm takes over 8 weeks!

Thus, diffusion is very rapid if only small distances need to be traversed, but excruciatingly slow for long distances. You can readily appreciate the importance of the cardiovascular system for transporting substances by convection (flow) from one part of the body to another. You can also see the importance of having thin endothelia in exchange vessels and very close proximity to tissue cells.

If you are interested in learning more about diffusion, especially across plasma membranes, click here. [Tutorial: Diffusion]

Topic 2: Metabolic Processes are Not Normally Limited by Transvascular Diffusion of Substrates

Exchange vessel networks provide large surface areas and short diffusion distances. Except for cerebral capillaries, their endothelia are very permeable to small molecules, ions, and water. Therefore, diffusion between blood and tissue cells is very fast.

Organic Substrates
The rate at which glucose, glutamine, fatty acids, amino acids, *etc.* are metabolized is normally limited by intracellular metabolic control processes, and in some cases by transport across the cell membrane rather than by the rate of substrate delivery from the blood by transvascular diffusion.

Maximal Oxygen Consumption in Skeletal Muscle
The maximal rate that an intensely exercising skeletal muscle can consume oxygen is not limited

by the oxidative capacity of the mitochondria. So what is the rate limiting step? Is it pulmonary ventilation? No. Is it oxygen diffusion from lung alveoli to pulmonary capillary blood? No. Is it oxygen dissociation from hemoglobin? No. Is it diffusion of oxygen from blood to cells? No. Is it blood flow? Yes. The maximum rate that the cardiovascular system can deliver arterial blood to an exercising muscle determines the maximal rate of oxygen consumption by the muscle. There is normally no diffusion problem.

What is the Effect of Edema?
If a tissue becomes edematous (*i.e.* its interstitial spaces become waterlogged), the average distance between blood and cells increases, and prolonged diffusion can retard metabolism.

What is the Effect of Myocardial Hypertrophy?
Concentric hypertrophy of cardiac muscle in response to chronic pressure overload is not accompanied by much of an increase in vascularization. Angiogenesis is minimal. Consequently, the average mitochondrion in a thickened cardiomyocyte is farther from capillary blood than it normally is. The increase in distance required for diffusion of oxygen is thought to be a factor in development of myocyte hypoxia and angina pectoris in concentric cardiac hypertrophy.

What about Unidirectional Fluxes?
In diffusion, the unidirectional fluxes of a substance are proportional to the concentrations on each side of the membrane and can be far greater than net flux, which is proportional to the concentration difference. This is especially true for water, which has an extremely high concentration on both sides of the endothelium (nearly 55.5 molar!). It has been estimated that the lateral unidirectional flux of water out of a capillary is roughly 40 times the rate of linear blood flow within the capillary. This is impressive but unidirectional efflux is almost balanced by unidirectional influx since the concentration of water is nearly the same on both sides.

> **Topic 3: Respiratory Gases in the Lungs Normally Equilibrate Between Alveolar Gas and Capillary Blood with Plenty of Room to Spare**

Consider the diffusional barrier in the lungs between alveolar air and pulmonary capillary blood. It consists of the alveolar epithelium, the capillary endothelium, their basement membranes, and a little interstitial connective tissue. These structures are very thin, very permeable to O_2 and CO_2, and have large surface area. The result is that by the time blood traverses about 1/3 of the capillary length it is already equilibrated with the O_2 and CO_2 in alveolar air. Even during intense exercise, when the rate of pulmonary blood flow has increased several-fold, equilibration occurs within 75% of capillary length. In pulmonary edema and/or fibrosis, this happy relationship may not persist, and problems with diffusion of O_2 can lead to arterial hypoxemia.

> **Topic 4: Rapid Equilibration of Small Ions across Endothelia**

Small ions equilibrate extremely rapidly across all but cerebral capillaries, allowing the kidneys to control not only the ionic composition of the blood plasma, but also that of the interstitium. Consequently, the ionic environment of most cells almost equals that of blood plasma and is nearly constant over location and time. The constancy of this so-called internal environment (dubbed the *milieu intérieur* by the great 19th century French physiologist, Claude Bernard) is known as homeostasis.

The Donnan Equilibrium
The ionic equilibrium that is reached between blood plasma and interstitial space is not a simple equilibrium in which each ionic species becomes equally concentrated on both sides of the endothelium. This is impossible since some of the anions involved, the plasma proteins, cannot readily pass most endothelia. Instead, a Donnan equilibrium (sometimes called Gibbs-Donnan) is established. In a Donnan equilibrium, a small transendothelial electrical potential is generated by ion diffusion, and the electrochemical potential of each ion, rather than simply its concentration, becomes equal on both sides of the membrane. The result is that the Na^+ concentration in interstitial space is about 0.97 times its concentration in blood plasma, and the Cl^- concentration is about 1.03 times its concentration in blood plasma.

To learn more about the Donnan equilibrium, click here. [Tutorial: Donnan Equilibrium]

Part 3: Transendothelial Fluid Flow

Topic 1: The Starling Hypothesis

The abundant pores in the endothelia of exchange vessels are essential for rapid exchange of nutrients and wastes. Their presence inevitably leads to another process – bulk flow of fluid between blood and interstitial space.

The hydrostatic pressure is normally much greater in capillary blood than it is in interstitial spaces. This pressure difference tends to drive a continuous flow of water, accompanied by small solutes, through endothelial pores from blood to interstitial spaces. Obviously, something must counteract this tendency or the interstitial spaces would progressively fill with water until interstitial pressure equaled capillary pressure and we would be tight-skinned contoured balloons, all puffed up with water. If a little isotonic NaCl solution is injected into an interstitial space, it is very quickly absorbed into the blood against a hydrostatic pressure difference. If we can explain this phenomenon, we have the explanation for why we ordinarily don't get grossly edematous. In the 1890s, some important physiologists thought that osmotic forces could not provide the explanation since total osmotic pressure is nearly the same in isotonic saline and blood plasma, and it was suggested that there was active absorption of fluid from interstitial spaces.

Ernest Starling provided the correct explanation in 1896. It is not active absorption. Even though plasma and isotonic saline have nearly the same total osmolarity, plasma has something that isotonic saline doesn't have – proteins. Starling measured the osmotic pressure due to plasma proteins. Of course, it is only a small fraction of total plasma osmotic pressure, which is mainly due to small electrolytes. But Starling found that the osmotic pressure due to plasma proteins is quantitatively similar to that of capillary hydrostatic pressure. He pointed out that plasma proteins do not equilibrate between blood and interstitial space since most capillaries are not very permeable to them. He proposed that the difference in osmotic pressure due to plasma proteins draws water into capillary blood from interstitial spaces, thereby counteracting the tendency of the hydrostatic pressure difference to drive water out. This proposal is known as Starling's hypothesis. The component of plasma osmotic pressure that is due to proteins is called the oncotic pressure (also called colloid osmotic pressure even though we now know that plasma proteins are not colloids). Plasma albumin is by far the most important protein that creates plasma oncotic pressure.

Topic 2: Contribution of the Donnan Equilibrium to Oncotic Pressure

One of the characteristics of a Donnan equilibrium is that the total concentration of small ions is larger on the side having the higher concentration of impermeant ions than on the other side. This means that the total concentration of Na^+, K^+, Cl^-, HCO_3^-, etc. is slightly higher in blood than it is in the interstitial space. Osmotic pressure is determined by the concentration of water, which is reduced by dissolved particles. The more dissolved particles, the less the concentration of water. Therefore, the osmotic pressure in plasma is higher than that in interstitial fluid, not only because the plasma proteins directly reduce water concentration, but also because of the Donnan effect that they induce. About a third of the total oncotic pressure in plasma is due to this Donnan effect.

Topic 3: A Note on Osmosis and Osmotic Pressure

The concentration of water is very high on both sides of the endothelium, but slightly less on the blood side than the interstitial side because of plasma proteins. Therefore, there is net diffusion of water molecules from interstitium to blood. Net diffusion of water down its concentration gradient is called osmosis. The hydrostatic pressure difference required just to stop osmosis is called the osmotic pressure difference.

When osmosis occurs through water filled pores, it sets up a hydrostatic pressure gradient through the pores that helps drive fluid even faster in the direction of water diffusion. Hence, osmosis through pores is not simply a water diffusion process, but also a water flow process. Flow of water through pores carries along any solute molecules that are small enough to get through the pores; therefore, it is called bulk flow.

When the hydrostatic pressure difference (ΔP) across the endothelium exceeds the osmotic pressure difference ($\Delta \pi$), there is net water movement out of the exchange vessel; this is called filtration (in many engineering applications, this is known as reverse osmosis). When the hydrostatic pressure difference is less than the osmotic pressure difference, there is net water movement into the exchange vessel; this is called reabsorption. Remember, ΔP drives fluid out of exchange vessels while Δπ sucks it back in.

To learn more about osmosis and osmotic pressure, click here. [Tutorial: Osmosis]

Topic 4: The Rate and Direction of Net Fluid Movement

The rate of net fluid movement from blood to interstitial space is given by the following equation:

$$J_V = Lp\left[(P_c - P_i) - (\pi_c - \pi_i)\right]$$

- J_V is net volume flux out of blood into interstitial space per unit of endothelial surface area (*e.g.* ml/min/cm^2)
- Lp is the hydraulic permeability coefficient (don't ask why it's called Lp – the answer is irrelevant)
- P_c is the hydrostatic pressure in exchange vessel blood (c is for capillary)
- P_i is the hydrostatic pressure in interstitial space
- π_c is the oncotic pressure in exchange vessel blood
- π_i is the oncotic pressure in interstitial space

The four influences that drive fluid movement across the endothelium (P_c, P_i, π_c, and π_i) are often called the Starling forces.

The term in brackets is the net filtration pressure, P_{net}. Thus,

$$P_{net} = (P_c - P_i) - (\pi_c - \pi_i)$$

Reasonable values for the Starling forces at the arterial end of an exchange vessel network are as follows:

P_c = 32 mmHg
P_i = 0 mmHg
π_c = 28 mmHg
π_i = 8 mmHg

These numbers are only approximate and they vary over location and circumstance. [Note: Some investigators believe the hydrostatic pressure in interstitial water is normally slightly negative compared to atmospheric (see Guyton and Hall, *Textbook of Medical Physiology, 10th Ed.*, 2000, Saunders, pp. 167-168).]

Using the above numbers:

$P_{net} = [(32 - 0) - (28 - 8)] = 12$

Since P_{net} is positive, we see that at the arterial end of the system, filtration into the interstitial space occurs.

As the exchange vessel network is traversed, P_c gradually declines due to viscous energy loss. The other Starling forces remain nearly constant. Reasonable values near the venous end of the system are:

P_c = 15 mmHg
P_i = 0 mmHg
π_c = 28 mmHg
π_i = 8 mmHg

$P_{net} = [(15 - 0) - (28 - 8)] = -5$

Since P_{net} is negative at the venous end of the system, we see that reabsorption from the interstitial space occurs here. In reality, filtration gradually gives way to reabsorption as the exchange vessel network is traversed. The result is that almost all of the filtered fluid is reabsorbed before the blood leaves the network. The small volume that is not reabsorbed enters lymph vessels together with small amounts of filtered plasma proteins (mainly albumin).

You might be wondering how a filtration pressure of 12 mmHg at the arterial end can be balanced by a filtration pressure of only -5 mmHg at the venous end. The answer is that the endothelium is considerably more permeable to water in the distal part of the system (postcapillary venules, etc.) than in the proximal part. With a larger Lp, the rate of reabsorption can almost match the rate of filtration even though the driving force is less.

There is a small complication. At any one time, not all pathways in an exchange vessel network have the same average pressures. There are vessels with relatively high pressure and those with relatively low pressure. Part of this disparity results from the phenomenon of vasomotion (rhythmic and apparently random constriction/relaxation cycles of terminal arterioles). The result is that at any one time, some capillaries/venules probably filter along most of their length while others reabsorb along most of their length.

You should get the picture of net fluid movements through the interstitium both longitudinally and transversely. It is possible, though not proved, that such percolation aids in the distribution of solutes to and from tissue cells.

The fraction of incoming plasma that is filtered varies widely from organ to organ – very high in renal glomeruli (about 20%) and extremely small in brain. A typical vascular bed might have a filtration fraction of roughly 0.03%. Except for renal glomeruli where the filtrate enters Bowman's capsule, about 90% of the filtrate is reabsorbed and the remaining 10% becomes lymph. Daily lymph flow is roughly equal to plasma volume.

The filtration fraction in renal glomeruli is so large that a significant increase in π_c occurs as blood traverses glomerular capillaries.

Do Filtration and Reabsorption Contribute Importantly to Exchange of Small Solutes Across the Endothelium?

The answer is no. The rate at which small solutes move across the endothelium by bulk flow is extremely slow relative to the rate at which they diffuse. Filtration causes net volume movements, but is of little importance in nutrient and waste exchange.

Topic 5: The Buffering Effect of the Interstitial Fluid

Plasma volume is about 5% of body weight while interstitial water is about 15% of body weight. Thus, about ¾ of total extracellular water is in the interstitium. Interstitial water is in dynamic equilibrium with plasma water. Any increase above normal plasma volume (*e.g.* excessive water drinking or overzealous IV infusion) is blunted by net filtration into the interstitium, due mainly to increased P_c, and (in the case of water drinking) decreased π_c.

Decreased plasma volume (*e.g.* hemorrhagic hypovolemia) is buffered by net reabsorption from the interstitium, due to decreased P_c. This process is a tremendously important automatic and quick compensation following acute hypovolemia. It is called transcapillary refill or mobilization of fluid (sometimes called autotransfusion). Transcapillary refill was discussed earlier in connection with circulatory shock (Chapter 15).

Topic 6: Situations that Change the Starling Forces

Think through the following situations. [We will refer to the difference between filtration and reabsorption as net filtration].

Situations that Lead to Decreased Interstitial Fluid

- **Hemorrhage.** During hypovolemic shock, precapillary resistance increases and mean arterial pressure may decrease. These changes lead to decreased P_c. The result is decreased net filtration with mobilization of fluid from the interstitial spaces (transcapillary refill). This is an important physiological compensation.
- **Dehydration.** A decrease in blood water results in decreased P_c and increased π_c. The result is mobilization of fluid from the interstitial space. Again, this is an important physiological compensation.

Situations that Lead to Increased Interstitial Fluid – The Causes of Edema

- **Exercise.** During exercise, mean arterial pressure increases, and in the exercising muscle precapillary resistance decreases. Both of these changes lead to increased P_c in the exchange vessels. Capillary recruitment due to relaxation of terminal arterioles increases the functional surface area of exchange vessels. The result is increased net filtration with increased lymph flow and some local edema. [The acute effect of "pumping up" with weights in the gym is mostly a matter of interstitial and cellular edema].
- **Right Heart Failure.** The general increase in systemic venous pressure that accompanies right heart failure backs up into the exchange vessel networks and results in increased P_c, which leads to edema.
- **Standing, Pregnancy, Tight Garters.** All these situations can lead to increased venous pressure in the legs, which in turn causes

increased P_c in exchange vessels. The result is increased net filtration and edema.
- **Deep Venous Thrombosis.** Obstruction of a vein leads to increased local venous pressure and, therefore, increased P_c and local edema.
- **Nephrotic Syndrome, Hepatic Cirrhosis, Protein Malnutrition, Protein-Losing Gastroenteropathy.** All these situations lead to decreased plasma albumin concentration with consequent decrease in π_c. The result is increased net filtration, increased formation of lymph, and edema.
- **Renal Retention of NaCl and Water.** If the kidneys retain too much salt and water, blood volume increases, which leads to an increase in P_c and edema.
- **Inflammation.** In inflammation, there is decreased precapillary resistance due to the action of various vasodilatory agents such as histamine and bradykinin. This causes an increase in P_c and capillary recruitment. There is also an increase in capillary permeability to water and, more importantly, an increase in permeability to albumin. The concentration of albumin in the interstitial space increases and, consequently, π_i increases. These effects all increase net filtration and result in local edema.
- **Lymphatic Obstruction.** Interstitial edema can also result from blockage of lymphatic drainage. This type of edema is called lymphedema.
- **Myxedema.** This is the edema of hypothyroidism. It is caused by a large increase in interstitial hyaluronic acid and, therefore, π_i.

The above examples of edema are given here to emphasize the importance of imbalances in the Starling forces. Please consult a pathology text for a more thorough discussion of edema.

Compensations

The responses to changes in the Starling forces are, to some degree, self-limiting. Consider an increase in P_c, which causes increased net filtration. The resulting increase in interstitial fluid causes an increase in P_i and a decrease in π_i, both of which attenuate the effect of the original increase in P_c.

A decrease in π_c also causes increased net filtration. Again, the resulting increase in P_i and decrease in π_i limit the magnitude of the edematous response.

Topic 7: Nature of the Interstitial Spaces

The interstitial spaces – the connective tissue regions between cells – are mostly in the gel state rather than the liquid state. Interstitial cells (*e.g.* fibroblasts), collagen, and other fibrous proteins are set in a proteoglycan (glycosaminoglycan) gel. The proteoglycan is mostly hyaluronic acid with a little protein. Hyaluronic acid is negatively charged and, therefore, induces a Donnan effect that partially balances the Donnan effect of the plasma proteins. The interstitial oncotic pressure, π_i, is caused partly by this Donnan effect. Plasma proteins that have leaked across the endothelium on their way to lymph contribute the remaining component of π_i.

The hyaluronic acid gel is normally somewhat dehydrated and is constantly trying to swell. The network of collagen fibers resists this tendency; *i.e.* the collagen network decreases the compliance of the interstitial spaces.

Diffusion of small solutes occurs almost as readily through the interstitial gel as it does through liquid water. Bulk flow through the interstitial spaces, however, is restricted to very small, ungelled regions that are present as narrow paths coursing through the gel.

Topic 8: Active Adjustments in Endothelial Permeability

Endothelial cells can actively contract. The contraction mechanism is similar to that of smooth muscle, involving crossbridge formation between actin and myosin triggered by phosphorylation of myosin light chains. When endothelial cells contract, the tight junctions between cells dissociate and the width of intercellular gaps increases. The endothelium becomes more permeable to everything, most importantly to plasma albumin.

Agents that induce active contraction of endothelial cells include histamine, bradykinin, substance P, leukotrienes, and thrombin. This response is especially marked in venules. It is very important in the edema associated with inflammation.

Oxygen free radicals also induce endothelial contraction. This response may be important in the edema that occurs following reperfusion of previously ischemic tissues.

Topic 9: How does Increased Endothelial Permeability Cause Edema?

The obvious answer is that, owing to increased flux of plasma proteins (mainly albumin) into the interstitial space, π_i increases and draws water from plasma. This is certainly the most important mechanism. There are, however, two additional contributions. The first is simply that when Lp increases, net filtration becomes faster for any given value of P_{net}. The second additional contribution is more interesting; its explanation requires a restatement of the equation for fluid flux:

$$J_V = Lp\left[(P_c - P_i) - \sigma(\pi_c - \pi_i)\right]$$

Notice that $\Delta\pi$ is now multiplied by σ, which is the reflection coefficient of the endothelium with respect to plasma proteins. Osmotic effectiveness of any solute is diminished to the degree that the membrane is permeable to the solute. The reflection coefficient indicates the degree to which effective osmotic pressure difference is diminished with respect to ideal osmotic pressure difference. It is 1.0 if the membrane is impermeable to the solute and, normally, this is essentially the case for most endothelia toward plasma proteins.

The reflection coefficient is zero when the membrane is just as permeable to the solute as it is to water. After all, how much osmotic pressure difference do you think a large solute gradient would express across a fish net? Answer: zero, because the reflection coefficient would be zero.

When endothelial permeability is increased by active separation of cells, the reflection coefficient for albumin decreases below 1.0, and effective $\Delta\pi$ becomes appreciably less than ideal $\Delta\pi$.

Summary of Topic 9

Edema develops when net filtration exceeds lymph flow rate. Active increase in endothelial permeability results in increased net filtration in three ways:
- Decreased $\Delta\pi$
- Increased Lp
- Decreased σ

Topic 10: Active Adjustments in Interstitial Compliance

The degree to which increased interstitial fluid volume changes interstitial fluid pressure (P_i) is determined by interstitial compliance, which can change in various circumstances. This is possible because of two important features of interstitial spaces:
1. The collagen network is tethered, via β_1-integrins, to long cellular processes of fibroblasts.
2. These long cellular processes are contractile.

When the fibroblast processes contract, interstitial compliance decreases; when they relax, compliance increases. Certain cytokines (interleukin-1 and TNFα) reduce contraction. So does cAMP. Inflammation is associated with a marked reduction in contraction of fibroblast processes, making edema formation a much faster and extensive process than it otherwise would be. It is estimated that in burn-injured skin, increased interstitial compliance with resulting reduction in P_i is a more important contributor to local edema than is increased endothelial permeability.

Part 4: The Lymphatic System

There is a system of tenuous endothelial tubes in most tissues that converge centrally into thicker vessels, and eventually empty into the left innominate and right subclavian veins. This system of tubes conveys net filtered fluid and proteins back to venous blood. The major central lymph vessel from the lower body is the thoracic duct, and it empties into the left innominate vein. [For the anatomy of the lymphatic system, please consult an anatomy textbook.] [For the role of lymph nodes in immunity, please consult an immunology textbook.]

The tissue-terminal lymph vessels are like vascular capillaries having no smooth muscle, but they are *cul-de-sacs*, only leading in one direction – centrally. Their endothelial cells are extremely thin and are not joined to each other by tight junctions. Instead, the adjacent, overlapping edges of lymph endothelial cells act as valves, permitting passage of fluid into the terminal lymphatics when the pressure gradient is inward, but retarding passage out of the terminal lymphatics when the pressure gradient is outward. Proteins, particulate debris, and bacteria can also move into the lymphatic capillaries.

The small lymph vessels are held open by a system of fine tensile fibers attached radially to nearby connective tissue. The larger lymph conduits have one-way valves, permitting flow only centrally, toward the innominate and subclavian veins. Another important property of small lymph vessels is that their endothelial cells rhythmically contract. In larger lymph vessels, the surrounding smooth muscle cells rhythmically contract.

The Sequence of Events

Whenever vascular filtration exceeds reabsorption, interstitial fluid (including excess protein) moves into the lumen of lymphatic capillaries in which hydrostatic pressure is kept low by the outward force of the tensile fibers. Rhythmic contractions of lymphatic endothelial cells move the fluid centrally, which is the path of least resistance. Contractions of smooth muscle in larger lymph vessels drive lymph onward. Central rather than peripheral flow is favored because of the one-way valves in the larger lymph vessels. Compression of lymph vessels by skeletal muscle contractions, respiratory pressure changes, and gastrointestinal pressure changes help to move lymph centrally.

Total daily lymph flow is roughly equal to a person's plasma volume (about 4% of body weight).

Some Tissues do not have Lymphatics

There are a few tissues that do not have lymphatic drainage including cartilage, bone, and central nervous system. How do they get along? I don't know. ☺

Part 5: The Blood-Brain Barrier (BBB)

Topic 1: The Problem

Cerebral spinal fluid (CSF) is secreted from blood by the choroid plexus and is reabsorbed back into blood by the arachnoid villi. Many membrane transporters participate in these processes. As CSF percolates through the cerebral ventricles, sulci, Virchow-Robin spaces, etc., the interstitial spaces of the brain equilibrate with it so that the concentrations of ions and small organic molecules in interstitial spaces are about equal to those in CSF. These concentrations are optimal for brain functioning. They are appreciably different from those in non-brain organs. It would be no good if these concentrations were dissipated across a pervious vascular endothelium.

For example, compared to blood plasma, cerebral interstitial fluid has somewhat higher concentrations of Na^+ and Cl^-, but lower concentrations of K^+, Ca^{++}, HCO_3^-, and glutamate. Cerebral interstitial fluid also has a lower pH. Cerebral interstitial concentrations must be maintained constant against any variations in blood plasma concentrations that might occur. In addition, circulating hormones, cytokines, etc. must not be allowed to disturb cerebral functioning.

Topic 2: The Solution

Figure 5
Most cerebral blood vessels have a very tight endothelium that does not rapidly dissipate the special concentrations of ions and organic molecules in brain interstitial spaces, and does not allow ready entry of systemic hormones and cytokines.

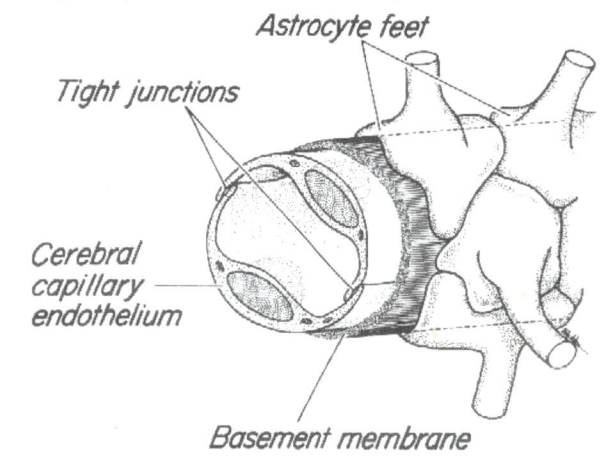

Figure 5. Cerebral continuous-tight capillary endothelium covered by astrocyte foot processes. Drawing by Dr. Donald Stubbs
The University of Texas Medical Branch
Dept. of Physiology & Biophysics
Galveston, TX

In addition to this barrier function, cerebral endothelium has a multitude of transporters that modify the composition of interstitial fluid and, therefore, of CSF. Thus, the composition of brain interstitial fluid and CSF is not only a function of the choroid plexus, but also of the vascular endothelium.

Topic 3: Transporters in Brain Vascular Endothelium

- **Na⁺-K⁺ pump:** Located in the abluminal membrane, it pumps Na⁺ into interstitial fluid and K⁺ out.
- **Glut 1:** This is one of the glucose facilitative transporters. Here it is responsible for getting most of the glucose required for cerebral metabolism from blood into the interstitial fluid of the brain.
- **Na⁺-coupled active transporters for amino acids:** There are several of these. They are responsible for supplying the brain with amino acids.
- **Na⁺-coupled glutamate transporter:** Responsible for transporting excess glutamate out of the brain.
- **Multi-drug receptors** (MDRs,): These are transporters that actively pump toxins out of the brain.

There are many other transporters. There are also many enzymes and receptors in the membranes of cerebral endothelial cells. Further details about membrane proteins and the composition of the CSF are beyond the scope of this chapter.

Topic 4: Some Substances Don't Need Transporters

O_2 and CO_2 are soluble enough in lipid bilayers to exchange rapidly across cerebral endothelial cells. Various lipid soluble drugs, including ethanol and heroin, can readily diffuse across cerebral capillaries. Water can diffuse rapidly enough through plasma membranes to maintain osmotic equilibrium between blood plasma and cerebral interstitial fluid.

Topic 5: Some Interesting Clinical Correlates

- In Parkinson's disease, we want to get more dopamine into the brain, but the BBB is practically impermeable to dopamine, so how do we deliver it? The answer is that we inject dopamine's metabolic precursor, L-DOPA (L-dihydroxy phenylalanine), which is transported across the BBB by one of the Na⁺-amino acid cotransporters.
- It would be nice if we could treat meningitis with penicillin. But the BBB is normally impermeable to penicillin. Nevertheless, penicillin is effective. How come? Answer: One of the problems in meningitis is a deterioration of the BBB. The BBB becomes permeable to all sorts of things, including penicillin. Meningitis' maliciousness is its defeat.

Topic 6: Some Exceptions

There are a few small regions where there is no BBB, and for good reason. These regions sense physical properties and chemical concentrations in blood plasma. They are called the circumventricular organs and include certain parts of the hypothalamus, the area postrema, and the pineal gland. In these regions, the vascular endothelium is fenestrated and very permeable to small solutes. The endothelium in these regions is even permeable to various circulating humoral agents such as cytokines.

Topic 7: Role of Astrocytes

See Figure 5 again
The basement membrane of cerebral capillaries is encased by the foot processes of astrocytes. These cellular elements are rather tightly packed around capillaries, and for a time it was thought that they might be responsible for the impermeability of the BBB, which we now know to be caused by the tight junctions between endothelial cells.

The astrocytes have a trophic role. They send signals to the endothelium that induce expression of various membrane transporters, enzymes, and receptors. These signals are not yet understood, but their existence implies that various cerebral endothelial functions must be up and down regulated according to need.

Chapter 18

Cardiovascular Effects of Aging

In this chapter, we discuss the effects of aging on cardiovascular functioning with emphasis on aging in healthy people.

Part 1 is an introduction.

Part 2 describes a small set of fundamental changes that occur with age and explains how these fundamental changes can explain many additional aging processes that occur in the arterial system, the venous system, and the heart in resting healthy people.

Part 3 extends the previous discussion to various measurable hemodynamic variables at rest.

Part 4 discusses age-related cardiovascular changes that are seen during exercise, and describes some important cardiovascular effects of exercise training.

Part 5 discusses effects of aging on the physiological responses to postural changes and hypovolemia.

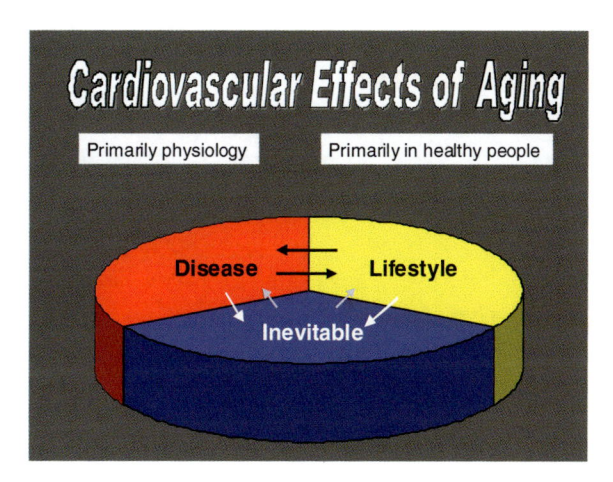

Part 1: Introduction

Topic 1: Perspective

Some gerontology textbooks define a "rule of thirds." One third of the aging process is inevitable. One third is due to destructive lifestyles (mainly physical inactivity and poor nutrition). One third is due to disease. The proportions are rough but the concept is useful. These three factors influence each other. Physical inactivity and poor nutritional choices increase the risk of cardiovascular diseases. Cardiovascular diseases often lead to decreased physical activity. Cardiovascular diseases and physical inactivity can both accelerate the inevitable physiological aging processes.

Aging processes are not necessarily linear with time. Some progressively accelerate; others occur early and then level off. Aging in the cardiovascular system follows various patterns; however, most cardiovascular declines are roughly linear with age beyond about 20 years, with some exceptions mentioned below.

The good news is that primary cardiovascular aging processes in healthy people are so well compensated by secondary changes that, at rest, very little compromise of cardiovascular functioning is apparent. The situation is not as rosy during exercise, but here the good news is that exercise training can help a lot.

As this chapter proceeds, take note of the compensations that help maintain adequate functioning of the cardiovascular system as we grow older.

This chapter treats aging from about 20 to 85 years of age. Scientific studies are sparse beyond 85.

Topic 2: Inevitable Aging Processes

Inevitable aging processes are presumably genetically programmed designs that limit life span selectively for each individual species. Progressive wear and tear also contributes. We don't know what the genetically programmed designs are. We do know that certain fundamental properties of the

cardiovascular system change with age, including the following:
- Decreased responsiveness of β adrenergic receptors
- Decreased availability of endothelial nitric oxide (NO)
- Increased stiffness of the walls of arteries and veins

These are extremely important changes, and there might be others yet undiscovered. But we don't yet understand the molecular genetics of inborn aging processes – or what to do about them.

Topic 3: Physical Activity Declines with Age

For various reasons, the amount and intensity of physical activity tends to decline with age. Decreased regular physical exertion contributes importantly to age-related cardiovascular changes. To the degree that the decline in physical activity is voluntary, it can often be voluntarily increased. There is now abundant evidence that physical training can, for a time, reverse and forestall some of the deterioration in cardiovascular functioning associated with aging. The age-related cardiovascular effects of exercise training are discussed in Part 3 of this chapter.

Topic 4: The Probability of Acquiring Major Cardiovascular Diseases Increases with Age

Atherosclerosis, hypertension, and heart failure are progressive diseases. Their incidence and severity increase with advancing age. So do the incidence of cardiac arrhythmias and valvular disorders. These diseases contribute importantly to age-related cardiovascular deterioration in the general population. Whether deterioration due to disease should be considered part of the "normal" aging process is an old and largely semantic argument. Since discussion of cardiovascular diseases would take us beyond the scope of this chapter, we will restrict the coverage mainly to aging in "healthy" people.

Topic 5: Common Abbreviations

CO = cardiac output
HR = heart rate
SV = stroke volume
EF = ejection fraction
LVED = left ventricular end diastolic
LVES = left ventricular end systolic

MAP = mean arterial pressure
PP = arterial pulse pressure
CVP = central venous pressure
TPR = total peripheral resistance

$\dot{V}O_{2\,max}$ = maximum rate of oxygen consumption

Part 2: Effects of Aging on Some Basic Properties of the Cardiovascular System in Healthy People at Rest

Topic 1: β Adrenergic Responsiveness Diminishes with Age

The ability of β adrenergic receptors to modulate the cardiovascular system decreases with age. Decreased β adrenergic influence is not caused by decreased numbers of sympathetic neurons, decreased action potential frequencies, or decreased norepinephrine release. Nor is it caused by decreased numbers of β adrenergic receptors on the cells of target organs. Instead, it is caused by decreased responsiveness of β receptors [due to decreased affinity for catecholamines and also due to receptor desensitization]. In addition, the effectiveness of various post-receptor membrane and cytoplasmic signaling processes involved in β adrenergic responses diminishes with age. The decline in β adrenergic responsiveness affects both $β_1$ and $β_2$ receptors.

The decline in β adrenergic responsiveness is not limited to the cardiovascular system but is a general phenomenon, occurring even in lymphocytes (which have often been studied in this regard).

The concentration of norepinephrine circulating in blood actually increases with age. The major cause is augmented "spillover" into blood from sympathetic nerve endings. Increased spillover results mainly from an age-dependent decrease in the rate of reuptake of norepinephrine back into the postganglionic nerve endings. It is also likely that more norepinephrine is released from sympathetic nerve terminals with each nerve impulse, partly compensating for decreased receptor responsiveness.

Decreased β_1 adrenergic influence results in a small reduction of resting heart rate and a marked decrease in the maximum heart rate achievable during intense exercise. It also limits the degree to which cardiac contractility can be increased during exercise.

Decreased β_2 adrenergic influence results in less catecholamine-mediated relaxation of vascular smooth muscle. This effect contributes to increased vascular smooth muscle tone, decreased arterial and venous compliances, and increased TPR (discussed below).

On the other hand, α_1 adrenergic responsiveness does not decrease with age (although α_2 responsiveness does). Cholinergic, muscarinic changes with age are not well defined and presumably not very important.

> **Topic 2: Endothelium-Dependent Relaxation of Vascular Smooth Muscle Declines with Age**

The availability of nitric oxide (NO) from vascular endothelium decreases with age. The probable main cause of this effect is decreased expression of endothelial nitric oxide synthase (eNOS). Decreased endothelial NO is partly responsible for increased vascular stiffness and the decreased vasodilatory response to exercise discussed later in this chapter. The usual decrease in physical activity with age is thought to underlie much of the decrease in endothelial NO.

> **Topic 3: Arterial Changes**

The Walls of Arteries Become Stiffer with Age

The walls of arteries get less distensible with age. In other words, they get harder to stretch. They get stiffer. This effect occurs even in the absence of atherosclerosis, although atherosclerosis commonly makes it worse.

Increased arterial wall stiffness is caused mainly by the following biochemical and ultrastructural changes that occur in the interstitial matrix of large arteries during aging:

- Decreased amounts of hyaluronic acid and chondroitin in the proteoglycan gel of the interstitial matrix, together with increased amounts of heparin sulfate and chondroitin sulfate
- Decreased elastin and increased collagen in the interstitial matrix, and various changes in their chemical composition
- Increased mineralization of elastin (Ca^{++} and phosphate deposition)

Another contribution to increased arterial wall stiffness is increased tone of vascular smooth muscle, which is thought to result from decreased β_2 adrenergic responsiveness and from decreased availability of endothelial NO.

Compliance of the Arterial System Decreases with Age

The direct consequence of increased arterial wall stiffness is decreased compliance of the arterial system, especially after about 60 years of age. [Remember that a decrease in compliance means a decreased volume change for a given pressure change or, conversely, an increased pressure change for a given volume change (Chapter 13).] Decreased compliance leads to increased PP and, therefore, increased systolic arterial pressure.

The Arterial Walls Thicken and Arterial Capacity Increases

Increased arterial stiffness is accompanied by increases in wall thickness and internal diameter. For example, internal diameter of the ascending aorta during systole increases nearly 1% per year from age 20 to age 60. Thus, at normal arterial pressures arterial capacity and arterial blood volume increase.

With respect to compliance, increased arterial volume tends to compensate slightly for decreased wall distensibility (since compliance is the product of volume and distensibility). In other words, the decrease in compliance would be even greater if there were not an increase in arterial capacity. [The effect of age on arterial capacity and arterial compliance are apparent in Figure 6 of Chapter 13.]

Arterial Pulse Wave Velocity Increases

The arterial pulse wave was described in

Chapter 13. Its velocity increases as distensibility of the arterial wall decreases and as wall thickness increases. Therefore, the velocity of the arterial pulse wave increases with age. Measurement of pulse wave velocity can be used to assess the status of the arterial tree. The slower the pulse wave velocity, the healthier and more youthful is the arterial system. This measurement is fairly simple and in the author's opinion should be more commonly used in clinical practice.

It was mentioned in Chapter 13 that reflected waves from peripheral arterial branches and constrictions interact with each outgoing pulse wave and contribute to its shape. When pulse wave velocity increases, reflected waves come back quicker on the main wave and their effect on the shape of the main wave changes. Thus, the shape of the pulse wave changes with age. Principally, earlier reflected waves cause an extra hump in the late systolic part of the main wave. This effect contributes importantly to the increases in systolic pressure and pulse pressure that are observed with aging. It is most prominent in the root of the aorta.

Aortic Impedance Increases

In previous chapters, we have related left ventricular afterload mainly to MAP, which is directly related to TPR. However, a more sophisticated measure of afterload is often used that takes into account the pulsatile nature of cardiac output. This measure of afterload is called the aortic impedance. You probably recall from physics that the load on a source of alternating electrical current is appropriately given by the impedance of the external circuit rather than by its ohmic resistance. A similar situation exists for the hydraulic load on the left ventricle since it delivers an "alternating current" of blood to the aorta. The theory and calculation of vascular impedance is a very complex subject that, fortunately, does not need to be tackled here. It's OK simply to view vascular impedance as a function of the amplitude of the pressure pulse divided by the amplitude of the flow pulse. Aortic impedance increases as TPR increases; it also increases as arterial wall stiffness increases.

Aging is associated with an increase in aortic impedance. This effect results primarily from the increase in arterial wall stiffness discussed above.

Consequently, aging is associated with an increase in afterload to the left ventricle even in people whose TPR does not increase. Chronically increased afterload induces a moderate degree of left ventricular hypertrophy in healthy old people.

Summary of Arterial Changes   Figure 1

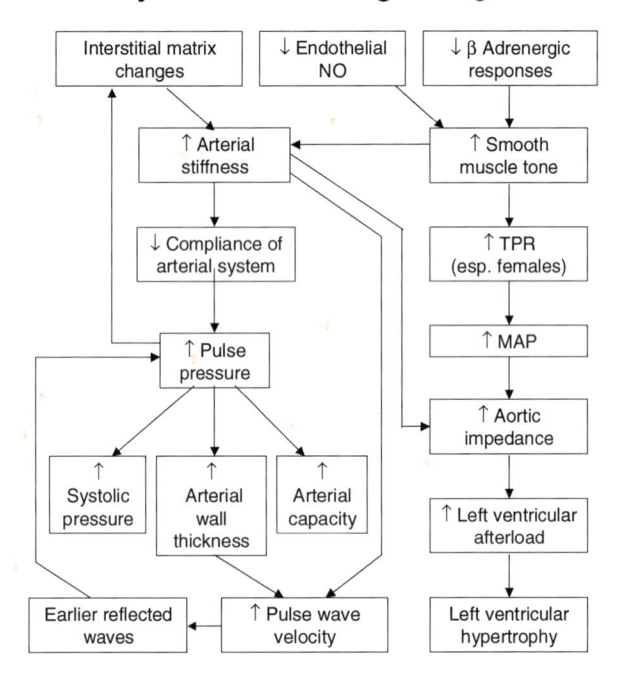

Figure 1. Summary of age-related changes in the arterial system.

Topic 4: Venous Changes

Just like arteries, the walls of veins get stiffer with age and, therefore, venous compliance decreases. Unlike arteries, venous capacity does not increase with age in healthy people, probably because venous pressures do not normally increase sufficiently to induce such a response. On the contrary, venous capacity decreases with age. Decreased venous capacity maintains CVP and, therefore, preload to the heart, at normal or slightly elevated values.

Biochemical changes similar to those described above for arteries probably also occur in the walls of large veins, although this has not been studied thoroughly. In addition, as with arteries, the tone of venous smooth muscle increases with age.

Cardiovascular Effects of Aging

Summary of Venous Changes   Figure 2

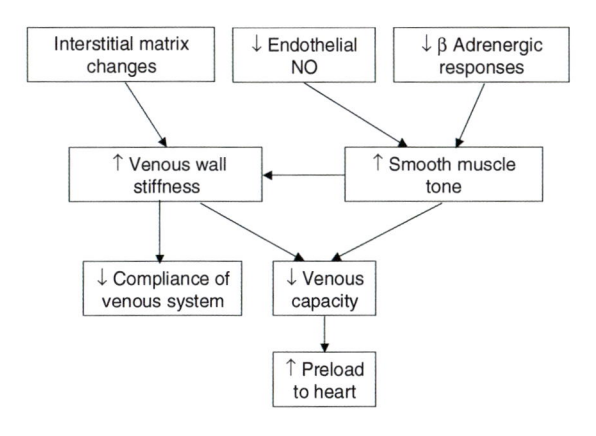

Figure 2. Summary of age-related changes in the venous system.

Topic 5: Cardiac Changes   Figure 3

Structure
The total number of cardiac myocytes decreases with age. The remaining myocytes tend to hypertrophy. The net result is a moderate increase in left ventricular wall thickness and total mass of the heart. Age-related hypertrophy occurs even in people without cardiovascular disease, but is accentuated by arterial hypertension. Left ventricular hypertrophy is a response to increased wall tension, which results from increased left ventricular afterload (aortic impedance) and, in males, from increased ventricular preload (see below).

Ca^{++} Movements During Cardiac Excitation
The events of excitation-contraction coupling in the heart (see Chapter 3) are affected by age in two ways:
1. The Ca^{++} pump in the network sarcoplasmic reticulum (SR) operates more slowly with advancing age. The probable cause is less phosphorylation of phospholamban, the SR protein that exerts an inhibitory effect on the Ca^{++} pump. This effect of age can be explained by the decrease in β_1 adrenergic responsiveness described above.
2. L-type Ca^{++} channels in working myocardium inactivate more slowly with advancing age. Remember that L-type Ca^{++} channels conduct the inward Ca^{++} current that keeps the membrane depolarized during phase 2 of the action potential. This inward current also supplies the Ca^{++} for Ca^{++}-induced Ca^{++} release from the junctional SR.

The immediate consequences of these changes in excitation-contraction coupling are:
- The duration of action potentials in working myocardium increases with age. Phase 2 gets longer. In other words, repolarization is delayed.
- Removal of Ca^{++} from the cytoplasm after each excitatory event is slowed. The duration of the Ca^{++} transient is increased.
- The duration of contraction is increased.

Ca^{++}-Overload Arrhythmias
Aging is associated with a higher risk of cardiac arrhythmias. One contributor is an increased incidence of so-called Ca^{++}-overload arrhythmias. Changes in the duration of Ca^{++} release from the SR and its rate of reuptake by the SR alter the coordination between these processes and can lead to spontaneous oscillations in cytoplasmic Ca^{++} concentration, which increase the probability of Ca^{++}-overload arrhythmias.

Changes in Oxygen Need and Oxygen Supply
Increased afterload, increased preload, and myocardial hypertrophy all result in an increased rate of oxygen utilization by the heart. The longer duration of contraction leads to a shorter diastolic period. Since most coronary flow to the left ventricle occurs during diastole (Chapter 16), the briefer diastolic period slightly compromises coronary blood flow. Thus, in old people, cardiac need for oxygen is increased while the ability to supply oxygen is reduced. Therefore, there is an increased propensity for myocardial ischemia especially during exercise.

Topic 6: Blood Volume

In some studies, total blood volume has been found to decrease slightly and in others not to change significantly. We can at least conclude that total blood volume does not increase with age.

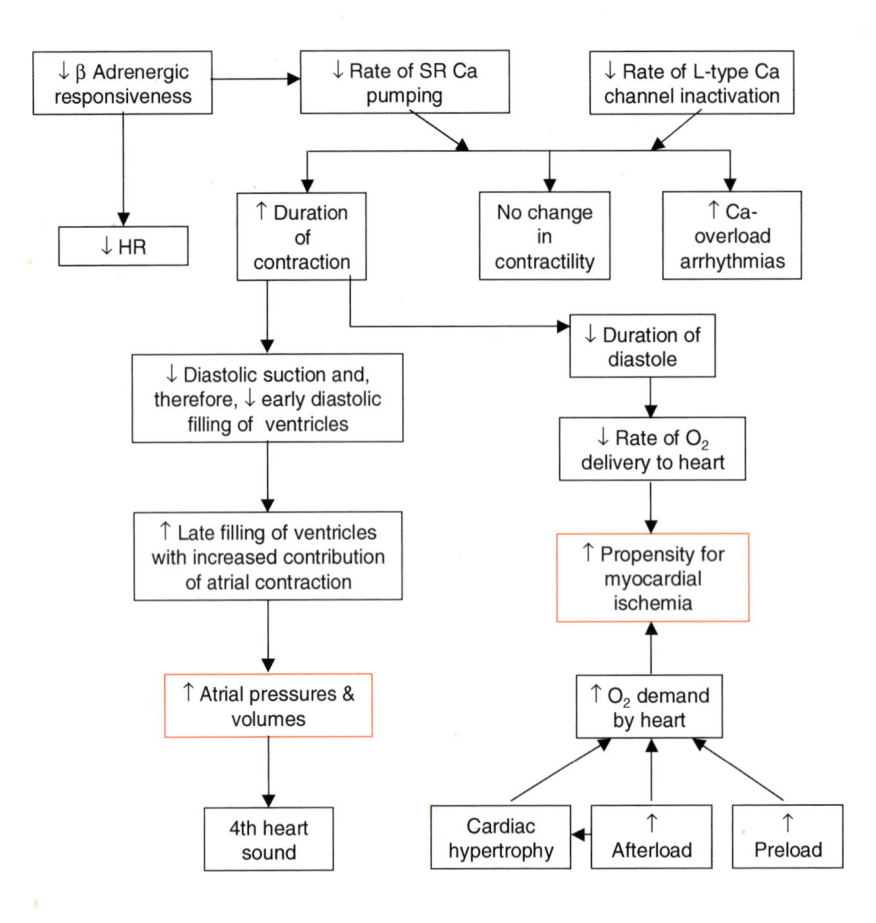

Figure 3. Summary of age-related changes in the heart.

Part 3: Hemodynamic Changes in Healthy People at Rest

Topic 1: Preview Table 1

The conclusions listed in Table 1 are largely from Lakatta (Selected References 1-4), based on the Baltimore Longitudinal Study of Aging. The comparisons are from age 20 to age 80. Very brief explanations for the changes are given in the table. Explanations that are more thorough are given below.

Topic 2: Arterial Pressures

Decreased arterial compliance causes increased PP and increased systolic pressure. Early-returning reflected waves contribute to these increases, especially in the ascending aorta. Increases in PP and systolic pressure occur even in healthy aging people who are not diagnosed with hypertension. In this normal group of people, MAP and especially systolic pressure increase moderately with age, but diastolic pressure does not increase significantly.

You should recall that as the arterial pulse wave travels distally away from the heart, systolic pressure and PP increase (Chapter 13, Figure 7). This distal augmentation in systolic and pulse pressures declines with age and cannot be observed in very old people. The reasons for this change have to do with the increase in pulse wave velocity; early returning reflected waves increase systolic pressure more in the ascending aorta than in more distal parts of the arterial tree. There is an interesting clinical consequence. In young people, systolic pressure in the ascending aorta is considerably less than that measured in the brachial artery, but in old people it is about the same. Thus, when systolic pressure measured at the brachial artery is the same in an old person as it is in a young person, the old person's left ventricle and ascending aorta must contend with a greater systolic pressure.

Table 1. Changes in Cardiovascular Variables with Age in Sedentary Healthy People at Rest (Sitting)

MAP	Increased slightly due to increased TPR
Arterial PP	Increased due to decreased arterial compliance and earlier reflected pulse waves
Systolic arterial pressure	Increased due mainly to increased PP and also to increased MAP
Diastolic arterial pressure	No change
TPR	Increased (especially in women)
LV afterload	Increased due to increased aortic impedance
Cardiac contractility	No change
Duration of cardiac contraction	Increased
SV	Increased about 10% in men by age 80 due to increased end-diastolic volume, no change in women
EF	No change
Starling effect	Increased
Anrep effect	Decreased
Cardiac preload	Increased end-diastolic pressures in men, no change in women
Early diastolic ventricular filling	Decreased due to less diastolic suction
Late diastolic ventricular filling	Increased
Atrial contraction	Increased contribution to ventricular filling
Left atrial pressure	Increased
Left ventricular mass	Increased due to increased afterload
Heart rate	Decreased about 10% by age 80
Sinus arrhythmia	Decreased
Cardiac output	No change in men, slight decrease in women due to decreased HR without corresponding increase in SV
Total blood volume	No change, or perhaps sometimes a small decrease

The increases in arterial wall thickness and vessel diameter mentioned above are probably responses to the increases in systolic pressure and PP. The biochemical changes in the walls of arteries that contribute to increased stiffness might also (at least in part) be responses to increased PP and systolic pressure.

Topic 3: Total Peripheral Resistance, TPR

TPR at rest may or may not increase because of aging (although it certainly does increase markedly when arterial hypertension is present). The very important Baltimore Longitudinal Study of Aging (see Selected References 1-4, which are reviews by E.G. Lakatta) demonstrated a large increase in healthy women with aging (about 50% increase in TPR from age 20 to age 85), but a much smaller, statistically insignificant change in healthy men. Increased TPR with age, when it occurs, probably results from decreased β_2 adrenergic relaxation of smooth muscle in resistance vessels, and from decreased availability of endothelial NO.

Topic 4: Cardiac Function

Systolic Function

In spite of increased aortic impedance, systolic ventricular function in people at rest is remarkably well preserved during aging. There is no change in left ventricular EF in either healthy men or healthy women, and there is no evidence for a decrease in contractility. The decrease in rate of SR Ca^{++} pumping, which would be expected to decrease contractility, is apparently compensated by slower inactivation of sarcolemmal Ca^{++} channels, which results in more Ca^{++} entry into each myocyte during excitation.

In men at rest, LVED volume increases moderately with age while LVES volume increases only slightly. Thus, in men at rest, SV increases with age (roughly 20% from age 20 to 85). The increase in LVED volume is a compensation that helps cope with increased afterload (along with the small amount of ventricular hypertrophy mentioned above). This compensation has not been demonstrated in women. In the Baltimore Longitudinal Study on Aging, women's resting end-diastolic, end-systolic, and stroke volumes did not change significantly with age, while men's SV increased. Undoubtedly the increase in TPR observed in the women in that study was responsible for the failure to elevate preload. Lakatta suggested that this gender difference relates to a difference in physical fitness levels between the men and women in that study – the men being more fit.

It is likely that the prolongation of ventricular contraction discussed in Part 2 of this Chapter helps to maintain youthful SV, end systolic volume, and EF during aging. Prolonged contraction increases effective contractility.

Recall the Anrep effect; it was discussed in Chapter 7. An acute increase in afterload to the left ventricle leads to a gradual increase in contractility over the next minute or two. This effect is thought to contribute importantly, at least in some circumstances, to the ability of the left ventricle to cope with changes in afterload. There is evidence that the Anrep effect is diminished with aging. Thus, in order to maintain normal SV against an acutely elevated afterload, the left ventricle of an old person must depend more on the Starling effect than does the left ventricle of a young person.

Diastolic Function
The drop in left ventricular pressure that occurs during the isovolumetric relaxation period and the early part of the rapid filling period becomes less steep with advancing age. This change follows from the fact that relaxation of ventricular myocytes is delayed. Consequently, the isovolumetric relaxation period gets longer with age and, more importantly, the rate of early diastolic filling of the left ventricle decreases. In other words, diastolic suction is less forceful and contributes less to diastolic filling.

Since there is no decrease in SV at rest during aging, it is obvious that total diastolic filling is not compromised and that more filling takes place later in the filling period. This can happen only if left atrial pressure increases. Of course, a reduction in early diastolic suction automatically leads to increased left atrial pressure, which then drives filling during the later parts of the filling period. There is no convincing evidence for an age-related decrease in left ventricular compliance during the reduced filling

and atrial contraction periods, so only a minor elevation of filling pressure is necessary.

In fact, resting LVED pressure, left atrial pressure, and pulmonary wedge pressure all increase slightly with advancing age in healthy men and women. The left atrium enlarges somewhat, and this often results in a 4th heart sound in healthy elderly people. Atrial contraction contributes a greater fraction of total diastolic filling with advancing age.
This all works just fine at rest and SV is not compromised.

Heart Rate
Resting HR decreases with advancing age in both men and women – at least a 10% decrease from age 20 to age 80. The most important cause of this decrease is the age-related decrease in sympathetic effect on the SA node discussed above.

The number of P cells in the SA node decreases with age, markedly past age 65. By age 75 only about 10% of the original number of P cells remains. The degree to which this anatomic decline contributes to the negative chronotropic effect of aging is not known.

Another factor that might be involved here is the intrinsic frequency of SA node rhythmicity; *i.e.* without any cholinergic or adrenergic input. Intrinsic frequency drops from about 104 cycles/min at age 20 to about 92 cycles/min at age 50.

The oscillations in HR that are related to breathing, called sinus arrhythmia, diminish in amplitude with age, probably due to decreased sympathetic, and perhaps parasympathetic, effectiveness.

Topic 5: Cardiac Output

In women, there is a slight decrease in resting CO with age due to the decrease in HR. In men, the increase in SV, due to an increase in end-diastolic volume, balances the decrease in HR and there is no decrease in resting CO. These are conclusions from the Baltimore Longitudinal Study on Aging.

Remember that arterial capacity increases with age and there is no increase in total blood volume. Therefore, venous volume decreases. It might be expected that a decrease in venous volume would lower CVP and the preload to the heart. The common increase in resting TPR would contribute to the decrease in preload. So SV might be expected to decrease with age in healthy people at rest – but it doesn't. In fact, as we have seen, resting SV increases slightly with age in men. This compensation is accomplished by an age-related decrease in venous capacity. There is less volume in the veins, but the veins constrict down so that the pressure doesn't fall and, in aging men at rest, youthful CO is maintained. In aging women, CO is not maintained quite at its youthful level, because TPR increases more in women that it does in men (Baltimore Longitudinal Study of Aging).

Biochemical changes in the interstitial matrix of veins and increased tone of venous smooth muscle are both thought to contribute to the age-related decrease in venous capacity.

Topic 6: Summary of Hemodynamic Changes with Aging in Healthy People at Rest — Figure 4

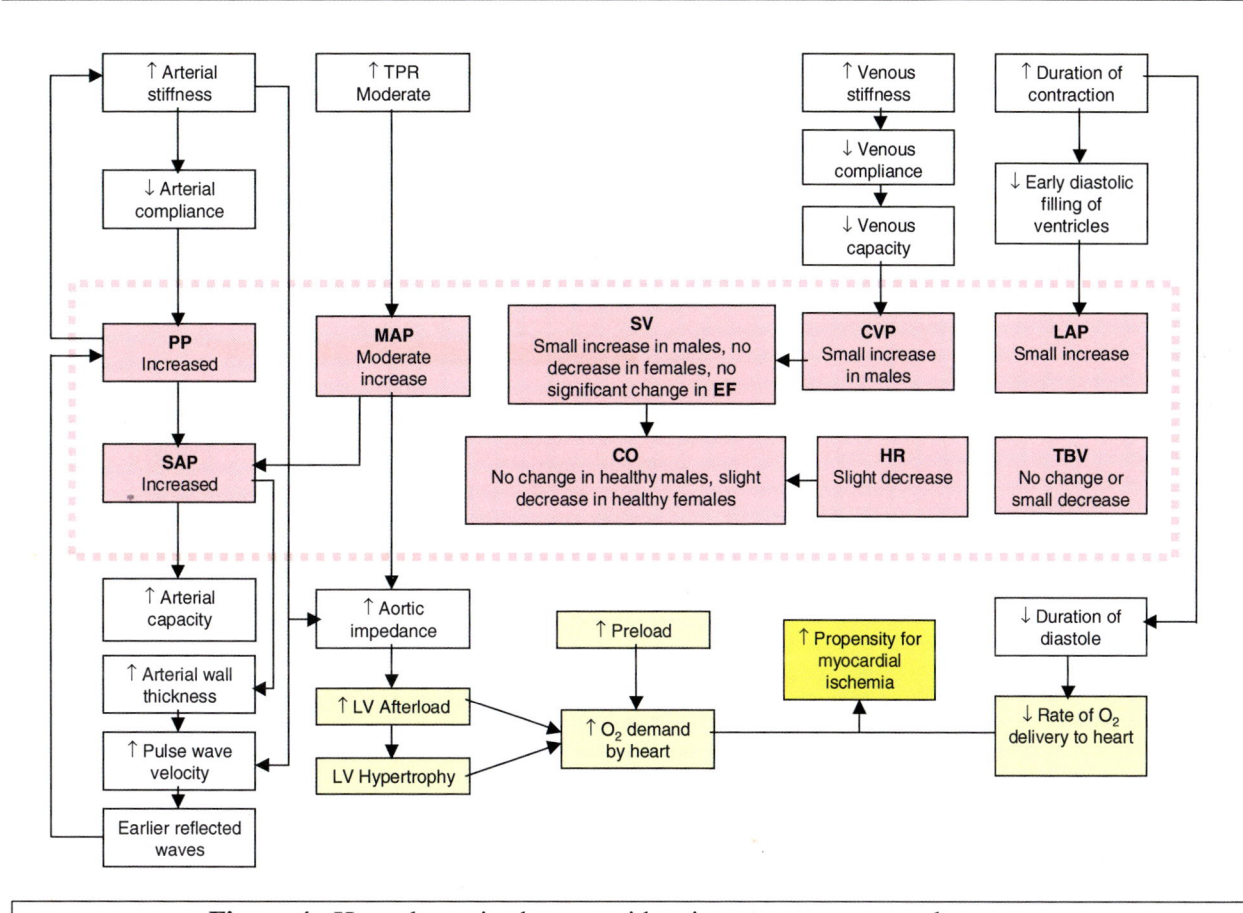

Figure 4. Hemodynamic changes with aging at rest: causes and consequences.

Part 4: Exercise in Aging and the Effects of Exercise Training

Topic 1: Preview   Table 2

Table 2. Effects of Aging on Cardiovascular Variables at Maximum Exercise Intensity in Healthy Sedentary People

Variable	Qualitative Effect of Aging
Maximum exercise intensity	Decreased
$\dot{V}O_{2\,max}$	Decreased
HR increase	Decreased
SV increase	Decreased only slightly
Cardiac contractility increase	Decreased
CO increase	Decreased
LVES volume decrease	Decreased
LVED volume increase	Increased
Starling effect	Increased
EF increase	Decreased
TPR decrease	Decreased
MAP increase	Not much change
PP increase	Not much change
Systolic pressure increase	Not much change
Aortic impedance	Increased

Topic 2: Maximum Rate of Oxygen Consumption and Maximum Aerobic Exercise Intensity

The rate of oxygen consumption increases as exercise intensity increases. It can increase roughly nine-fold in young sedentary people during prolonged exercise. Eventually a maximum is reached, called $\dot{V}O_{2\,max}$, which is a measure of the ability to perform aerobic exercise. It can be increased by appropriate training and is greatest in elite endurance athletes.

Figure 5
In cross-sectional studies of healthy people, $\dot{V}O_{2\,max}$ decreases with age. It also decreases with age in longitudinal studies of sedentary people, both men and women. A parallel observation is that the maximum achievable intensity of aerobic exercise decreases with age. All of this comes as no surprise to most of us older folks who are well aware of our decreasing exertional capacities.

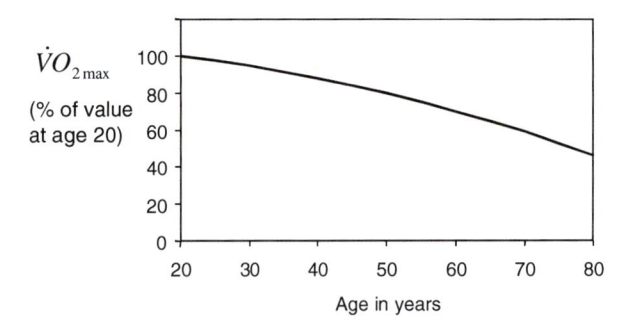

Figure 5. Effect of aging on maximum rate of oxygen utilization during exercise, relative to that at 20 years old.

When $\dot{V}O_{2\,max}$ is divided by urinary creatinine (a measure of muscle fiber mass), the decline with age is considerably reduced. This is because skeletal muscle fiber mass also decreases with age in sedentary people due to fewer motor units and skinnier fibers. The decrease in number of motor units (motor neuron plus its innervated muscle fibers) is especially marked after about age 60. In addition, age-related orthopedic problems and early fatigue often limit exercise frequency and intensity. Clearly, the decline in $\dot{V}O_{2\,max}$ with age is not entirely a cardiovascular problem. It reflects, to a considerable degree, a decrease in the ability to perform intense exercise due to neuromuscular, orthopedic, and other declines, even in clinically healthy people.

The decrease in $\dot{V}O_{2\,max}$ with age can contribute to the decrease in maximal exercise capacity. Conversely, decreased exercise capacity resulting from muscular and skeletal deteriorations can contribute to the decrease in $\dot{V}O_{2\,max}$. Sorting out these directional cause and effect relationships is a difficult problem in this area of research.

The decrease in $\dot{V}O_{2\,max}$ and maximal exercise intensity with age have three general causes.
1. Maximum CO achievable at high exercise intensity decreases with age. This effect of aging will be discussed in Topic 3.
2. The degree of oxygen extraction from blood flowing through maximally exercising skeletal muscle decreases with age. Decreased O_2 extraction results mainly from decreased numbers of skeletal muscle fibers and, to a

lesser degree, atrophy of the remaining fibers. It is possible that decreased capillarization in skeletal muscle contributes to decreased O_2 extraction with age in sedentary people; however, this has not been proved. Decreased ability of mitochondria to use O_2 is apparently not involved.

3. The proportion of maximum CO that is captured by exercising muscle decreases with age due to decreased local vasodilation. This is an expected consequence of decreased O_2 extraction according to the circulating NO mechanism for local blood flow control (see Chapter 16), and of decreased availability of endothelial NO.

Topic 3: Cardiac Output, Heart Rate, Stroke Volume, and Ejection Fraction during Strenuous Exercise

Figure 6

In sedentary people, the increase in CO that can be induced by strenuous exercise declines with age. This effect results mainly from a decrease in the ability to increase HR. The maximum HR that can be achieved during strenuous exercise roughly equals 220 minus the age in years. This decline in maximum HR is due mainly to decreased β adrenergic effectiveness at the SA node.

In young people, strenuous exercise results in a small increase in LVED volume and a marked decrease in LVES volume (see Figure 16 in Chapter 7). SV and EF both increase. In fact, EF can increase from about 65% at rest to more than 85% during maximal exercise. The increases in SV and EF result mainly from increased contractility induced by increased $β_1$ adrenergic activity.

In old people, SV increases during strenuous exercise nearly as much as it does in young people. However, since old people's capacity for β adrenergic modulation is diminished, the increase in SV is mostly due to increased LVED volume rather than reduced LVES volume, and EF does not increase much. In other words, exercise-induced increases in old people's SV must rely much more on the Starling mechanism than on increased contractility.

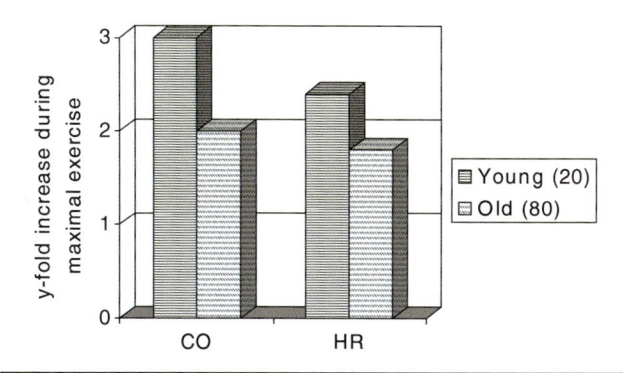

Figure 6. Effect of maximal exercise on CO and HR. Both young and old people were healthy and sedentary. Responses in males and females were roughly the same and are lumped together here. Data are from E.G. Lakatta (see Selected References).

Topic 4: Arterial Pressures, TPR, and Arterial Impedance during Strenuous Exercise

During dynamic exercise, CO increases while TPR decreases. The increase in CO exceeds the decrease in TPR and, therefore, MAP increases. It increases by an amount that is dependent upon the intensity of exercise. There is also an increase in SV during dynamic exercise. The increase in SV, together with a briefer rapid ejection period, causes PP to increase. The increase in PP causes systolic pressure to rise more than MAP rises and diastolic pressure to rise less than MAP rises (see Chapter 13).

At any given relative intensity of exercise, MAP and systolic pressure increase at least as much in old people as they do in young people. TPR, however, does not decrease as much in old people as it does in young people, probably due mainly to decreased availability of endothelial NO. [Interpretation is difficult, however, since maximal exercise intensity for the oldsters is not as great as it is for the youngsters.]

As discussed in Chapter 8 and elsewhere in this book, changes in TPR are of major importance for regulating CO during exercise. Decreased TPR leads to increased preload to the heart and, therefore, greater SV. The deficit in TPR reduction when old people exercise strenuously contributes to the deficit in maximal CO.

In youngsters, dynamic exercise, although it raises MAP and systolic pressure, does not result in an increase in aortic impedance. In other words, left ventricular afterload is not increased. This happy circumstance apparently results from relaxation of aortic smooth muscle by β₂ adrenergic stimulation, with consequent increase in aortic volume and reduction of aortic stiffness. In oldsters, however, aortic impedance does increase during dynamic exercise because of less β₂ adrenergic responsiveness and increased interstitial stiffness.

Topic 5: Summary of Aging and Exercise Figure 7

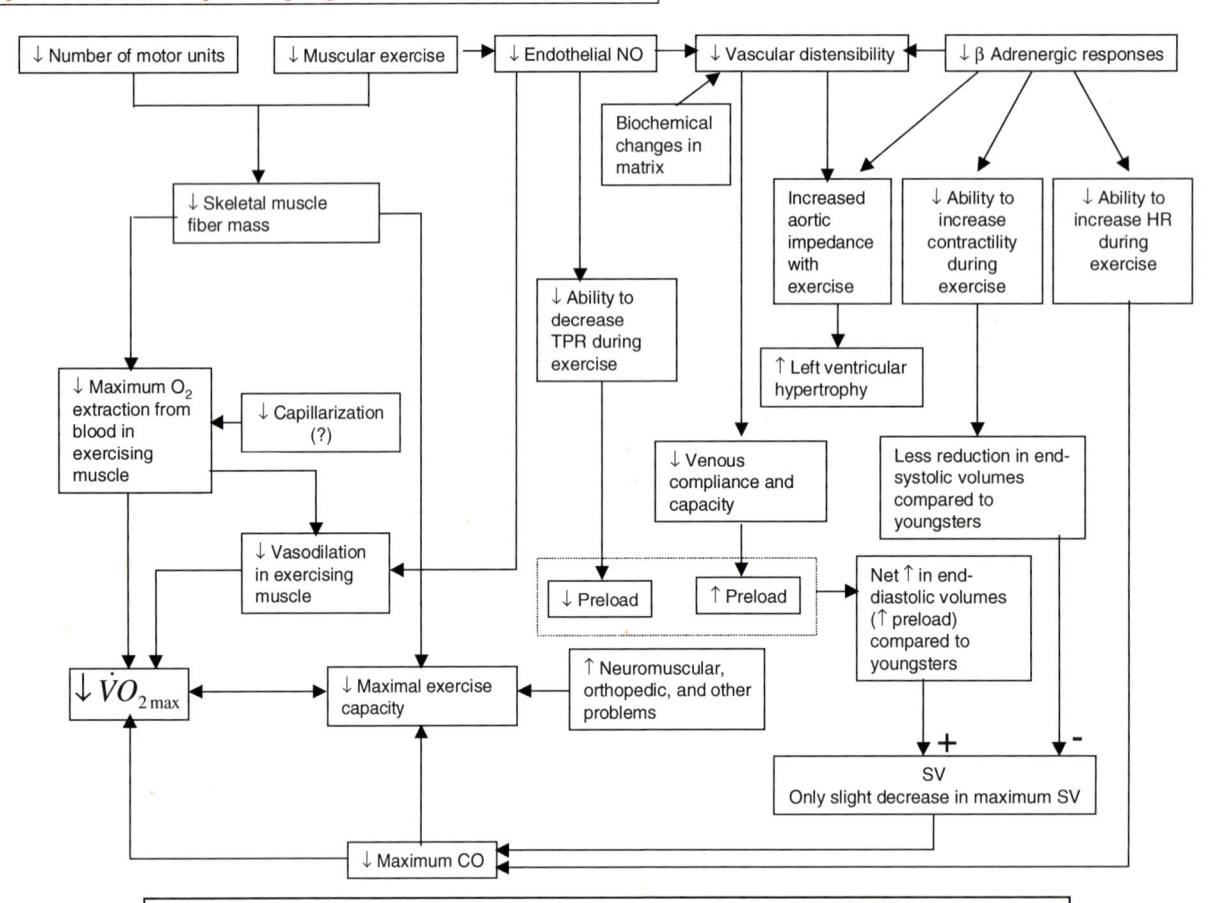

Figure 7. Effects of age on the cardiovascular responses to intense exercise.

Topic 6: Effects of Training

Life-long exercise training can prevent, or rather forestall, much of the exercise-related functional decline with age. Not all, but much. In addition, healthy older people who were previously sedentary can regain much of their lost functionality with regular exercise regimens. A sedentary lifestyle is a risk factor that can hasten cardiovascular and other declines. Most studies on this subject have been done using endurance training, *i.e.* aerobic exercise. Recent evidence shows that strength training can also be of profound benefit in elderly people and even in people with heart failure.

One thing that doesn't improve with training is the ability to increase HR with exercise. The rough 220 minus age rule holds for maximum HR whether a person trains or not. Apparently, β adrenergic responses diminish with age regardless of physical fitness.

Nevertheless, maximum CO increases with training. In old people, this increase is entirely due to an increase in SV. The increase in maximum SV with training in old people results mainly from an increase in LVED volume rather than a decrease in LVES volume. In other words, in old people, training-induced increases in SV must rely mainly on the Starling effect.

There are two probable causes for the increase in LVED volume and, therefore, SV with training

1. Training results in a greater drop in TPR during intense exercise and, therefore, a greater rise in preload to the heart. The cause of this training effect is greater metabolic hyperemia in exercising muscle due to increased O_2 extraction. This effect follows from the training-induced increase in ability of skeletal muscle to perform intense exercise and consume O_2, which, in turn, results from increased skeletal muscle fiber size, increased activity of various mitochondrial enzymes, increased capillarization, and increased availability of endothelial NO.
2. Training results in an increase in total blood volume and, consequently, an increase in preload to the heart.

The bottom line here is that endurance training leads to increased preload to the heart during exercise as a result of greater vasodilation and increased circulating blood volume. The heart responds by the Starling effect. Thus, training increases maximum SV. But there are additional training effects that help the heart cope with increased preload.

- Training promotes a partial reversal of the age-related changes in excitation-contraction coupling. Specifically, the rate of Ca^{++} reuptake by the network SR increases with training. The result is a return toward earlier and faster relaxation. This is called a positive lusitropic effect. Ventricular pressure drops more abruptly during the isovolumetric relaxation period and the y descent in the atrial pressure curve re-steepens. Early suctional filling of the left ventricle increases. The reliance on atrial contraction lessens.
- Arterial wall stiffness decreases. Consequently, arterial compliance increases. Pulse wave velocity decreases. Resting arterial impedance decreases. It becomes easier for the left ventricle to eject blood.
- The exercise-induced increase in EF with exercise is augmented and may approach that seen in young people
- Physiological cardiac hypertrophy occurs (see Chapter 10). Thus, there is an increase in contractility during exercise and a small decrease in LVES volume. This effect may be the primary cause of the increase in exercise-augmented EF. In addition, it is possible that there is a positive inotropic effect of training due to increased β adrenergic responsiveness.
- In rat hearts, the fast V_1 isoform of the myosin heavy chain is gradually replaced by the slower V_3 isoform with aging. This may also be true in other small mammals, but apparently not in humans. We have mainly the V_3 isoform all along. Exercise training in rats does not reverse the trend toward V_3 but this finding is irrelevant for people.

Additional information about the effects of exercise training on the cardiovascular system can be found in a review by S. Gielen *et al.*, *Circulation*, 122: 1221-1238, 2010.

Topic 7: Summary of Training Effects Figure 8

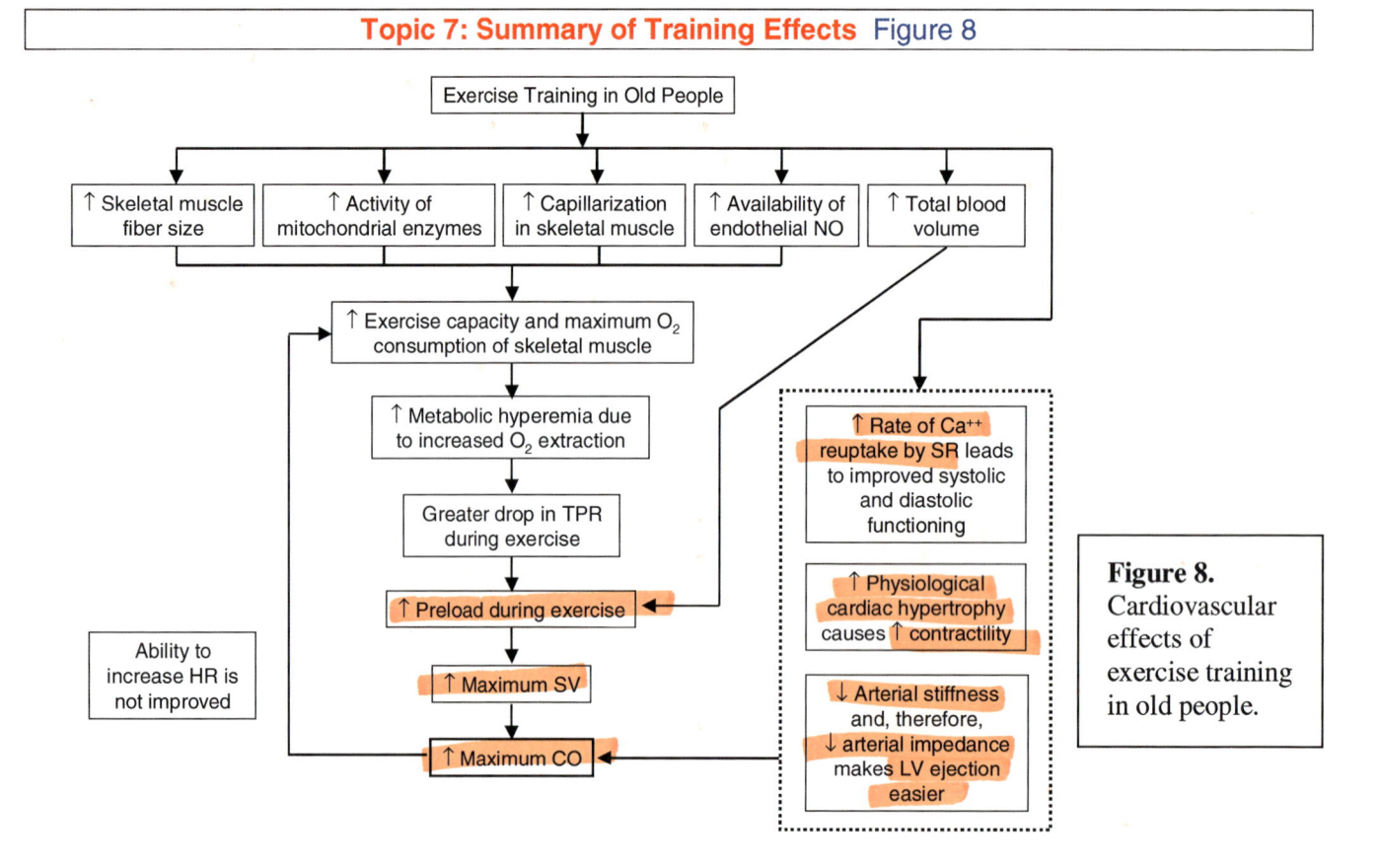

Figure 8. Cardiovascular effects of exercise training in old people.

Flow chart:
- Exercise Training in Old People →
  - ↑ Skeletal muscle fiber size
  - ↑ Activity of mitochondrial enzymes
  - ↑ Capillarization in skeletal muscle
  - ↑ Availability of endothelial NO
  - ↑ Total blood volume

- ↑ Skeletal muscle fiber size, ↑ Activity of mitochondrial enzymes, ↑ Capillarization in skeletal muscle, ↑ Availability of endothelial NO → ↑ Exercise capacity and maximum O₂ consumption of skeletal muscle → ↑ Metabolic hyperemia due to increased O₂ extraction → Greater drop in TPR during exercise → ↑ Preload during exercise → ↑ Maximum SV → ↑ Maximum CO

- ↑ Total blood volume → ↑ Preload during exercise

- Ability to increase HR is not improved

- ↑ Rate of Ca⁺⁺ reuptake by SR leads to improved systolic and diastolic functioning
- ↑ Physiological cardiac hypertrophy causes ↑ contractility
- ↓ Arterial stiffness and, therefore, ↓ arterial impedance makes LV ejection easier
→ ↑ Maximum CO

Part 5: Responses to Postural Changes and Hypovolemia

Topic 1: Orthostatic Stress

A major problem with old people is falls. One contributor to the propensity for old people to fall is an abnormally large drop in CO and MAP upon standing. A large drop in arterial pressure with standing is called orthostatic hypotension. It can lead to fainting.

Old people who are healthy and who have remained reasonably active have no particular problem with orthostatic hypotension. On the other hand, old people who, for one reason or another, are very inactive do tend to have problems with orthostatic hypotension.

Sudden standing from a reclining or sitting position elicits various responses that were described in Chapter 8, Part 3. Here is a brief review. Upon standing, blood tends to pool in the veins of the lower extremities. Venous pressure decreases in proportion to height above the so-called hydrostatic indifference point (a little below the diaphragm). Thus, right atrial pressure decreases. Decreased preload to the heart results in smaller ventricular end-diastolic volumes and a smaller SV. The direct effect is reduction of CO and, therefore, reduction of MAP. In the absence of appropriate compensations, CO and MAP can drop enough to cause fainting.

The immediate compensations that ordinarily re-elevate right atrial pressure and prevent orthostatic hypotension are:

- Venous compression by contraction of skeletal muscles in the legs.
- Baroreceptor reflexes that cause increased HR, increased contractility, increased TPR, and decreased venous capacity.

These compensations normally return CO nearly to its supine value, but SV remains lower (unless exercise is begun).

The baroreceptor reflexes that affect the heart depend mainly on β_1 adrenergic responses. Those that affect vascular smooth muscle (to raise TPR and lower venous capacity) depend mainly on α_1 adrenergic responses. Since β adrenergic responsiveness diminishes with age, orthostatic stress results in a smaller reflex increase in HR in old people than in young people.

However, the decrease in SV that occurs upon standing is less in old people than it is in young people. This is because venous compliance decreases with age and, therefore, there is less venous pooling of blood upon standing in old people. It has also been suggested that the reflex decrease in venous capacity might be greater in old people than in young people since this α_1 adrenergic effect on venous smooth muscle (constriction) might be counteracted less by the β_2 effect (relaxation) that has diminished with age. The bottom line is that the weaker HR increase that occurs when an old person stands is approximately balanced by less drop in SV, and the decrease in CO upon standing is no more severe in healthy old people than it is in healthy young people.

As mentioned above, completely sedentary or debilitated old people tend not to cope well with orthostatic stress. The reasons are probably decreased blood volume and decreased reactivity of the baroreceptor reflexes, as discussed in Chapter 15, Part 5 for the situations of bed rest and space flight.

Topic 2: Acute Hypovolemia

The responses to acute hypovolemia (hemorrhage) were discussed in Chapter 15, Part 4. Fast reflex responses cause increased HR, increased contractility, increased TPR, and decreased venous capacity. Since the cardiac responses (mainly β_1 adrenergic) are attenuated with age, old people tend not to cope as well with blood loss as do young people.

Selected References for Chapter 18

- Lakatta, E.G., Cardiovascular Regulatory Mechanisms in Advanced Age, *Physiological Reviews* 73:413-467, 1993.
- Lakatta, E.G., Y.Y. Zhou, and R.P. Xiao, Aging of the Cardiovascular System, Chapter 42 in *Heart Physiology and Pathophysiology, 4th Ed.*, Edited by N. Sperelakis, *et al.*, Academic Press, 2001.

Index

Index

A

A band(s), 11, 13
a wave, 49, 133
Acetylcholine, 37, 39, 40, 116, 139, 157
Acetyl-CoA, 82, 83
Actin, 13, 15-18, 22, 24, 25, 34, 108, 109, 111, 114, 175
Actinin, 13, 15, 16, 108
Action potentials
    cardiac, with aging, 183
    pacemaking cells, 29
    T cells, 31
    vascular smooth muscle, 110
    working myocytes, 27
Active hyperemia, 155-157, 160, 161
Active relaxation of smooth muscle, 115
Active state, 17, 24
Active tension, definition, 33
Acyl-CoA synthetase, 82
Adenosine, 90, 114, 117, 119, 156, 157, 163
    diphosphate (ADP), 17, 18, 83, 84
    monophosphate (AMP), 37, 85, 117, 156
    triphosphate (ATP), 17, 18, 32, 81-87, 89, 108, 110, 113, 116, 117, 156, 157, 161, 163
Adenylyl
    cyclase, 37, 40, 114
    kinase, 85
ADP-ATP transferase, 84
Adrenal
    cortex, 41, 144, 145
    medulla, 37, 39, 115, 138, 139, 147, 148, 162
Adrenalin, 36
Adrenergic, 14, 37-39, 109, 115, 119, 127, 139, 160, 161, 180, 181, 183, 185, 186, 189-193
    receptors, 37-39, 109, 115, 139, 160, 161, 180
Afterload
    a determinate of stroke volume, 6, 63, 64
    aortic impedance and, 182
    conpensations for changes in, 69
    definition, 33
    effect on shortening velocity, 35
    performance curves for the heart, 70
Aging
    aortic impedance, 182
    arterial changes, 182
    arterial pulse wave velocity, 181
    Chapter 18, 179
    exercise, 188
    hemodynamic changes, 184, 187
    hypovolemia, 147, 193
    nitric oxide, 181
    orthostatic stress, 192
    venous changes, 182, 183
Albumin, 172, 173, 175, 176
Aldosterone, 143-146
Amlodipine, 120
Amyl nitrite, 120
Anaerobic metabolism, 149, 159
Anemia, 102
Angina pectoris, 87, 89, 91, 119, 120, 158, 171
Angiogenesis, 165
Angiotensin, 93, 113, 115, 116, 119, 120, 124, 141, 143-149
Angiotensin converting enzyme, 115-117, 120, 124, 144
Angiotensinogen, 115, 144
Anrep effect, 63, 69, 70, 159, 185, 186
Anterior cardiac veins, 162
Antidiuretic hormone (ADH) (vasopressin), 113, 115, 119, 138, 141, 142, 144-147, 149
Antihypertensive drugs, 120
Aortic
    impedance, 182, 183, 185, 190
    pressure, 33, 49
    stenosis, 5, 70, 88
Area postrema, 138, 144, 146, 147, 178
Arrhythmia(s), 27, 53, 54, 59, 61, 90, 180, 183, 185
Arterial
    baroreceptors, 137, 138, 140, 145, 146, 152
    blood volume, 6, 49, 124, 134, 142, 144, 145, 181
    capacity, 79, 181, 186
    changes with aging, 181
    compliance, 5, 73, 105, 107, 123, 125, 127, 131, 132, 181, 184, 185, 191
    hypertension, 70, 88, 91, 124, 127, 183, 185
    impedance, 107, 191
    pressure, 2, 5, 49, 73, 123
        determined by, 123, 124
        exercise and, 189
    pulse wave, 49, 128, 129, 181, 184
    pulse wave velocity, 181
    Systemic Arterial System, Chapter 12, 123
    wall stiffness, 181, 182
Arteriolar
    constriction, 148
    resistance, 134
    smooth muscle, 103, 121, 124, 139, 147, 160, 162
    wall tension, 160
Astrocytes, 178
Atenolol, 120
Atherosclerosis, 158, 165, 180, 181
Atherosclerotic, 88, 101, 158
Atmospheric pressure, 124
Atrial
    action potential, 20, 27, 37
    baroreceptors, 138
    conduction, 20
    contractility, 37
    contraction, 43, 47-49, 50, 52, 133, 186, 191
    contraction period, 47
    depolarization, 20, 55, 56
    diastolic gallop, 51
    dysrhythmias, 60
    fibrillation, 60

flutter, 60
hypertrophy, 93
kick, 44
myocardium, 20, 29, 31, 37
myocytes, 9
natriuretic peptide, 114, 117, 142, 145, 146, 148
premature contractions, 60
pressure, 43, 45, 46, 49, 50, 51, 66, 67, 77, 78, 132, 133, 185, 186, 191, 192
pulse, 132
tachycardia, 60
Atrioventricular (AV)
conduction defects, 61
node, 19-22, 28, 29, 31, 37, 39, 40, 54, 56, 60, 61, 138, 139, 152
Augmented unipolar limb leads, 55, 59
Automaticity, 19-21, 29, 31, 32, 107
Autonomic nervous system, 36, 39, 137, 138, 152
Autoregulation, 70, 106, 160, 163
Autoregulatory range, 106, 160
Autotransfusion, 134, 147, 174
Axial accumulation of red cells, 101
Axis deviation, 58

B

Bainbridge reflex, 152
Baltimore Longitudinal Study of Aging, 184, 185, 187
Baroreceptor reflexes, 78, 137, 139-141, 148, 151, 152, 154, 192, 193
Bed rest, 151, 193
Bernard, Claude, 171
Bernoulli
effect, 101
equation, 98
Bezold-Jarisch reflex, 152
Blood flow
cerebral, 159
coronary, 163, 164
principles of, *Chapter 11*, 95
regional control, 155
velocity of, 3
Blood pressure
aging and, 184
arterial, 43, 72, 87, 123, 126, 131, 137, 138, 147, 153, 154, 160, 180, 181, 185, 192
central venous, 5, 67, 70, 72-78, 109, 119, 123, 124, 132, 137-147, 151-153, 180, 182, 186
conversion factors, 7, 95
diastolic, 49, 67, 125-128, 153, 184, 189
hypertension, 70, 88, 91, 124, 127, 183, 185
mean arterial, 5, 6, 41, 66, 70, 73, 78, 100, 105, 106, 109, 115, 117, 120, 123-127, 134, 135, 137-153, 155, 160-163, 174, 180, 182, 184, 185, 188-190, 192
pulse, 49, 78, 125-128, 137, 149, 152, 180-182, 184, 185, 188, 189
systolic, 4, 52, 88, 125-128, 133, 153, 182, 184, 185, 189, 190
table of normal values, 7

venous, 5, 6, 73, 75, 77, 78, 106, 123, 131, 132, 174, 175, 180, 182
Blood volume
aging and, 183
distribution of, 3
long-term control of, 141
one of the primary adjustable parameters of the cardiovascular system, 5
Blood-brain barrier, 144, 167, 168, 177
Blushing, 151
Bowditch effect, 26
Brachial artery, 5, 88, 125, 184
Bradycardia, 7, 59, 152
Bradykinin, 116-118, 149, 152, 157, 158, 175
Breathing, 59, 132, 135, 149, 186
Bruits, 99, 101
Bulk flow, 167, 172, 174
Bundle branch(s), 21, 29, 32, 56, 60
Bundle of His, 10, 19, 20, 21, 56, 60

C

c wave, 49, 133
Calcitonin gene-related peptide, 117
Calcium release channels, 109, 112
Calcium-induced calcium release, 24, 28, 34, 38, 40, 109, 112, 121, 183
Calcium-overload arrhythmias, 183
Caldesmon, 111, 114
Calmodulin, 111-113, 115, 118, 119
Calponin, 111, 114
Calsequestrin, 14, 23
Capacitance vessels, 103
Capillary recruitment, 105, 106, 156, 161, 175
Captopril, 120
CapZ protein, 13
Cardiac
action potentials, 19
changes with aging, 183
contractility, 5, 37, 38, 52, 73, 112, 137, 150, 181, 185, 188
adrenergic effects, 37
definition, 5
cycle, 5, 43, 46, 47, 49, 50, 54, 123, 127, 133, 164
Chapter 5, 43
events, 47
phases, 46
effectiveness, 73-76, 78, 79
efficiency, 88
excitation, *Chapter 3*, 19
function curves, 67, 73-76, 78
glycosides, 40
hypertrophy, 88, 91-93, 165, 171, 183
index, 4, 7
muscle, 9, 18, 19, 33
force-velocity relationship, 36
length-tension relationship, 33
Regulation of Contraction, Chapter 4, 33
Structure and Mechanism of Contraction, Chapter 2, 9

myocytes, 9
output
   regulation of, *Chapter 8*, 73
   definition, 4
   heart rate effect, 72
   metabolic demands and, 6
   postural changes and, 76
remodeling, 159
reserve
   inotropic, 68
   intrinsic, 63
tamponade, 68, 153
Cardiac contractility
   one of the primary adjustable parameters of the cardiovascular system, 5
Cardiogenic shock, 149
Cardiomyopathies, 69, 159
Cardiopulmonary baroreceptors, 138, 139-141, 146, 147, 150, 152
Cardiovascular center, 138, 141, 144-148, 150, 151, 153
Carotid sinus, 78, 137, 138, 148, 152
Catecholamines, 76, 147, 180
Caveolae, 108, 112, 167, 168
Central command, 150
Central ischemic response, 148, 152
Central veins, 72, 73, 132, 135
Central venous pressure (CVP), 5, 67, 70, 72-76, 78, 109, 119, 123, 132, 137-143, 145-147, 151-153, 180, 182, 186
   definition, 5
   determination of, 5
   Guyton diagrams and, 73
   in the calculation of mean arterial pressure, 123
   Starling curves and, 67
   venous pressure gradient and, 132
Cerebral blood flow, 78, 152, 159-161
Cerebral spinal fluid, 41, 177, 178
Chemoreceptors, 138, 148
Chest leads, 58
Cholinergic receptors, 186
Chordae tendineae, 43
Choroid plexus, 177
Chronotropic effect, 37, 114, 158, 186
Circle of Willis, 159
Circulating depolarizing factor (CDF), 150
Circulatory shock, 149
Circumventricular organs, 178
Circus movement, 61
Cirrhosis, 175
Clonidine, 120
Collagen, 16, 35, 116, 175, 176, 181
Colloid osmotic pressure, 150, 172
Compensatory pause, 61
Compliance
   aortic, 125
   arterial, 123
   aging and, 181
   importance of, 127
   definition, 5
   distensibility and, 124

   interstitial spaces, 176
   venous, 131
   ventricular, 67
      in hypertrophy, 91
      in pathological conditions, 68
Concentric hypertrophy, 88, 91, 93, 171
Conduction velocity, 21, 30, 31, 36, 37, 139
Congestive heart failure, 40, 52, 68, 70, 72, 79, 91, 112, 115, 123, 174, 180
Constrictive pericarditis, 68, 153
Continuity equation, 97
Contractility
   adrenergic effects, 37
   Anrep effect and, 69
   cardiac glycosides and, 40
   definition, 36
   effect on stroke volume, 68
   in aging, 185
   in determination of stroke volume, 6
   in exercise, 71
   muscarinic effects, 39, 40
   myocardial stunning and, 89
   oxygen cost of, 86
   Starling curve and, 67
Contracture, 89
Coronary
   artery disease, 87, 115
   sinus, 162
Coronary circulation
   adenosine, 117
   anatomy and physiology of, 162
   collaterals and angiogenesis, 165
   nitroglycerine, 120
   sympathetic effects, 37
Costameres, 16
Creatine, 81, 84
Creatine kinase, 84
Creatine kinase shuttle, 84
Creatine phosphate, 81, 84
Creatinine, 188
Crossbridge
   adrenergic effects, 38
   asynchrony, 18
   cycle, 17, 24, 25, 93
   cycling, 81, 84, 85
   definition, 17
   latch state in smooth muscle, 109
   mechanism in smooth muscle, 109
Cushing reflex, 152
Cyclic AMP, 37, 39, 40, 114, 118, 176
Cyclic GMP, 114-119, 121, 156
Cytoskeleton in smooth muscle, 108

D

Deep venous thrombosis, 175
Dehydration, 149, 174
Delayed K^+ channels, 28, 31, 39, 110
Dense bodies, 108
Dense plaques, 108

Index

Desmosomes, 10
Diacylglycerol, 111-114, 119
Diastasis, 47
Diastole
   definition, 1
Diastolic
   depolarization, 29-32, 39, 40, 60
   dysfunction, 35, 68, 89, 92
   effect of aging on diastolic function, 186
   filling, 11, 33, 35, 46, 47, 66, 70, 72, 91, 186
   period, 44, 183
   pressure, 49, 67, 125-128, 153, 184, 189
   suction, 45, 47, 91, 92, 185, 186
   untwisting of the ventricles, 44
   ventricular end-diastolic pressure, 4, 52, 63, 67, 92, 185
   ventricular end-diastolic volume, 47, 51, 52, 65, 67-72, 92, 185, 186
   volume, 70, 71
Diazoxide, 121
Dicrotic notch, 128
Dicrotic wave, 49, 125, 128
Diffusion
   coefficient, 170
   principles of, 170
Digitalis, 40
Digoxin, 40
Dihydropuridine receptors, 23, 24, 38, 110-113, 115
Diltiazem, 120
Dioxygenation reaction, 157
Dipole, 53
Discontinuous endothelia, 169
Distal tubules, 142, 144, 145
Distensibility, 68, 124, 128, 181
Diuresis, 41, 142
Diuretic(s), 121, 124
Donnan equilibrium, 171, 172
Dopamine, 178
Double product, 88
Dromotropic effect, 37
Dystrobrevin, 15
Dystroglycan/Dystrophin Complex, 15
Dystrophin, 15, 16, 159

E

Eccentric hypertrophy, 92, 93
Echocardiography, 47
Ectopic foci, 29, 32, 60, 61
Edema, 77, 78, 117, 171, 174, 175, 176
   cellular edema, 91, 174
   interstitial edema, 117
   myxedema, 175
   pulmonary edema, 171
Eicosanoids, 118
Einstein, Albert, 170
Einthoven
   limb leads, 55, 58
   Willem Einthoven, 55
Ejection fraction, 5, 7, 47, 69, 180
Elastance, 67, 68

Elastic recoil, 48, 49, 128, 132
Electrical axis of the heart, 57, 58
Electrocardiogram, 47, 53-62
Electrocardiography (*Chapter 6*), 53
Electrochemical potential, 27, 171
Electrogenic, 32
Electromechanical coupling, 112
Enalapril, 120
End pressure, 98, 99
End-diastolic pressure-volume relationship, 63, 67
Endocardial, 10, 21, 27, 54, 56, 164
Endogenous ouabain, 41
Endothelia
   continuous, 167
   discontinuous (sinusoids), 169
   fenestrated, 168
Endothelial
   cell retraction, 117, 118
   effects on vascular smooth muscle, 118
   nitric oxide, 76, 116, 127, 156, 180, 181, 185, 189, 191
   nitric oxide synthase, 116, 156, 181
   permeability, 175, 176
   structure, 167
   transendothelial diffusion of solutes, 170
Endothelin, 93, 113, 115, 119
Endothelium-derived hyperpolarizing factor, 118
End-systolic, 49
   elastance, 63, 64, 69
   pressure, 52, 63-65, 69
   pressure-volume relationship, 63-65, 68, 69
   volume, 47, 51, 52, 64, 65, 68-71, 92
Epicardial, 10, 21, 27, 36, 54, 56, 162, 164
Epinephrine, 36, 37, 39, 113, 115, 119, 139, 148, 162
Equilibrium potential(s), 27, 28, 110
Erythrocyte (red blood cell) (RBC), 104, 157
Essential hypertension, 145
Essential myosin light chain, 12
Events of the cardiac cycle, 51
Exchange vessels, 103, 162, 167-170, 172-175
Excitation-contraction coupling, 22
Exercise
   active hyperemia, 161
   adaptation of baroreceptor responses, 140
   adjustments in sympathetic nerve activity, 150
   and the skeletal muscle pump, 135
   cardiac hypertrophy, 91, 92
   edema of, 174
   effect on duration of diastole, 47
   effects of training in aging, 190
   effects on arterial pressures and total peripheral resistance, 126
   effects on stroke volume, heart rate, cardiac output, end-systolic volume, and end-diastolic volume, 70
   epinephrine-induced arteriolar dilation, 162
   Guyton diagram, 76
   in aging, 188
   receptors, 138, 150
   role of venous reservoir, 134
   the primary cardiovascular effects of, 76
Exocytosis, 36, 109, 117, 168

Expiration, 50, 59, 135, 152, 153

F

Fahraeus-Lindqvist effect, 104, 105, 157
Fainting, 151, 160, 192
Fatigue, 188
Fatty acids, 81, 82, 170
Femoral artery, 101, 128
Fenestrated endothelia, 168
Fibrillation, 60, 61
Fibronectin, 16
Fibrous skeleton of the heart, 10, 43
Fight or flight reaction, 79, 140, 151, 162
Filtration, 77, 146, 173-177
First degree AV block, 61
First heart sound, 50
Foot processes, 177, 178
Force-velocity relationship, 36
Fourth heart sound, 50
Foxglove, 40
Frank, Otto, 64
Frank-Starling Law, 66
Frontal-plane electrocardiography, 55

G

Gap junctions, 10, 20-22, 53, 107
General static pressure, 74, 75
Gibbs-Donnan equilibrium, 171, 172
Glomerular filtration rate, 142-146
Glut 1, 178
Glutamate, 177, 178
Glutamine, 170
Glycogenolysis, 148
Glycolysis, 82, 84, 85
G-proteins, 112
    G_{12}, 112, 113, 115, 119
    G_i, 40
    G_q, 111-115, 118, 119
    G_s, 37, 39, 112, 114, 115, 117-119, 156
Gravity, 72, 76, 95, 132, 141, 151
Guanethidine, 120
Guanosine triphosphate, 112-114
Guyton
    Arthur C. Guyton, 73
    diagram(s), 73-77, 79, 141

H

Hageman factor, 116, 117
Heart
    actions of autonomic nervous system on, 36
    block, 61
    electrical axis of, 57
    excitation of cardiac muscle, *Chapter 3*, 19
    heart-lung preparation, 63, 65, 66
    regulation of contraction, *Chapter 4*, 33
    responses to chronic overload, *Chapter 10*, 91
    sounds, 47, 50, 101, 133
    Starling curves, 67
    Starling's Law of, 35, 65
    structure and mechanism of contraction, *Chapter 2*, 107
    the cardiac cycle, *Chapter 5*, 43
Heart failure
    and aging, 180
    and edema, 174
    and inotropic reserve, 69
    causes, 35, 52, 67, 70, 89
    treatment, 5, 23, 119, 120, 190
Heart rate
    and duration of diastole, 47
    determination of, 20, 30
    effect of high heart rates on stroke volume, 72
    effect on baroreceptor firing, 137
    effect on contractility (staircase phenomenon), 26
    effect on myocardial oxygen consumption, 87
    effects of $\beta 1$ adrenergic stimulation, 39
    in aging, 181, 186
    in atrial tachycardia, 60
    in AV block, 29
    in exercise, 70, 189
    in the Bainbridge reflex, 152
    in the diving reflex, 151
    in vasovagal faint, 151
    in ventricular tachycardia, 61
    one of the primary adjustable parameters of the cardiovascular system, 5
    sinus arrhythmia, 59
Hematocrit, 101, 102, 104, 105
Hemoglobin, 76, 116, 157, 161, 163, 167, 171
Hemoglobin-based oxygen carriers, 157
Hemorrhage, 134, 147, 148, 149, 174, 193
Hemorrhagic shock, 149
His-Purkinje system, 19, 20, 21, 29, 32
Histamine, 116, 117, 149, 157, 175
Homeostasis, 171
Hyaluronic acid, 175, 181
Hydralazine, 121, 124
Hydrostatic indifference point, 77, 78, 192
Hydrostatic pressure, 77, 95, 132, 172, 173, 177
Hypereffective heart, 67, 70, 76
Hyperemia, 151, 155-158, 161, 162
Hyperplasia, 91
Hyperpolarization, 27, 29, 112, 115, 118, 156
Hypertension, 41, 89, 112, 115, 117, 119, 120-123, 127, 140, 145, 160, 180, 184
Hypertrophy
    and chronic overload, 91
    and myocardial oxygen consumption, 87
    and ventricular compliance, 68
    concentric, 88, 91, 93
    eccentric, 91, 92
    electrical axis deviation, 58
    in aging, 182, 183
    mechanisms of, 91, 93
    physiological, 92, 191
Hyperventilation, 161
Hypoeffective heart, 67, 70

Hypothalamus, 41, 138, 139, 151
Hypothyroidism, 175
Hypovolemia, 134, 149, 192
Hypovolemic shock, 150, 160, 174
Hypoxia, 32, 84, 88-90, 112, 115, 148, 149, 155, 165, 171
Hypoxic vasodilation, 155

I

I band, 11-13, 35
Incisura, 49, 125, 128
Inflammation, 116, 118, 157, 175, 176
Inositol trisphosphate (IP3), 109, 111-114, 117-119, 121
Inotropic cardiac reserve, 68
Inotropic effect, 36, 37, 40, 63, 68, 114, 139, 158, 159, 191
Inspiration, 50, 59, 135, 153
Intercalated disk, 9, 10, 20, 21
Internodal tracts, 20
Interstitial spaces
   and edema, 77
   and transcapillary refill, 147, 174
   and transcytosis, 168
   and transendothelial fluid flow, 172
   and transvascular exchange, 167
   nature of, 175
Intracranial pressure, 152
Intrathoracic
   arteries, 152
   blood vessels, 153
   space, 132
   veins, 5, 44, 74, 132, 152
Intrinsic cardiac reserve, 63
Inwardly rectifying K^+ channels, 110, 112
Ion channels
   background, 28
   BK_{Ca}, 110, 112, 114
   chloride, 109, 110
   delayed K^+, 28, 31, 39, 110
   f, 30-32, 39, 40
   K_1, 28, 30, 31
   K_{ATP}, 110, 112, 156
   K_{IR}, 110, 112
   K_V, 110
   L type Ca^{++}, 14, 23, 24, 28-32, 38, 39, 40, 109-115, 120, 158, 183
   nonselective cation, 109, 110, 113, 115, 157
   T type Ca^{++}, 30, 32, 109
   transient outward, 28
   voltage-gated Na^+, 14, 27, 30-32
IP_3 receptor, 109, 112, 121
Iron, 157
Irreversible shock, 150
Ischemia, 32, 89, 90, 92, 150, 152, 158, 159
Ischemic, 89, 90, 91, 148, 165, 175
   preconditioning, 90
Isometric
   contraction, 33
   force, 34, 35
   tension, 12, 35, 36
Isosorbide dinitrate, 120

Isotonic, 142, 145, 150, 172
Isovolumetric contraction, 46-49, 85, 164
Isovolumetric relaxation, 45, 46, 48, 49, 85, 133, 186, 191

J

Junctional SR, 14, 15, 23, 24, 26, 28, 34, 38, 40, 183
Juxtaglomerular
   apparatus, 115, 120, 144, 145
   cells, 124, 143, 144, 146

K

Kallikrein, 116
Kinetic energy, 98, 99
Kininases, 116
Kininogen, 116, 117
Krebs cycle, 82, 83, 84

L

Lactate, 81, 82, 84, 85
Lactic acid, 149
Laminar flow, 99-101, 105
Laminin, 15, 16
Laplace relationship, 45, 85, 86, 92, 124
Latch state, 109
Lateral pressure, 98, 99
Left
   anterior descending artery (LAD), 162
   circumflex artery, 162
   coronary artery, 162
Length-tension relationship, 34, 158
Limb leads, 55, 57, 58
Losartan, 119
L-type Ca^{++} channels, 23, 24, 28-32, 38-40, 109, 110-115, 158, 183
Lusitropic effect, 37, 158, 191
Lymph, 173-177
Lymphatic, 167, 175-177
   obstruction, 175
   system, 176

M

Macula densa, 143, 144
Malnutrition, 175
Maximum rate of oxygen consumption, 170, 188
Mayer waves, 154
Mean arterial pressure (MAP)
   and afterload performance curves, 70
   and pressure-flow autoregulation, 106, 155, 160
   definition, 5
   estimation of, 125
   in estimating stroke work, 66, 87
   main discussion of, 123
Mean circulatory filling pressure, 74
Mean electrical axis of the QRS complex, 57, 58
Mechanism of contraction, 17, 109

Index

Medullary cardiovascular center, 138, 141, 144-148, 150, 151, 153
Meningitis, 178
Metabolic autoregulation, 155, 157, 163
Metabolic hyperemia, 155, 163, 191
Metarterioles, 103
Metoprolol, 120
Microcirculation
    definition, 1, 103
    Fahraeus-Lindqvist effect in, 105
    in skeletal muscle, 161
    low hematocrit in, 104
    pressure drop through, 4
    resistance to flow through, 103
Microvascular networks, 167
Minoxidil, 121
Mitochondria, 9, 23, 81, 85, 92, 155, 161, 163, 165, 171, 189
Mitral
    insufficiency (regurgitation), 91, 92
    prolapse, 43
    stenosis, 5
Motor units, 22, 188
M-protein, 14
Multi-drug receptors, 178
Murmur(s), 50, 99, 101
Muscarinic acetylcholine receptors, 37, 40, 139
Muscle pump, 131, 135
Muscular dystrophy, 16, 18, 159
Myocardial
    action potentials, 27, 28, 38
    cells, 9, 28, 81, 88, 155
    contractility, 89
    depressant factor, 150
    energetics, 81
    hibernation, 89
    hypertrophy, 171
    hypoxia, 52, 81, 88, 89
    infarction, 53, 69, 87, 89, 91, 152, 164
    ischemia, 32, 53, 68, 69, 87, 88, 91, 117, 158, 183
    oxygen consumption, 87, 88, 158
    stunning, 89
Myocarditis, 69
Myocardium
    action potentials in, 27
    atrial, 20, 29, 31, 37
    structure of, 9
    ventricular, 10, 19, 21, 27, 37, 52, 56, 91, 162
Myofibrils, 9-12, 14-16, 21, 23, 81, 91, 92, 108
Myofilaments, 24, 26, 38, 91, 108, 158
Myogenic, 19, 107, 160
Myoglobin, 85
Myomesin, 14
Myosin, 12-14, 17, 18, 22, 25, 34, 38, 89, 93, 108-114, 175, 191
Myosin heavy chain, 12, 93, 191
Myosin light chain, 109, 111-114, 175
Myosin light chain kinase, 111-114
Myosin phosphatase, 111, 113, 114
Myosin-binding protein C, 14, 38
Myostatin, 93
Myxedema, 175

N

Nephrotic syndrome, 175
Network SR, 14, 23, 191
Neuropeptide Y, 117
Neurotensin, 117
Newton, 96
Newtonian, 99-102
Nicotinic, 139
Nifedipine, 23, 120
Nitric oxide
    and adenosine, 156
    and atherosclerosis, 158
    effect of shear rate on release, 157
    in exercise, 76
    main discussion, 156
    mechanism of action, 114
    overview, 116
    scavenging, 157
    synthase, 158
Nitroglycerin, 120
Nitroprusside, 120, 124
Noradrenalin, 37
Norepinephrine, 37, 115, 119
Normal values for the cardiovascular system, 7
Nucleus ambiguous, 138
Nucleus tractus solitarius (NTS), 137

O

Operating point, 66, 67, 73-78, 142, 143
Orthostatic stress, 192
Osmolarity, 139, 143-145, 147, 148, 172
Osmoreceptors, 139, 147
Osmosis, 167, 172, 173
Osmotic, 172, 173, 176, 178
Ouabain, 40, 41
Overshoot, 19, 30
Oxidative phosphorylation, 81-84
Oxygen
    cost of contractility, 86
    delivery, 85, 88, 155, 161, 163
    extraction, 88, 155, 163, 164, 188
    free radicals, 89

P

P cells, 20, 28-31, 37, 39, 40, 139, 155, 186
P wave, 51, 55-57, 60-62
Pacemaker, 19, 29, 30, 32, 39, 59, 60
Pacemaker potential(s), 19, 29, 30, 32, 39
Pacing, 20, 21, 29, 30, 60
Pain, 89, 117, 151
Papillary muscles, 10, 21, 43
Parasympathetic
    effects on heart, 37

nerve endings, 39
stimulation of P cells, 40
tone, 37, 39, 59, 92
Passive length-tension relationship, 35
Passive tension (definition), 33
Passive vascular beds, 105
Penicillin, 178
Peripheral resistance
and nitric oxide scavenging, 157
in aging, 185
in anemia, 102
in exercise, 126, 134, 150
in Fahraeus-Lindqvist effect, 105
in simple model of circulatory system, 6
target of many antihypertensive drugs, 124
total (TPR), one of primary adjustable parameters, 5
unit (PRU), 7, 96
Permeability
capillary, 117, 149, 175
coefficient, 173
pH, 148, 150, 161, 177
Pharmacomechanical coupling, 113
Phases of cardiac action potentials, 27, 29, 30
Phospholamban, 15, 38, 39, 183
Phospholemman, 14, 38, 39
Phospholipase, 111-114
Physiological hypertrophy, 92
Pituitary, 138, 139, 144-147
Plasma skimming, 104
Plateau
of myocardial action potential, 28, 29
of P cell action potential, 30
of venous return curve, 74
Plug flow, 104
Poiseuille equation, 99
Polycythemia, 102
Postural changes
effects on cardiac output and MAP, 76, 192
Power stroke, 17, 18, 33
PR interval, 56, 61, 62
Prazosin, 119
Precapillary
resistance, 2, 41, 96, 100, 124, 127, 129, 139, 155-158, 161, 174, 175
resistance vessels, 2, 41, 96, 100, 124, 127, 129, 139, 155-158, 161
sphincters, 103
Precordial leads, 58
Preload
definition, 33
Premature atrial contractions, 60
Premature ventricular contractions, 60
Pressure
atmospheric, 124
hydrostatic, 77, 95, 132, 172, 173, 177
interstitial, 172, 176
intracranial, 152
intrathoracic, 74, 135, 152, 153, 164
oncotic, 150, 172, 173, 175
osmotic, 172, 173, 176

overload, 91, 92, 165, 171
transmural, 74, 86, 124, 127, 131, 132
Pressure-flow autoregulation, 106, 149, 155, 160, 161
Pressure-volume
curve(s), 64
loop(s), 87
relationship, 5, 52
Primary adjustable parameters of the cardiovascular system, 5, 6, 63, 73, 75, 123, 124, 132, 137
Propranolol, 37, 120
Prostacyclin, 116
Prostaglandin(s), 117
Protein kinases
myosin light chain kinase, 111-114
protein kinase A, 37, 39, 114
protein kinase C, 113
protein kinase G, 114, 156
Proximal tubules, 142, 143
Pulmonary
artery, 4, 43, 46, 99, 101, 106, 138
circulation, 105, 106, 155
microcirculation, 2
pressures in pulmonary system, 7
venous system, 2
Pulmonic valve, 46, 50
Pulse
jugular, 132, 133
pressure, 49, 78, 125-128, 137, 149, 152, 180-182, 184, 185, 188, 189
wave, 49, 123, 128, 129, 182, 184, 185
wave velocity, 128, 182, 184
Pulsus paradoxus, 153
Purkinje cell(s), 21, 27, 29-32
Purkinje fibers, 21, 27, 56, 60
Pyruvate dehydrogenase complex, 82

Q

Q wave, 51, 56
QRS complex, 56, 57, 60-62
QT interval, 56

R

R wave, 51, 56-59, 61
Rapid ejection period, 46-50, 85, 125-127, 133, 164, 189
Rapid filling period, 46-50, 52, 133, 186
Rate-pressure product, 88
Reactive hyperemia, 158
Reactive vascular beds, 106
Receptors
A_2 (adenosine), 114, 117
adrenergic, 37-39, 109, 115, 139, 160, 161, 180
AT_1 (angiotensin II), 113, 115, 119
dihydropuridine, 23, 24, 38, 110-113, 115
IP_3, 109, 112, 121
muscarinic, 37, 40, 139
nicotinic, 139
purinergic, 113

ryanodine, 15, 23, 109, 112
Red blood cells, 104, 157
Reduced ejection period, 46-51, 85, 164
Reduced filling period, 47-50, 52, 133
Reentry, 27, 59, 60, 61
Reflection coefficient, 176
Refractory period, 27-29
Regulatory myosin light chains, 12, 38, 110, 114
Remodeling, 91, 92, 159
Renal
    control of NaCl and water output, 142
Renin, 115, 120, 124, 142-146
Renin-angiotensin-aldosterone system, 142, 143, 145, 146
Reperfusion injury, 89
Repolarization, 20, 28, 51, 54, 56
Reserpine, 120
Resetting of baroreceptor reflexes, 140
Resistance
    conversion factors, 7
    to flow (distribution in systemic system), 3
Respiratory
    cycle, 59, 153
    gases, 1, 103, 171
    pressure changes and lymph flow, 177
    pump, 135
Resting potential, 19, 27-29, 110
Reynolds number, 100, 101
RhoA, 113, 114, 119
Rho-kinase, 113-115, 119
Right
    coronary artery, 162
    heart failure, 174
    ventricular ejection, 45
Rigor bond, 17, 18
Rigor mortis, 18
Rouleaux, 105
Ryanodine receptor(s), 15, 23, 109, 112

S

S wave, 51, 56, 57
Sarcoglycans, 15
Sarcolemma, 9, 10, 14-16, 22, 23, 26, 38, 40, 108, 112, 113, 115, 121
Sarcomere(s), 5, 10-14, 16-18, 22, 23, 33, 34-36, 64, 65, 70, 81, 91, 92, 108, 158, 159
Sarcoplasmic reticulum, 9, 14, 23-26, 29, 34, 36, 38, 39, 40, 68, 70, 89, 91, 108, 109, 111-113, 121, 158, 183, 185
Sarcospan, 15
Second degree AV block, 61
Second heart sound, 50
Semilunar valves, 50
SERCA, 14, 15, 26, 38-40, 108
Series elasticity, 22
Serotonin, 116, 157
Shear rate, 96, 99, 101, 102, 157, 158
Shear stress, 96
Shock, 149
Sigma effect, 103, 105

Sildenafil (Viagra), 121
Sinoatrial (SA) node, 1, 19-22, 28-31, 37, 39, 40, 54, 56, 59, 60-62, 92, 139, 152, 155, 158, 186, 189
Sinus
    arrhythmia, 59, 153, 186
    bradycardia, 59
    rhythm, 20, 59, 152
    tachycardia, 59, 60
Skeletal muscle
    action potentials, 27
    adenosine as vasodilator, 117
    and venocompression, 76
    asynchronous firing of motor units, 22
    Ca^{++} release from SR, 24
    contraction upon standing, 77
    contractions and lymph flow, 177
    control of blood flow in, 161
    in aging, 188
    length-tension relationship, 33
    maximum oxygen consumption by, 170
    myocytes, 9, 163
    oxygen extraction from blood, 164
    pressure-flow autoregulation, 106
    pump, 162
    reduced TPR in exercise, 126
    rigor mortis, 18
    series elasticity, 22
    titin, 35
Slack length, 11, 33, 35, 45, 46
Smooth muscle
    and venous capacity, 2
    Chapter 12, 107
    of precapillary resistance vessels, 2, 103
S-nitroso-hemoglobin, 157
Sodium-potassium pump, 14, 32, 40, 41, 81, 85, 109, 178
Space flight, 151
ST segment, 56, 61
Staircase phenomenon, 26
Standard limb leads, 56, 57
Starling
    curves, 63, 66, 67, 73
    effect, 63, 66, 67, 69, 70, 76, 86, 92, 124, 135, 158, 185, 186, 188, 190, 191
    Ernest Starling, 65, 172
    forces, 173, 175
    hypothesis, 172
    Starling's Law of the Heart, 65
    Starling work curve, 66
Stenosis, 33, 91, 101
Streamline flow, 99
Stroke index, 4, 7
Stroke volume, 4-7, 46, 47, 51, 52, 63-72, 76, 87, 91, 92, 125, 126, 128, 135, 149, 153, 158, 159, 180, 186
    control of, 52
    definition, 4
    regulation of, *Chapter 7*, 63
Stroke work, 66, 69, 87
Substance P, 116, 117, 157, 158, 175
Supraventricular tachycardia, 60, 72, 152
Sympathetic

activity, 37, 39, 76, 78, 79, 133, 134, 138, 139, 143, 145-148, 150-153, 160-162
   effects, 37, 143
      on the heart, 37
      on venous blood volume, 133
   mechanisms of action, 37
   tone, 37
   tracts, 138
Syncope, 40, 151, 160, 192
Syncytium, 10
Syntrophins, 15, 159
Systemic vascular resistance, 5
Systole, 1, 5, 43-47, 49-52, 64, 85, 86, 88, 89, 91-93, 101, 127, 158, 164, 181
   atrial, 1
   ventricular, 2, 43, 44, 46, 49, 50, 125, 132, 133
Systolic, 4, 7, 44, 49, 52, 68, 70-72, 88, 89, 91, 125-128, 133, 153, 180-182, 184-186, 189, 190
   dysfunction, 89
   ejection, 44, 88
   function in aging, 185
   motions of the heart, 44
   pressure, 4, 52, 88, 125-128, 133, 153, 182, 184, 185, 189, 190
   suction, 45, 133
   twisting of the ventricles, 44

T

T cells, 20, 29, 31, 37, 40
T tubules, 9, 14, 22, 23, 26, 108
T wave, 51, 55-57
Tachycardia, 7, 60, 152
Thebesian veins, 162
Thick filaments, 12
Thin filaments, 13, 34, 35
Third degree AV block, 62
Thirst, 142, 144, 145
Thoroughfare channels, 103-105
Threshold, 27, 29-32, 39, 40
Thrombin, 175
Tight junctions, 167-169, 175, 176, 178
Time-tension index, 88
Titin, 13, 14, 35, 45, 46, 93
Tone
   G_{12}/Rho-kinase pathway for increasing, 113
   G_s/cGMP pathway for reducing, 114
   parasympathetic, 37, 39, 59, 92
   sympathetic, 37
   thin filament pathway for increasing, 113
   vascular smooth muscle, 109, 110
   venous, 149
Total blood volume, 5, 6, 63, 73, 75, 124, 134, 137, 141-149, 151, 183, 185, 186, 191
   a determinant of cardiac output, 6
   and diuretics, 124
   distribution, 3
   in Guyton diagrams, 75
   in long term control of MAP, 145
   one of the independently adjustable parameters of the cardiovascular system, 5
Total peripheral resistance (TPR)
   and Guyton diagrams, 75
   definition, 5
   in aging, 127, 185
   in calculating MAP, 123
   in determining MAP, 124
   in exercise, 126, 134, 161
   one of the primary adjustable parameters of the cardiovascular system, 5
Trabeculae carnae, 10
Training, 92, 165, 179, 180, 188, 190, 191
Transcapillary refill, 149, 174
Transmural pressure, 74, 86, 124, 127, 131, 132
Transvascular exchange, 167
Transverse tubules, 9, 14, 22, 23, 26, 108
Treppe, 26
Tricuspid valve, 20, 50, 133
Triple product, 88
Tropomyosin, 13, 17, 18, 22, 24-26, 34, 38, 108, 111, 114
Troponin, 13, 17, 24, 25, 26, 34, 38, 108, 110, 111
T-type Ca^{++} channels, 30, 32, 109
Turbulence, 99-102

U

Unipolar limb leads, 55
Urinary, 142, 146, 188
Urine, 141-145

V

v wave, 49, 50, 133
Vagal, 40
Vagus, 138
Valsalva maneuver, 152
Valsartan, 119
Varicosities, 36, 109
Vascular smooth muscle, 107, 108, 156, 181
   Chapter 12, 107
Vasoactive intestinal peptide, 117
Vasoconstriction, 115, 119, 139, 144, 149, 155, 158, 160-162
Vasodilation, 112, 117, 119, 158, 161, 162, 189, 191
Vasodilator drugs
   agents that hyperpolarize the plasma membrane, 121
   agents that influence the cGMP signaling mechanism, 120
   agents that inhibit Ca^{++} release from the sarcoplasmic reticulum, 121
   agents that reduce norepinephrine release from sympathetic nerve endings, 120
   central nervous system adrenergic inhibitors, 120
   Chapter 12, Part 5, 119
   inhibitors of renin secretion and angiotensin II production, 120
   smooth muscle receptor blockers, 119
Vasodilator metabolites, 156-158, 160, 161, 163
Vasomotion, 174

Index

Vasopressin (antidiuretic hormone) (ADH), 113, 115, 119, 138, 141, 142, 144-147, 149
Vasovagal
  faint, 151
  syncope, 151
Venae cavae, 43, 45, 47, 99
Venocompression, 76, 135
Venoconstriction, 76, 135, 147
Venous
  capacity, 2, 5, 6, 63, 73, 75, 76, 78, 100, 103, 107, 123, 24, 132, 133, 137, 139, 141, 144, 145, 147, 149, 161, 182, 187, 192, 193
    one of the primary adjustable parameters of the cardiovascular system, 5
  compliance, 75, 107, 131-133, 181, 182, 193
  pooling of blood, 77, 78, 193
  pressure, 5, 6, 73, 75, 77, 78, 106, 123, 131, 132, 174, 175, 180, 182, 192
  pulse, 132
  pumps, 135
  reservoir, 133
  return curve, 74-78
  valves, 77, 135
Ventricular, 49
  afterload, 88, 182, 183, 190
  afterload performance curves, 70
  compliance, 52, 63, 66-68, 186
  contractility, 69
  depolarization, 51, 56
  diastole, 2, 44, 47, 125
  diastolic gallop, 50
  dysrhythmias, 60
  ejection, 47, 125
  end-diastolic pressure, 49
  end-diastolic volume, 4, 5, 47, 192
  end-systolic pressure, 49
  end-systolic volume, 4, 47
  extrasystoles, 61
  fibrillation, 61
  filling, 35, 44, 46-48, 50, 153, 185
  function curves (Starling curves), 66, 67
  hypertrophy, 58, 68, 88, 93, 182, 183, 186
  myocardium, 10, 19, 21, 27, 37, 52, 56, 91, 162
  myocytes, 9, 14, 19, 27, 39, 44, 139, 186
  myofibril, 11
  preload, 67, 183
  premature contractions, 60
  pressure, 43, 46-52, 63-65, 67, 68, 91, 186
  pressure-volume loops, 43, 51, 52, 63, 64, 65, 67, 68
  repolarization, 56
  suction, 46
  systole, 2, 43, 44, 46, 49, 50, 125, 132, 133
  tachycardia and flutter, 61
  untwisting, 45, 46, 48
  volume, 47
Venules, 1-3, 103, 118, 119, 132, 134, 139, 162, 165, 167, 173-175
Veratridine, 152
Viagra, 121
Viscosity, 96-105

Voltage-gated ion channels, 23, 27, 28, 30, 109
Voltage-gated Na^+ channels, 28, 109
Volume conductor, 53, 54
Volume overload, 91, 92, 159
Volume receptors, 138
Volume work, 87

W

Wall stress, 86, 88
Waller, Augustus, 55
Wedge pressure, 186

X

x wave, 49, 133

Y

y wave, 49, 133
Yield pressure, 105

Z

Z lines, 11, 13-17, 34, 35, 108
z point, 49

Made in the USA
Charleston, SC
26 June 2013